Epi Info™ and OpenEpi In Epidemiology and Clinical Medicine

Health Applications of Free Software

Andrew G. Dean

Kevin M. Sullivan

Minn Minn Soe

February 2010

Rights And Acknowledgements

Legal Mantra

"The use of registered names, trademarks etc. in this publication does not imply that such names are exempt from the relevant laws and regulations and therefore free for general use. The authors make no representation, express or implied, with regard to the accuracy of the information contained in this book and deny legal responsibility or liability for any errors or omissions that may be made. Statistical results in particular should be checked with at least one other program and/or with a statistician to verify important conclusions. Drug dosages and medical advice are for illustration only, and should be checked against other sources"

The chapters on statistics and on OpenEpi were made possible, in part, by a grant from the Bill and Melinda Gates Foundation.

We have tried to adhere to the medical adage, "First of all, do no harm," and would be grateful for your comments, corrections, and suggestions. The authors' email addresses can be found at www.openepi.com.

Authors

Andrew G. Dean, MD, MPH, FACE, began his public health career as Peace Corps Physician for Somalia in 1965, then was an international health researcher, President of the Council of State and Territorial Epidemiologists, and avocational computer programmer before joining the US Centers for Disease Control and Prevention(CDC) in 1984. He led the Epi Info development team for 18 years. Beginning in 2002, he programmed the Javascript framework and interface of OpenEpi, and developed Epi Info applications for patient records and antiretroviral dose calculations in an HIV/AIDS clinic in the Dominican Republic. He has 70 publications, including a blog and websites at www.openepi.com and www.epiinformatics.com .

Kevin M. Sullivan, PhD, MPH, MHA, was a member of the Epi Info Development Team, and supervised the statistical programming in the current version of Epi Info. He is co-designer, statistical prime mover, and publicist for OpenEpi, as well as Associate Professor in the Departments of Epidemiology and Global Health, Rollins School of Public Health at Emory University, and a consultant in the Nutrition Branch at CDC. His life list includes 82 peer-reviewed publications, 25 books, manuals, or book chapters, and 39 invited articles or letters to the editor. He has a website at http://www.sph.emory.edu/~cdckms/ Kevin is the author of the chapter on nutritional anthropometry, and he and Minn Minn Soe authored the chapters on analysis and statistical methods.

Minn Minn Soe, MD, MPH, MCTM, was born in Burma (Myanmar), and worked with migrants in conflict zones along the Thai-Burma border., before emigrating to the U.S in 2001. He tested Epi Info analytical functions and developed statistical code for parts of Open Epi while working in the Rollins School of Public Health at Emory University. He participated in several epidemiological research studies and population-based surveillance systems at Emory University and the Division of HIV/AIDS, CDC. He is currently a medical epidemiologist at the Tennessee State Health Department. Outside of working hours, Minn and his family are busy raising funds to support poor orphans in Burma.

Taha Kass-Hout, MD, MS, is Director, Division of Emergency Preparedness and Response, Biosurveillance Program Manager, CDC, and a member of the InSTEDD (Innovative Support to Emergencies, Diseases, and Disasters) team (www.InSTEDD.ORG.) He and Eduardo Jezierski are coauthors of Chapter 27, describing a demonstration of an Epi Info database on the Internet "Cloud"

Eduardo Jezierski, MsC, Vice President, Engineering, of InSTEDD, spent nine years in software development at Microsoft, first supporting large-enterprise customers, then later as Program Manager and Solutions Architect.

Consuelo M. Beck-Sagué, MD, FAAP, infectious disease specialist, pediatrician, and medical epidemiologist, worked for almost 20 years at CDC, and then four years as a pediatric clinical consultant for the Clinton Foundation HIV/AIDS program clinician in the Dominican Republic. She is author or co-author of more than 100 publications, a power user of Epi Info, and .co developer of the ARVCalc and Clinic applications described in Chapters 19 and 23.

We are grateful to **Roger Mir** of the Epi Info Development Team, CDC, who provided advice and the GUID example in 20, **Jinghong Ma,** Senior Systems Architect, Data Management Team, Global Immunization Division, CDC, who provided materials for Chapter 26 on the SAFE system, to **Dr. Pasquale Falasca**, Ravenna, Italy (www.epiinfo.it), for data and ideas for Chapter 29 on Clinical Auditing, and **Dr. Leonel Lerebours Nadal,** Santo Domingo, DR, for the spreadsheet report example.

Table of Contents

"Is that a stethoscope around your neck, or a flash memory stick?"

Introduction

Computing, data management, and analysis are essential to quality public health and clinical medicine. In the next few decades it will not be possible to practice either field without computing skills.

Should medical and public health professionals put their hands on keyboards and understand informatics? Ask a surgeon if he/she should give up hands-on operating and leave it to technicians, working through several layers of functionaries to get the job done. This is the model that is implicit in many data systems. The geeks in the back room, fresh from 2-year associates training in "Information Technology" are allowed to run the show because other professionals do not have interest or skills in working with data.

Politicians rightly wring their hands at "the cost of medical care," but who has the tools to discover the pressure points of cost, outcome, preventable risk factors, side effects of prevention, and lack of access to the system? Can we offer an interactive game in four dimensions showing all these elements in color for a given population? Can we make virtual improvements and see the results? Unfortunately, we are a long way from that point. But, for those who want to collect, manage, and analyze data with their own laptop or desktop computers, this book and programs available without cost from the Internet offer the opportunity to leap small or medium sized mountains of data.

Why Free Software?

In the best tradition of medicine and public health, scientific methods are free, and are shared without proprietary interest. Software for public health and medical computing can be considered a detailed methods statement for the computer; it should be freely available for evaluation and worldwide use. This book provides a guide to selected resources for do-it-yourself computing in medicine or public health. The programs mentioned have their own help files, but we will supplement these, and provide examples from public health and health care settings.

Even if you are entirely content with other software resources at your disposal, and/or have no alternative but to use the ones provided by your institution, you may still be interested in free software that you can provide to others, or use to do a survey or study outside the scope of the institution's software. You may have a dataset to explore that came from another source, or an emergency situation requiring quick tabulations, or need a statistical calculator for summary data-- perhaps in a paper you are preparing or reviewing.

The Need for Medical and Public Health Software

A few decades ago, computers were rarely used in medicine or public health except for billing, and epidemiology was done using tick marks on paper. In the 1980's a research project at a university with a $50,000,000 grant saved all its data in four refrigerator-sized hard disk drives that together provided almost a gigabyte of storage. Today, any computer store offers FOUR gigabyte flash-memory devices to put in a pocket with loose change. But most of us don't have our medical records on one of these, or know how to begin finding them in the multiple cities where we have lived, visiting doctors whose names are long ago forgotten.

Since the 1960s, a few dedicated visionaries have felt that medicine without computer assistance is both inefficient and dangerous.

"Where's the outrage?" cried Braithwaite, referring to medical errors as the fourth leading cause of death in the U.S. The outrage should come from how little interest we have in investigating medical errors compared to air disasters.
"Hospitals are the most dangerous place to go. What's the safest? An airplane," he said. The number that die from medical errors is equivalent to a jumbo jet crashing every day.

Dodge J, Health-IT World News, May 21, 2004.

"It is widely recognised that accessing and processing medical information in libraries and patient records is a burden beyond the capacities of the physician's unaided mind in the conditions of medical practice." Dr. Larry Weed, (Weed LL, Clinical Judgment revisited, Methods of Information in Medicine, F.K.Schattauer Verlagsgesellschaft mbH,1999, p. 279)

The US National Library of Medicine and its MEDLARS database led the way in 1964 in developing search capabilities for the medical literature. Today, using MEDLARS and Google.com it is possible to find summary information on almost any medical topic, but too many searches for full text come to a screeching halt at the web page of a publisher who offers to let you read a potentially lifesaving 4-page article, written gratis by another professional, for the price of a hotel room and a 15-minute struggle with an on-line credit card mechanism. Full text access to medical knowledge, and particularly mechanisms for publishers to receive a fair return from worldwide use, are key to the future of medicine, now that search engines are available to begin to make sense of the enormous volume of material.

How Should You Read This Book and Why?

It may be that you are in a university or hospital setting, surrounded by information resources and expensive software, but also restricted by the setting from doing your own computing, when on field trips in Timbuktu or door-to-door interviews in California. You may run a hospital in a developing country, or work as an epidemiologist in any setting, and you need to enter your own data and/or analyze data abstracted from large databases by others. Or you may have students or satellite organizations that cannot afford expensive software, or whose purchasing systems prevent their acquiring it.

We have tried to start from the beginning and enable any medical or public health professional with minimal computer skills to install and use Epi Info in Microsoft Windows(R). OpenEpi is a separate program that runs on the Internet and in Windows, the Macintosh, or Linux, using all the popular browsers. If you are already an experienced Epi Info user, the later chapters describe techniques for developing applications that others can use, and you may want to skip the first few chapters. When you need a particular HowTo, consult the index of this book and also the index for the Epi Info Help file and the examples and tutorials that come with both programs.

Resources

One reason to read this book is that the content is free, and can be distributed in digital form with the software. We know you won't weigh that argument very heavily, as the book may be free, but your time is not, and there are some 8 billion web pages you could also be reading, mostly without charge. If you find it useful, however, you can make as many copies as you like and give them to students or colleagues.

The Epi Info software can be downloaded from www.cdc.gov/epiinfo and OpenEpi from www.openepi.com. Examples given in this book and other teaching materials are available at www.epiinformatics.com. Epi Info comes with practice data sets in SAMPLE.MDB and REFUGEE.MDB. Tutorials are available on the Help menu and in each OpenEpi module.

CHAPTER 1: EPI INFO™ AND OPENEPI

This is a book about two free software packages, Epi Info™ and OpenEpi, and their use in public health and medical settings. Both may be downloaded from the Internet; instructions for downloading and installation are provided in Chapter 3. OpenEpi can also be used directly from the Internet without installation.

Epi Info™

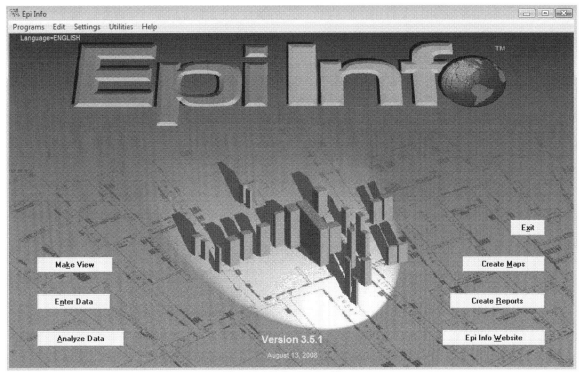

The Epi Info Main Menu

Epi Info is a suite of computer programs for Microsoft Windows(R), developed at the Centers for Disease Control and Prevention (CDC), the US national public health agency, and freely downloadable from the CDC website www.cdc.gov/epiinfo/ . Epi Info allows anyone with modest computer skills to develop a questionnaire or screen form that automatically creates a database and allows entry of as many records as desired. Analysis proceeds through simple commands such as LIST, FREQuency, TABLES, MEANS, MAP and GRAPH.

Results include statistics appropriate to the output. For example, the TABLES command with two yes/no variables representing Disease and Exposure, automatically calculates odds ratios and risk ratios with exact confidence limits, various types of chi-squares, and Fisher exact and mid-p tests of association with graphics of the table contents. The MEANS command offers Student t-tests, ANOVA, and Kruskal-Wallis results. More advanced statistics include linear and logistic regression, analysis of complex sample data, Kaplan-Meier and Cox proportional hazards analysis with graphs. A variety of graphs, including graphs automatically stratified by (for example) county, can be produced with the GRAPH command. The MAP command and the EpiMap program offer elementary, but rather extensive possibilities for Geographic Information Systems.

Commands used interactively are automatically available for saving as a program that can be run again later. A programmable menu is provided that can be used to develop complete applications that are entirely menu driven. Much of this book will describe methods of building on these features.

The first version of Epi Info for DOS was developed in 1985 and the Windows version in 2000. A brief history is available in the "Museum" in the Epi Info website http://www.cdc.gov/epiinfo/background.htm .

Because Epi Info was originally designed for epidemic investigation, epidemiologists and other public health and medical professionals used it on a laptop computer to rapidly develop a questionnaire and enter and analyze data, often in a motel room near the outbreak site.

Over the years, thousands of users have helped to shape Epi Info's features, and it has gradually been adapted for use in more permanent applications, such as surveillance systems or vital statistics at a district or small country level, research studies, record reviews, and even modest Electronic Medical Record systems. This book will describe the use of the Windows version of Epi Info that was first released in the year 2000.

In recent years the manual for Epi Info has given way to the electronic help file, which is less convenient for some purposes. The CDC Epi Info Development Team plans to release a printable manual in PDF (Adobe Reader) format. When available, this will be a valuable resource to be used in conjunction with this book. We will review the basics, but the present book will focus on building applications for long-term use.

Features of Epi Info™ for Windows

- MakeView – allows designing a questionnaire or form View on the screen. The data entry process can be guided by program statements called Check Code if desired

- Enter – displays Views created in MakeView to enter data into the database or retrieve records already entered

- Analysis – Reads, lists, imports, exports, and does tabulation and statistical analysis, mapping, and graphing of data from files in 20 different popular data formats

- Compatibility with industry standards, including:

- Microsoft Access and other SQL and ODBC databases

- Visual Basic, Version 6

- Output as HTML web pages

- Epi Report, a tool that allows the user to format data contained in Access or SQL Server. The generated reports can be saved as HTML files for easy distribution or web publishing.

- Epi Map, an ArcView®-compatible GIS

- NutStat, a nutrition anthropometry program that calculates percentiles and z-scores using either the 2000 CDC or the 1978 CDC/WHO growth reference

- Logistic regression and Kaplan-Meier survival analysis

- A program for comparing data entered by two operators as a check on accuracy

- Password protection, encryption, and compression of Epi Info™ data

- Teaching exercises

- Analysis, import and export of data in 20 different file formats

System Requirements

- Windows 98, NT 4.0, 2000, XP, or Vista is required.

- 32 MB of Random Access Memory. More RAM: 64 MB for Windows 4.0 and 2000, 128 MB for Windows XP, 1 GB for Vista.

- 200 megahertz processor is recommended - 300 for Windows XP., more for Vista

- At least 260 megabytes of free hard disk space (Drive C) to install; 130 megabytes after installation.

Who Uses Epi Info and What For?

Since 1998, there have been approximately 2,000,000 successful downloads of Epi Info from the CDC website in 180 of Earth's 193 countries. A Google search for EpiInfo produces more than a million references.

There has not been a proper survey of Epi Info use internationally, but it is used as the core of surveillance systems for immunizable disease in 27 African countries and 8 provinces in Kenya. An Epi Info system for Acute Flaccid Paralysis (possible poliomyelitis) surveillance in India functions in 300 district sites covering 25% of India's population.

Ma J, Otten M, Kamadjeu R, Mir R, Rosencrans L, McLaughlin S, Yoon S. New frontiers for health information systems using Epi Info in developing countries: Structured application framework for Epi Info (SAFE). Int J Med Inform. 2007 Mar 16;

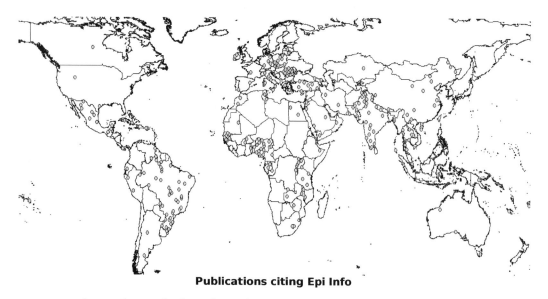

Publications citing Epi Info

The map above shows the location of more than 300 articles referenced in the MEDLARS system for which a country of origin and "Epi Info" could be extracted from the title or abstract. Note that this almost excludes the US and UK where country is seldom mentioned in article titles. Supplementary Google searches, however, turned up 85,900 references containing "Epi Info" and "United States" or US and 30,800 with "Epi Info" and "United Kingdom" or UK Examining the first 50 confirmed all to be relevant, although not all were formal, peer-reviewed publications.

Of the 1,060,000 documents found that mentioned Epi Info, (using the search term, Epiinfo, in www.Google.com (on September 28, 2009):

- 52.5% contained the word "epidemiology"
- 21.4% contained the word "surveillance"
- 14.3% contained the word "hospital"
- 14% contained the word "clinical"
- 11.3% contained the word "survey"
- 7.8% contained the phrase, "public health"

For pages classified by language, only 54% (149,000) were in English, the rest being in: Portuguese (45,400); Spanish (39,000); French (14,000); Simplified (People's Republic, Singapore) Chinese (7,7200); German (1,770); Italian (6,580); and Thai (2,620). Other languages with more than 200 web documents included Vietnamese, Japanese,Traditional (Taiwan, Hong Kong, Macau) Chinese, Arabic, Russian, Norwegian, Dutch, and Korean.

It should be noted that the number of hits in both the Google and Yahoo search engines is highly approximate, and should only be taken as a general guide. It is safe to conclude that Epi Info is widely used in public health and clinical medicine. You can perform your own searches to find web pages from or about a particular location and situation.

In Lima, Peru, data for a CDC and Partners in Health research project on Multidrug-Resistant Tuberculosis (MDRTB) was entered into an Epi Info questionnaire View with 16 related views. The paper data abstraction form comprises 45 pages, and many patients have scores or hundreds of x-rays, cultures, sputum smears, and drug-months of treatment. Customized menus prepare data tables entered in duplicate by different operators for comparison in the Data Compare module, disclosing and correcting hundreds of errors that otherwise would have entered the final database. A menu for Analysis allows graphing of cultures or smears over time for each patient and performs calculations like, "Duration from first MDRTB treatment regimen to first of at least two consecutive negative cultures, provided that a positive culture was obtained within 30 days before or xx days after the start of treatment." The latter makes extensive use of the new SUMMARIZE command in Analysis, which, when combined with RELATE, allows access to each patient's first (min date) or last (max date) record of the type that is selected.

The CDC Global AIDS Program (GAP) uses Epi Info forr the collection and analysis of data on HIV and AIDS in 27 Africancountries. GAP and the Global Immunization Division of CDC have collaborated to develop a structured application development framework called SAFE (Structured Application Framework for Epi Info)

SAFE uses a standard folder structure, modular programming, dynamic program creation from resource files, an application user interface, variable naming conventions, and a standard analysis and reporting format. It has been used for a data management system for prevention of mother-to-child transmission of HIV in Tanzania and Botswana, and Nigeria. It was used to build a Voluntary Counseling and Testing (VCT) application in Mozambique.

The HIV/AIDS applications share similar user interfaces and resource files, such as GIS shape files, code tables, and analytic programs. The structured framework will allow more rapid application development, easier support, and faster updates.

Because Epi Info may be freely distributed without licensing restrictions or cost, it is a useful resource for applications in developing countries. Since it incorporates many common Windows file formats, it can be combined with commercial programs such as Excel or Microsoft Access where these are available. Maps developed in ArcView at a central site can be used at all sites that have Epi Info and its Epi Map program. The Epi Info menu is programmable and can be used to unite elements of several programs into a single convenient application.

What is OpenEpi?

OpenEpi is a series of Internet programs providing online or offline calculation for epidemiologic summary data. It provides an alternative to the DOS program Statcalc that is provided with Epi Info. OpenEpi includes statistics for counts and person-time rates in descriptive and analytic studies, stratified analysis with exact confidence limits, matched pair analysis, sample size and power calculations, random numbers, chi-square for dose-response trend, sensitivity, specificity and other evaluation statistics, R x C tables, and links to other useful sites.

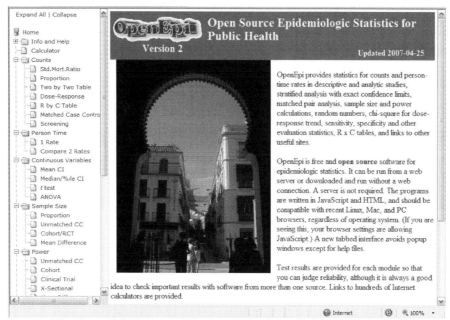

The OpenEpi Menu and Framework of Statistical Calculators

OpenEpi is free and open source software for epidemiologic statistics. It can be run from the web server at www.openepi.com or downloaded and run without a web connection. A server is not required. The programs are written in JavaScript and HTML, and should be compatible with recent Linux, Mac, and PC browsers, regardless of operating system. A new tabbed interface avoids popup windows except for help files. The open source license allows the programs to be downloaded, distributed, or translated. OpenEpi development and testing was supported in part by a grant from the Bill and Melinda Gates Foundation. Test results are provided for each module so that you can judge reliability, although it is always a good idea to check important results with software from more than one source. Links to hundreds of other Internet calculators are provided. A toolkit for creating new modules and for translation is included in the downloadable version.

The website registers over a million "hits" per year, from 155 countries, about two thirds being outside the US. There are currently (October 2009) 87,000 citations to "OpenEpi" in Google search.

References

www.cdc.gov/epiinfo/ The main Epi Info site, from which you can download Epi Info and find other resources

www.openepi.com The site for OpenEpi

www.epiinformatics.com A site for Epi Info and OpenEpi resources, including this book

CHAPTER 2: COUNTING DEATHS, DISEASES, AND MEDICAL CARE EVENTS

Public health surveillance and most medical care monitoring and research depend on counting or measuring something and summarizing the results. The pioneers who paved the way toward counting events and summarizing results for a population, include John Graunt for mortality, and John Snow for associating mortality with risk factors and introducing the use of Geographic Information Systems.

Counting of Cases by Person, Place, and Time

I N my Discourses upon the *Bills* I shall first speak of the *Casualties,* then give my Observations with reference to the *Places,* and *Parishes* comprehended in the *Bills;* and next of the *Years,* and *Seasons.*

Natural and Political Observations Made upon the Bills of Mortality (1662)

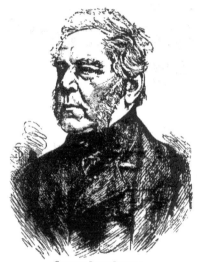

CAPTAIN JOHN GRAUNT

Person, Place, and Time, defined as in a modern epidemiology class, but three and a half centuries earlier.

[Portrait from http://www.york.ac.uk/depts/maths/histstat/people/graunt.gif but others doubt that this is the right John Graunt]

Risk Factors and Geographic Information Systems

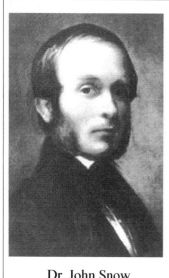

Dr. John Snow

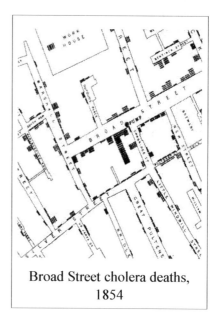

Broad Street cholera deaths,
1854

..in 1853, whilst the mortality in St. Saviour's was at the rate of two hundred and twenty-seven to one hundred thousand living, that of Christchurch was only at the rate of forty-three. Now St. Saviour's is supplied with water entirely by the Southwark and Vauxhall Company, and Christchurch is chiefly supplied by the Lambeth Company.

Dr. John Snow, the patron saint and founder of modern epidemiology, not only developed the plotting of data on maps ("Geographic Information Systems") with exquisite precision, but also furthered the analysis of epidemic data in terms of risk factors, such as consumption of water from particular sources. We now have the benefit of a century and a half of statistical development to do the same analysis, but the grand concept of finding ASSOCIATIONS between DISEASE and RISK FACTORS using RATES is well illustrated in Dr. Snow's work.

Electronic Medical Records

Electronic Medical Records have undergone a half-century of development since the 1950s, and been the subject of much enthusiasm, massive standardization efforts, and many books and articles. Although the adoption of electronic records is accelerating in the US and Europe, there are still relatively few hospitals with completely computerized record systems., and fewer still with regular analysis of medical conditions encountered.

http://en.wikipedia.org/wiki/Electronic_medical_record

Generally, the priorities of clinical computing are accurate recording and retrieval of individual patient events, billing, and, of course, legal integrity and confidentiality. Many programs have been written to assist in individual doctor-patient interaction, for example, in differential diagnosis, choosing and prescribing medication, and summarizing laboratory values.

Population Medicine vs Clinical Care—Two Faces of Medical Computing

Epidemiology, represented by John Graunt and John Snow, and tens of thousands of current epidemiologists and public health workers, proceeds by COUNTING or AVERAGING data for defined populations—the ill and the well, for example, or the exposed and the unexposed. As suggested by Graunt, the analysis usually includes PERSON, PLACE, and TIME.

Analysis by COUNTING in categories is usually known as a FREQUENCY DISTRIBUTION, for example, the numbers of males and females, and the data are described as CATEGORICAL. Measurements like blood pressure or weight (CONTINUOUS data) are averaged to determine the MEAN and other summary statistics.

At least since John Snow, epidemiologic analysis has included the search for associations between DISEASE (Graunt's "casualties," other's "adverse events" or just "events") and EXPOSURE to putative RISK FACTORS--the foods, airs, waters, and places of modern times. In its simplest form, this involves calculation of rates of DISEASE among the EXPOSED and UNEXPOSED cohorts or rate of EXPOSURE among the CASES and CONTROLS, usually done by cross tabulation in a two-by-two table.

The twentieth century saw the statistical tools refined to remove the influence of CONFOUNDERS, factors like age, sex, and pre-existing disease, that bias results by being associated with both disease AND exposure. For example, age is already known to be associated with higher rates of cancer. A citizen reports a high rate of cancer among workers in a factory, or residents of a certain block. It is important to correct for the effect of age (a possible confounder), particularly if the factory employs mostly older workers, or the block contains an old-persons' home. Statistical techniques for this include stratified analysis and logistic regression.

So far, we have suggested that clinical computing focuses more on collecting and preserving accurate records, and assisting with care of the patient. Aggregation is done for research purposes, and considerable extraction and processing is necessary for billing, insurance claims, and medical staff oversight, but the priorities rightly rest on care of the individual patient. In a later chapter, we will describe a clinical care system written in Epi Info that provides assistance in calculating doses of antiretroviral drugs for treatment of HIV and AIDS, a non-trivial task in pediatrics because doses are based variously on body weight or body surface area, and a number of extra conditions must be considered.

Aggregation and statistics can be done by a variety of software packages such as SPSS, SAS, and Stata, but outside organizational settings, they may be expensive, and extra features like mapping and graphing may cost extra. None of these programs offer customizable data entry forms to the extent provided by Epi Info. Microsoft Access provides programmable data entry and report generation, but does not do epidemiologic statistics. In the long run, we all tend to favor the tools with which we are familiar, but we hope to show in this book that many tasks can be done without professional programmers, without software cost, and without fear of violating proprietary restrictions, by using free programs such as Epi Info and OpenEpi.

CHAPTER 3: DATA CONCEPTS AND DEFINITIONS

What Is or Are DATA?

Data, now generally accepted as either singular or plural [1] consist(s) of information that can be stored or processed.

> "Print, film, magnetic, and optical storage media produced about 5 exabytes of new information in 2002. Ninety-two percent of the new information was stored on magnetic media, mostly in hard disks."
>
> ---
>
> http://www2.sims.berkeley.edu/research/projects/how-much-info-2003/execsum.htm

This is the equivalent of printed material from 40,000 trees (800 gigabytes) *for each person* of the 6.3 billion global population. One can now buy a disk drive to hold that much --one terabyte (1000. gigabytes)-- for two days' minimum wage in the US.

Most of the data is in the form of images, films, recordings, web pages, and documents, that have complex structures not easy to summarize, after ignoring the problem of more than 6000 languages on earth[2]. Even text documents vary so much that the Holy Grail of universal standardized medical records is not in hand after many decades on the Quest[3]

Epi Info, OpenEpi, and many other database and statistics packages organize data in rows and columns or records and variables to make summarization possible. If all the numbers in a column called AGE represent ages in years, it becomes possible for the computer to produce a count, a mean value, and other statistics. Most of this book concerns methods for placing data in rows and columns, and for doing analysis of such data to produce meaningful information.

What is a RECORD?

In both epidemiologic and clinical systems, the concept of RECORD is basic to computing. For clinicians, "records" are folders or clipboards containing various forms that describe interactions with a single patient. The clinical record as a whole is in a format that might be described as "semi-structured," although that term would be too generous for some of the handwriting and the loose papers protruding from the back.

---

1 http://www.askoxford.com/asktheexperts/faq/aboutgrammar/data

2 http://www.lsadc.org/info/pdf_files/howmany.pdf

Epi Info and OpenEpi

Most computer systems designed for statistical processing depend on records arranged in rows and columns, like a ledger or spreadsheet. Usually the columns are known as variables or fields, and there is one row for each RECORD with an identifying number included. Examples of RECORDS in clinical computing include:

- The admission record of one patient
- A prescription or medication order
- A visit or clinical encounter by a patient
- An operative record
- A discharge summary
- A laboratory report
- Emergency medical services record of one ambulance run

The concept of a single patient folder as a record still holds, but to preserve the neat row-and-column concept, it must be broken into a number of *related* records, each containing a record number or key to linked it to the main record--the face sheet or admissions record. Computer records, in order to allow easy processing, are generally in *structured* format, although in some software, images, documents, music, and videos are becoming part of the row-and-column structure. Epi Info allows images to be included within records.

Public Health records might include:

- A report of one (or many) cases of measles to a health department
- In interview with one case or control in an investigation or study
- An abstract of a hospital record in an investigation or study

Many records are collected primarily for the purpose of aggregation, and, without analysis, have very little value. Additional records may be produced as a result of analysis, for example:

- A summary of disease reports for the past week
- Frequency of recent salmon croquette consumption among cases and controls

Public health agencies often run clinics or conduct home care nursing, which gives rise to records similar to those in clinical care in general. Other records where the focus is on storage and retrieval might include:

- An immunization card
- A restaurant inspection result

---

3   http://en.wikipedia.org/wiki/HL7

Environmental monitoring gives rise to records that may be useful from time to time in public health, but whose primary purpose is monitoring and archival, for example:

- Hourly chlorine and turbidity levels at a water filtration station
- Ozone levels in the air at a particular place and time

Variables and Fields

Records, in turn, are usually broken into variables or fields. We use the terms interchangeably, although "field" is used when entering data, and "variable" is used as in algebra during data analysis so that one can refer to Age as the difference between DateOfBirth and TodaysDate in issuing commands.

In the row and column paradigm, Columns are Variables, with Rows being records, each of which has the same column components. Epi Info also allows you to DEFINE new variables that can be set to values by program commands, and optionally written into a new Data table.

Data Values

Given Rows and Columns or Records and Variables, the values in the grid cells are Data Values. If the left margin of the grid contains record numbers, then data values lie at the intersection of Row (record number) and Column (variable name) values.

Record Number	Age	Sex
1	13	Female
2	24	Male
3	56	Female

The Age for the record having Record Number 2, is 24. Sex in this record is "Male".

Forms, Questionnaires, or Views

Statistical programs and spreadsheets usually offer a grid similar to those above, into which Data Values can be entered. For some purposes, such as accounting, the grid format is the most convenient and efficient, although it favors those with good eyesight and a steady mouse.

Another method of data entry presents a questionnaire or form on the computer screen so that values can be entered with the keyboard, moving from field to field with the Enter or Tab key or with the mouse. Many such forms are custom programmed for a particular purpose, but Epi Info allows you to start with a form and build the database automatically. In Epi Info for Windows, the questionnaire or form is also called a View, since one can have several "views" of the same database.

In practice, this has not often happened, and the terms "Form" or "Questionnaire" may be more appropriate.

Database=Project=MDB

By now, you are wondering where the data are stored. In general, one or more collections of records is called a database. In Epi Info, the default database is of the Microsoft Access type, or MDB for Microsoft Database. We also chose to call it a Project in Epi Info because it can contain one or many View and Data combinations related to a particular topic.

An MDB, also called a Project, is a file having the extension .MDB. It contains TABLES of at least the following types:

- A Data table—simple rows and columns, compatible with Access and many other systems

- A View table—useful only to Epi Info, describes a screen View with details such as fonts, screen prompts, and locations of data entry fields

- (Optional) Code tables—containing choices to present to the user for a particular field, for example "Male" and "Female" for a Sex field.

Since an MDB can hold up to about a thousand tables, it is possible to put many Views and their corresponding Data tables in a single MDB or Project. In practice, it is probably better to start a new Project for each logical set of Views, for example, a single epidemic investigation or study.

Types of Tables in Epi Info Databases

The main types of tables in Epi Info are View Tables, Data Tables, and Code Tables. A View Table contains a row for each page and variable of the Epi Info questionnaire, form, or View. The columns contain information about the Prompt, the Variable Name, the Data Type, location of the entry blank and the prompt on the screen (x and y coordinates), the Check Code that belongs to the field, page or record, and lists of legal values. View Tables only have meaning to Epi Info, not to the average user, and not to Microsoft Access.

Data Tables, however, contain one row for each record (instance of a form/questionnaire/View) and can be read and processed by Epi Info, Microsoft Access, and many other programs. The columns correspond to variables or fields in the database, and each has a variable name.

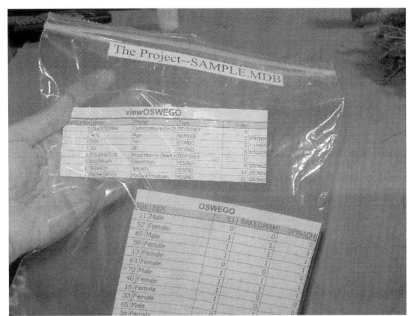

A View Table and a Data Table Inside an "MDB"

Imagine the MDB as a plastic bag, in which the Data tables and Views (and optional Code tables) reside. The View table, called viewOswego, is a table containing variable names, types, and screen prompts, with a number of columns to the right of those shown that indicate placement on the screen, fonts, Check Code, etc.

The matched data table called Oswego contains rows (records) of data values, shown here as Age, Sex, Ill, Bakedham, and Spinach. Each person can be identified as Ill or Well and a consumer or non-consumer of Baked Ham and Spinach before the foodborne outbreak. Other foods, times and dates would be shown in columns to the right.

Levels of Computer Use

Computer use can be divided into several levels:

1 Interactive computing--Enter some data, click a choice, and get results. Generally statistical calculators fall in this area, as does the interactive analysis of a data file in a statistics program like SPSS, Epi Info, SAS, or Stata.

2 Computer programming--Create a series of program statements that are saved in a file so that you can repeat the same operations some other time, or give the program to others to run. Epi Info constructs a program as you interact with the Analysis module, thus somewhat blurring the distinction between interactive computing and programming. Editing the resulting program and inserting new commands could be considered "programming."

3 Application or systems development--Create a number of programs, database definitions, help files, links to Internet sites, and other useful items, and make the programs accessible and easy to use by providing a menu system. Test the system with multiple users on different kinds of computer systems to be sure it can be as widely used as desired.

The book will provide examples of all three levels of use, using free resources--mainly Epi Info and OpenEpi. OpenOffice was used to write this book, and Google searching is the basis for most of our medical and computing decisions. The next chapter describes the two main programs and gives an example of how Google can be used to evaluate their distribution and use.

Concepts for Using Epi Info

Databases or Projects, also known as MDBs, can contain one or many data sets. Major data functions that you will encounter on the Epi Info menu are:

Make View

A dataset is described by designing a Questionnaire View on the screen. Optional Check Code commands can be inserted to guide the data entry process.

Enter Data

A Data table is automatically constructed from the Questionnaire View and data can be entered in the blank fields shown on the screen. The cursor moves automatically from one field to another and from page to page. Saving of data is automatic as soon as one leaves a page or record.

Analyze Data

The Analysis program can read, tabulate, and do statistics with data from the current dataset or from files in 21 other formats. Analysis commands are produced and saved as a program (PGM) as you click on and interact with dialog boxes for each command.

CHAPTER 4: INSTALLING EPI INFO AND OPENEPI

Skip this chapter if you have already installed Epi Info and wish to use OpenEpi directly from www.openepi.com. Local installation of OpenEpi is also described here as an option for use when there is no Internet connection.

Why do we insert a chapter on installation at the beginning of the book rather than buried in an Appendix at the end?

- Because this is a manual about *using* the software, it is important to use the software.

- Downloading and installing these two programs is quite simple, since they are not encumbered with advertisements, adware, and complicated configuration choices.

- OpenEpi can be used directly from the Internet and need only be installed for use where there is no Internet connection, or, in Microsoft Windows, if you wish to save output files to disk.

- One of our most successful classroom experiences required the students to install Epi Info on their own laptops prior to the class.

Installing Epi Info

Epi Info is a Microsoft Windows® program. You can run it in any Windows-based computer likely to be still running. If you have a Macintosh with Windows installed in a program like Parallels or Bootcamp, you can install and run Epi Info. under Windows. Windows emulators on the Mac and Linux platforms are available, but little testing has been done in these environments. Current versions (3.5.1) of Epi Info will not run directly in the Macintosh or Linux operating systems, but the upcoming Version 7 of Epi Info is designed to run in Ubuntu, a version of Linux.

Requirements for installation are given on the Epi Info website, but any reasonably modern computer with Windows will be fine. You do need to have appropriate user settings on your computer to install software (usually administrator or power user). To install Epi Info, point your browser to http://www.cdc.gov/epiinfo/ and click on the download button to choose Web Install or

Epi Info and OpenEpi

Download Setup.exe. Both work well, but downloading Setup provides a copy that you can put on a CD and give to others. We suggest changing the file name Setup.exe to something unique like EISetup35.exe, so that it is not confused with other "Setup.exe" files on your computer. It doesn't matter much where you save the setup file, as long as you have disk space.

Read the instructions about older versions, and uninstall them if necessary (Windows START | All Programs | Epi Info | Uninstall). The Web Install and Setup installations are nearly identical after you get started by clicking the Web Install button or double clicking the (hopefully renamed) setup file icon in My Computer. If you say OK or "Next" to all the choices, you should have a complete installation with an Epi Info icon on the desktop in a few minutes. The dialog to choose individual programs looks like only the first one is selected, but OK installs them all.

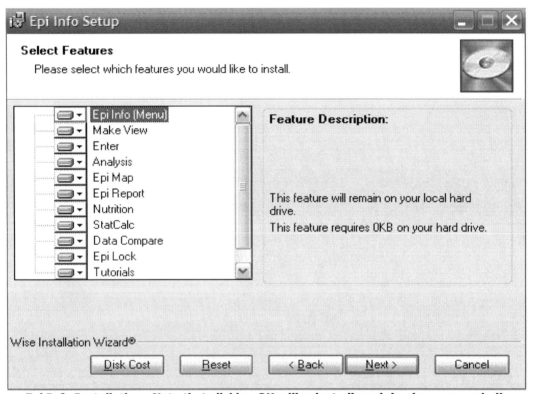

Epi Info Installation. Note that clicking OK will select all modules (recommended).

After this has been accomplished, you should see setup screen shown above. In most cases, you want to install all the programs, so just click the NEXT button, and accept the default settings while the programs install.

If things went well, click on the Epi Info icon and you should see the main menu and be ready for the next chapter. Help is available (epiinfo@cdc.gov) as described on the website and in the chapter on troubleshooting later in this book.

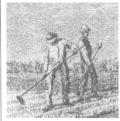

"You mean you just downloaded that new hoe for free without asking the systems overseer?"

(image: http://www.ortongardens.com/images/hoe.jpg, with permission)

Installing Epi Info in Microsoft Windows Vista®

Microsoft Windows Vista requires an additional module called the DHTML Editing Control for Applications, that, for mysterious reasons, must be downloaded directly from the Microsoft Website rather than from the Epi Info website. This step is easy but confusing. Just click on the link called "Download the DHTML Editing Control for Applications" at the bottom of the www.cdc.gov/epiinfo/ page, and you will arrive at the Microsoft site after a warning message about Microsoft being outside of CDC. Ignore the voluminous text on the page and click the rectangular "Download" button. Agree to any messages from Vista and allow the DHTML Editing Control to install. Installation and use of Epi Info should then similar in both Windows XP and Vista.

Installing Epi Info for Languages Other Than English

The Epi Info website (www.cdc.gov/epiinfo) currently offers language packages to run Epi Info in Spanish, Italian, or Russian rather than English. Unfortunately, the language packages must be downloaded and installed separately, as follows:

1. Go to www.cdc.gov/epiinfo and find the link to TRANSLATIONS. Click to this page and download one or more of the three translation files to a directory in your epi_info directory called TRANSEXE.

2. Run the Epi Info menu by clicking its icon on the desktop and choose MANAGE TRANSLATIONS from the SETTINGS menu. Most of this complicated dialog is for translators, not for users; you need only the INSTALL feature. You should see your downloaded language in the box on the left. Click to select it and then click INSTALL.

3. You should see a dialog from TSETUP about a slight delay, and then (with almost no delay), another message that says EXIT TSETUP. The latter means success, and you can now proceed to the SETTINGS menu again to use CHOOSE LANGUAGE and select your language. Now now until you choose ENGLISH or another language, Epi Info will operate in the chosen language.

4. Note: In versions of Epi Info prior to 3.4, Spanish is already supplied with the installation program, and you need only use the INSTALL LANGUAGE and CHOOSE LANGUAGE features of the SETTINGS menu to install and choose it.

Installing OpenEpi on a Local Computer

OpenEpi is easy to use directly from www.openepi.com on the Net , but, if you are traveling to those few remaining areas where there are no Internet cafes (usually with Internet, but no café), you can run the programs from your hard disk or even from a CDROM without an Internet connection. They are entirely constructed as web pages, and will run in any modern browser that supports JavaScript and HTML, in Windows, the Mac, or Linux. Even some cell phones will now run OpenEpi in their browsers (see the later chapter on OpenEpi).

To install OpenEpi on a local drive, first access http://www.openepi.com and find the menu item called Download OpenEpi, about two-thirds of the way down the list on the left side of the menu screen. Click this item and follow the instructions on the download page. If you have a Windows or Vista computer, choose the MSI download on the right side of the page. If you have Linux or a Macintosh but not Windows, then choose the ZIP file. In either case, clicking the link should download the file.

You may choose to save the file or to open and run it directly. The MSI file will install OpenEpi in a location that you choose, or in the default Windows Program Files folder. Linux and Macintosh systems will unzip OpenEpi.zip after allowing a choice of location.

To run OpenEpi, double click its icon in Windows, or run Index.htm in other systems. You can double-click the icon or Index.htm to bring up the default browser, or run the browser first and then choose Index.htm as the local file to be run.

The MSI installation places several icons on the desktop:

- OpenEpi, to run the local program

- OpenEpiSave, to run OpenEpi and save output to disk in a folder called RESULTS

- OE-EpiInfo Linker, to run a program that modifies the Epi Info menu and adds a link to OpenEpi under Utilities. After you have run this program once, you can delete its icon. Epi Info must be installed on the same computer before you run this program.

OE-EpiInfo Linker makes a copy of the EpiInfo menu, originalEpiInfo.MNU, before modifying EpiInfo.MNU, in case anything goes wrong.

Note::Unfortunately, there is a limitation in the Google Chrome browser that does not allow saving a language and other preferences when running OpenEpi from a local disk, and we cannot recommend that Google Chrome be used for this purpose, although it runs OpenEpi from the web very well.Having completed the desired installations, you are **armed and dangerous to unevaluated data and READY[4] TO ROCK-N-ROLL.**

4

CHAPTER 5: THE EPI INFO MAIN MENU

Getting Acquainted

To run Epi Info, find it's icon on the desktop, and double-click it. You should see the menu..

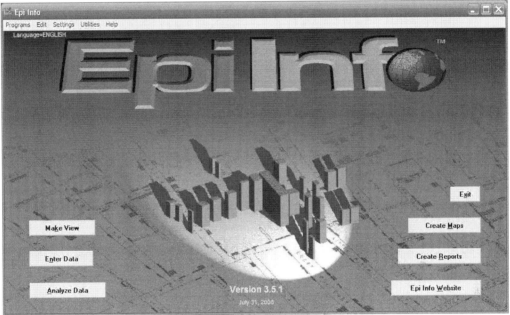

The Epi Info Main Menu

The screen image is John Snow's famous map of the location of cholera cases surrounding the Broad Street pump in London in 1854. Artistic license has been taken in representing cases near the pump as vertical solids rather than with Dr. Snow's neat tick marks.

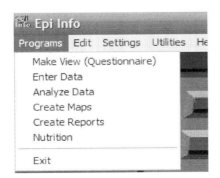

The main programs of Epi Info can be accessed either through the PROGRAMS submenu as shown to the left or by clicking on the menu buttons.

Epi Info and OpenEpi

MakeView is used to design a questionnaire or View. Epi Info automatically constructs a data table from the View so that data can be entered in the **Enter** program. **Analysis** is the data management and statistics program that reads any of 22 file formats, performs user-determined manipulations of the data, and produces tables, epidemiologic statistics, and graphs. **Epi Map** links geographically related data to maps, either from the Create Maps button or from Analysis.

On the EDIT menu, alternative pictures can be chosen from the PICTURE item. Edit This Menu displays the text behind the current menu. The SETTINGS menu provides for installation and choice of non English language translations of Epi Info, and a setting to determine whether new database files will be created in Microsoft Access 97 or Microsoft Access 2000/2002 format. Epi Info will read files in either format automatically, but needs to have a preference set for creating new files. (Note: A bug in Epi Info 3.5.1 prevents making a View from an existing data table unless the database type is Access 97.)

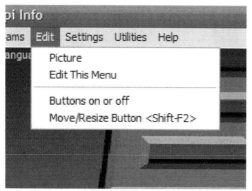

The Edit Menu

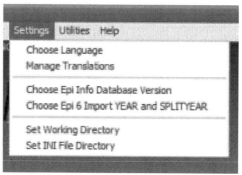

The Settings Menu

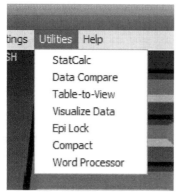

The Utilities Menu

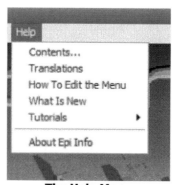

The Help Menu

Menu items under UTILITIES include the ***StatCalc*** epidemiologic calculator, and programs for comparing (validating) data in two different tables and for encryption (***EpiLock***). ***Table-to-View*** produces a questionnaire View from a Microsoft Access data table, and Visualize Data allows access to the inner details of database files for expert users.

The HELP menu contains the entire manual and help file rather modestly listed as CONTENTS. Tutorials include three interactive exercises in epidemiologic computing. The Epi Info Exercises are the basis of a week-long advanced course in Epi Info use. They are best used as printed material. What's New describes features introduced in the most recent Epi Info for those already familiar with Epi Info. A README.TXT file downloadable from the CDC website provides further information about recent improvements.

To gain confidence and to see that your system is functioning well, you might click on each of the buttons on the main menu and briefly examine the program that appears. After you run a program, return to the menu by the Exit button, the small "x" box in the upper right corner, or EXIT in the FILE menu. We will visit each program again in more detail, as described below.

The Menu (MNU) File

If you are interested in the details of the file behind the menu, the item called EDIT THIS MENU on the EDIT menu will display it in the Wordpad editor. This text file is responsible for both the appearance and the function of the menu. Other MNU files can be created to develop customized menus for other purposes.

CHAPTER 6: MAKEVIEW AND ENTER

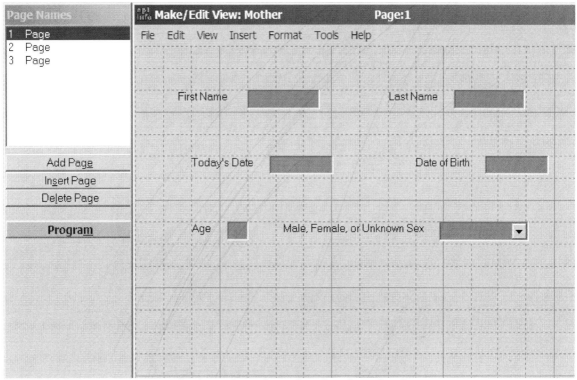

Designing a Questionnaire View in MakeView

Concept

A Microsoft Access® *database* or Epi Info *project* is a file that contains multiple tables.
An Epi Info questionnaire is stored in a View table, and Epi Info automatically creates a
Data table for storing entries.

Designing A Questionnaire View

To run MakeView, click on the MakeView button on the main menu screen. You should see a blank page for constructing a View. Questionnaires are called Views in Epi Info because there can be more than one View of a database or data table. A database table with the prefix "view" stores the screen appearance of the questionnaire, the characteristics of the fields, and any Check Code that gives special instructions for the data entry process. Data values entered in the Enter program are stored in another table, the Data table, without a special prefix.

To make a View, from the FILE menu choose NEW…. The dialog CREATE OR OPEN PROJECT appears. Enter a name for your project database, such as your name or initials, and click OPEN.

A project or database (.MDB for "Microsoft Database") file can hold as many Views and data tables as you wish (well, up to 1000, anyway). Generally it is best to create a new MDB file for each project you develop, as an MDB containing hundreds of tables will be hard to manage. Analysis programs for processing the data can be stored in the same MDB with the data, making a convenient project package, although they are easier to edit if stored separately as text files.

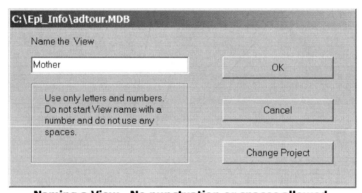

Naming a View. No punctuation or spaces allowed.

In the "Name the View" dialog, enter MOTHER as the name of the View within the MDB, and then click OK. Place the cursor near the upper left corner of the blank screen and click the *right* mouse button. The field dialog box that appears offers options for entering the prompt, the field type and length, and a number of others like Repeat Last.

See Chapter 16 for a discussion of "How Many Fields is Too Many," and precautions to take if your View exceeds 200 fields.

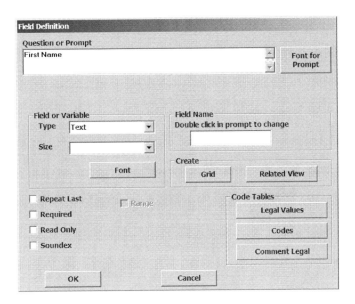

For the first field, enter the prompt "First Name" (without the quotation marks) and press Enter twice. This makes a text field that can hold up to 255 characters.

Concept

A *Field* is a place on the screen for entering data. It usually has a question or prompt and one of various types of entry blanks. The Field Name is the same as the name of the variable or column in a separate data table that stores the data.

For the next field, you could move the cursor and right-click with the mouse on a suitable location, but, to see a shortcut method, press Enter instead while the cursor is in the FIRST NAME field. The field dialog pops up again and you are ready to enter "Last Name" as the prompt. After doing so, press Enter twice, and note that the second field is now automatically positioned on the View.

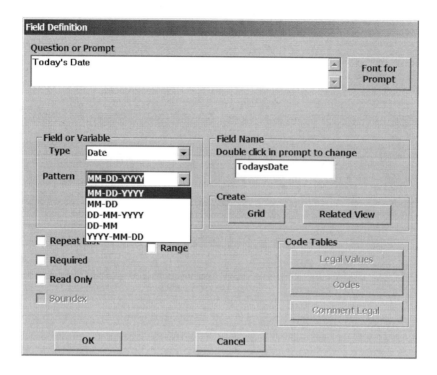

Below First Name, right-click to add another field. Enter the prompt "Today's Date," and use the scroll bar to the right of the field types to see the other types. Choose the DATE type and the appropriate date format as MM-DD-YYYY or DD-MM-YYYY in the dialog. Click OK. Add another field for "Date of Birth," using the same field type and pattern. Click OK.

Right-click on the form to make a field for AGE. Type "Age" as the prompt. Choose NUMBER for the TYPE and then choose ### or ## from the PATTERN list. You can also type patterns into the pattern window. Click on OK at the bottom of the dialog.

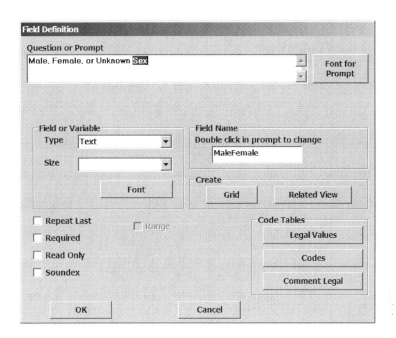

The next field is "Sex." We will use it to illustrate how variable names are constructed. Right-click where you would like to place the field. Type "Male, Female, or Unknown Sex" in the prompt window, press Enter, and note what appears in the Field Name window on the right. Now click again in the prompt window, and with the left mouse button held down, select just the word "Sex". Double-click on the selected word, "Sex," in the prompt window. Note that the variable name becomes SEX. (In Epi Info 6, we would have enclosed "Sex" in curly brackets.)

Specifying Legal Values

It is often important to limit the valid entries in a given field to prevent misspellings, upper-and-lower case combinations, and other freelancing. An examination of surveillance records at CDC, for example, revealed 10 different ways to indicate that a "bat" was involved in a rabid animal report, including entries in Latin.

Hence, let's create legal values for SEX by clicking the LEGAL VALUES button. In the dialog box that appears, choose CREATE NEW, and then enter suitable values (Male, Female, Unknown) in the list that appears, pressing Enter after each to obtain a new blank line. Click OK, and then OK again in the field dialog box. Note the button on the right side of the SEX field. Left-click on the button to show the list of legal values from which to select during data entry.

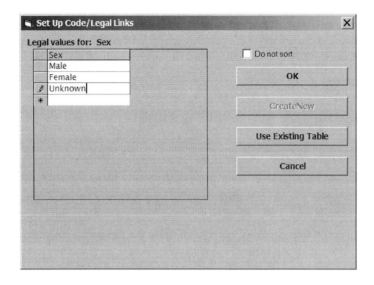

Arranging the Screen

To move a field on the screen, click on the prompt for the field and drag it to a new location while holding the left mouse button down. Use this method to space the fields on the page. Most types of fields can be resized by clicking in the field and then clicking and dragging the colored "handles" that appear. Text fields are limited to one line, but we will add a multiline field later.

Let's *group* the fields together for esthetic reasons and to make them easier to move. To do this, first select the fields on this page by left clicking in the upper left corner and dragging the dotted rectangle that appears until it includes all the fields (or just a few). Now go to the INSERT menu and choose Group. Give the group the name "Demographics,"and click OK. If you hold down the left mouse button over the word Demographics, you will be able to drag and reposition the entire group and its contained fields as a unit.

The first page should look like this:

It is time to save the page and add another one. Click on the ADD PAGE button under the page window on the left side of the screen. The first page is saved automatically and a blank page appears.

Large (multiline) Text Fields

Make a field of the MULTILINE type having the prompt, "Comments of Interviewer." Click OK and then click on the field, adjusting its size as you did with the grid to make it large enough to enter a number of comments. There is no practical limit on the amount of text that can be entered in MULTILINE fields. Add a text field for "Interviewer's Initials," and save this page with the SAVE command on the FILE menu. This completes the questionnaire View.

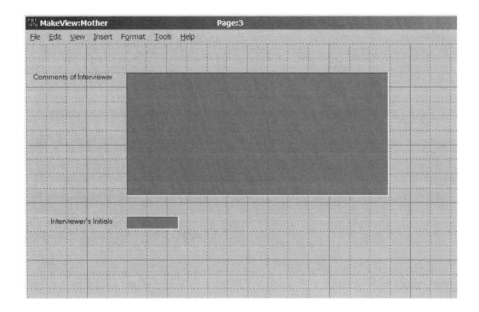

Making a Data Table from a View and Entering Data

Concept
A Data table in Epi Info is constructed automatically from information in the View table. Editing the View causes the structure of the table to be updated before the next data entry.

Still within *MakeView*, choose ENTER DATA from the FILE menu and respond "OK" to have the program construct a database from the View. The data table will have the name displayed ("Mother"), unless you choose to edit the name. When you click OK, the *Enter* program displays the View for data entry. Try entering first and last names, today's date, and a date of birth, pressing the Enter or Tab key after each field. Note that the cursor moves on to the Age field and allows entry without performing any automatic calculations. Because we would like AGE to be calculated automatically after entering Today's Date and a Date of Birth, we will return to the *MakeView* program and add Check Code commands to do the calculation and skip over AGE if the dates are entered.

Check Code Programming for Data Entry

Return to the *MakeView* program by choosing EDIT VIEW from the FILE menu. Bring up the Check Code environment by clicking the PROGRAM button on the left. The Check Commands panel appears at the top of the screen. Below it is the program editor.

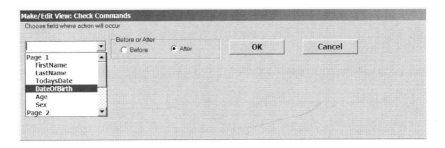

Click on the arrow under "Choose Field Where Action Will Occur" to pull down the choices. Since we want Age to be calculated after DateOfBirth is entered, choose the DateOfBirth field. In the tree of commands on the left side of the screen, click on the ASSIGN command. Display the list of available variables for the ASSIGN VARIABLE by clicking on the arrow. Choose AGE. Since it is not immediately clear how we should calculate the age from two dates, click on the FUNCTIONS button, and then choose DATES and then YEARS from the list of functions in the help window. Information appears about the YEARS function:

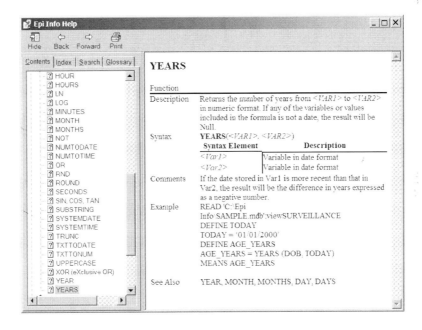

YEARS is a function that calculates the interval between two date fields in years rather than days, weeks, or months. The starting date is listed first and the ending date second in the parentheses, separated by a comma. A list of functions is contained in the Functions and Operators section of the Epi Info help file and later on in this book.

The help window provides enough information so that we can type

Years(DateOfBirth,TodaysDate)

for Expression. Choose the field names from AVAILABLE VARIABLES if you do not know them in advance. Exact spellings are required, but upper and lower case are not important. Do not put a space after YEARS

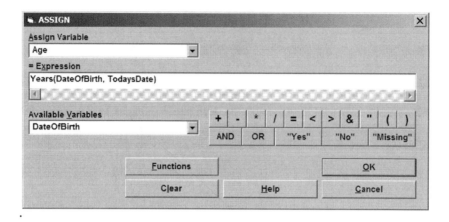

Click on the SAVE button and note that the command,

      ASSIGN Age=Years(DateOfBirth, TodaysDate)

appears in the program editor.

Now from the Command tree, choose the IF command. In the IF CONDITION box, type (or select from the pull-down list and the buttons) the condition, AGE>=0. In the window under the THEN button, type GOTO SEX. (If you click the THEN button instead, you will have access to the available commands, but only on the tabbed dialog, not in the command tree).

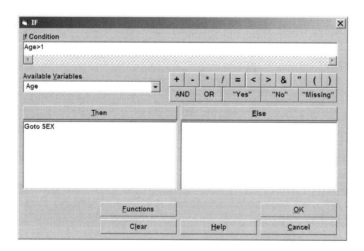

Click OK, and you should see in the program window, the commands:

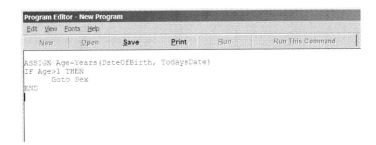

You have written your first Epi Info Check program. Exit from the Check programming facility by clicking on the OK button. This completes the View.

Concept

Check Code in Epi Info spells out what should happen before or after the cursor enters a field during data entry. The Check Code for each field is stored in the View with that field. Complex conditions and actions can be specified to impose "business rules" on the data being entered, and minimize the amount of editing needed later. See Chapters 19 and 20 for more extensive examples of Check Code.

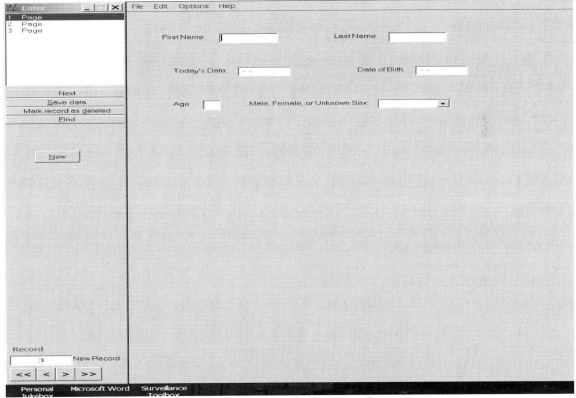

A Questionnaire View in the Enter Program

Although you could exit from MakeView at this point and run the Enter program from the Epi Info menu, it is more convenient to run Enter from within MakeView so that you can return and make changes. Choose ENTER DATA from the FILE menu once again to return to Enter.

Entering Data and Verifying that Your Check Code Works

You should have the MOTHER questionnaire on the screen. If not, go back to the main menu and choose ENTER DATA, OPEN on the File menu, and then the database that you created and the MOTHER View. Enter data in the fields displayed. After you enter Date of Birth, the age should be calculated automatically, and the cursor should jump to the Sex field. At the end of each page, the entries will be saved automatically.

After entering the data for page 2, press the Enter key. You can also click on the NEW button to save the current record and move to page 1 of a blank record. You should then see an empty record, ready for entry. Note that the record number appears at the lower left. To see previous records, click on the single back arrow button next to the record number. Be sure to enter at least three records so that we can do analysis of the results.

As a preview of the Analysis program, close the Enter program by choosing Exit from the FILE menu or clicking on the red X on the top line, and click ANALYZE DATA in the Main menu. Click the READ command at the top of the first panel, and, if necessary, Choose Project, to migrate to the project MDB containing Mother. Click on Mother and OK to load the data you have just entered, and you should see the number of records displayed. Then choose LIST from the command tree, Grid View, and OK to see the data. You will use Analysis much more in later chapters, but, for now, it is enough to verify that you have created a database and entered several records. Exit from Analysis by clicking on EXIT.

Opening Another View in ENTER

To load another View containing more data, choose the ENTER button from the main menu, then OPEN from the FILE menu and then CHANGE PROJECT. Choose the database SAMPLE and the View OSWEGO. Note the record number at the lower left is 76, representing the 75 records in the table plus the empty record now on the screen.

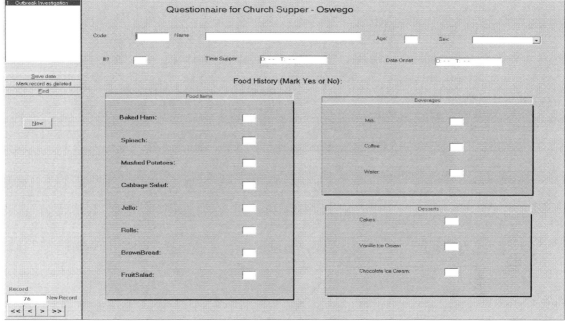

The Oswego View. The First Empty Record is Number 76.

Moving From Record to Record

Examine the records in the file by moving from record to record with the arrow buttons on the lower left. The double arrows move to the first and last records; single arrows move one record at a time. To move to a new empty record, click on the double right arrows twice, or on the NEW button.

Finding and Retrieving Records

To find records matching specified criteria, click on the FIND button on the left. A dialog box appears. Choose the AGE field and then type "11" (without quotation marks) in the field that appears. Click on the OK button to find all the records in which AGE is 11. To choose one of these records for editing, double-click on the left side of its row until the entire row is highlighted and the selected record appears on the screen. If you prefer not to select one of the records shown, but to continue with the current record, click on the BACK button.

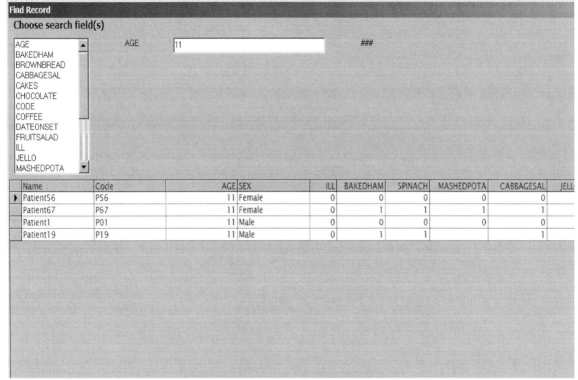

Searching for Records with Age = 11

A More Complicated View with Groups of Variables and Related Views

Open the View called SURVEILLANCE in the SAMPLE.MDB database. Note that the variables are arranged in groups. Find record number 1 using the arrow keys in the lower left corner. Now click page 3 of the pages represented at the top left.

Related Views are shown as buttons on the questionnaire View, in this case, below the other questions. Because each of the related Views is designed for a particular disease, they are inactive and do not respond to mouse clicks when you first open SURVEILLANCE and a new, blank record is displayed.

Note that the Disease in record 1 is "Hepatitis," and that the HEPATITIS button is therefore active. Click on this button to see the special form for Hepatitis. In this usage of related forms, only one record can be entered for the Hepatitis Details for a given case, but with other forms of related records (e.g., for children in a household), multiple records can be entered. Use the Back button to return to the main Surveillance form.

Related views can be used to capture more detail for particular cases, as here for Hepatitis. In a later chapter, we show how to insert a related View for "Child" in the records for "Mothers", so that each mother can have links to the records of any number of children. The use of related records for linking repeating data is common.

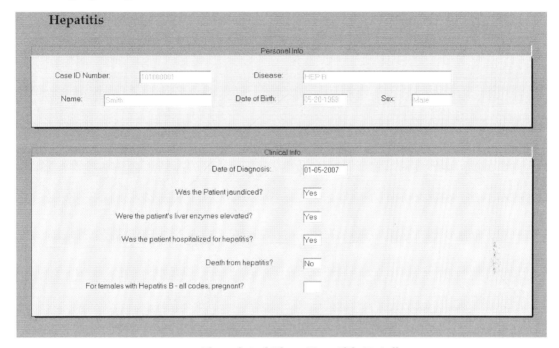

The related View, Hepatitis Details

After experimenting with SURVEILLANCE and perhaps entering one or more records, choose EXIT from the FILE menu to return to the main menu.

CHAPTER 7: A TOUR OF ANALYZE DATA

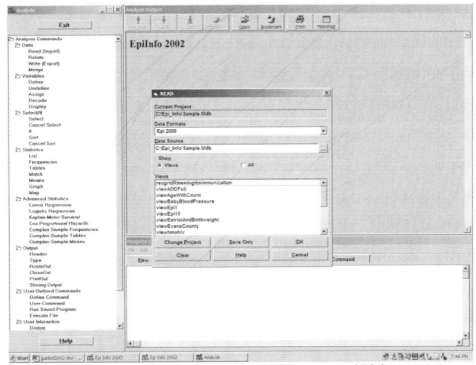

The Analysis Program and the READ Command Dialog

To run the Analysis Program, click the ANALYZE DATA button on the main menu screen. Note that all commands are shown in the tree view on the left. Clicking on a command will bring up a dialog that places the command in appropriate form in the program editor at the bottom of the screen. Results appear in the Output window, a simplified version of the Microsoft Internet browser.

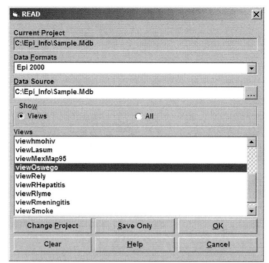

The READ Command Dialog

READing a View in Analysis

Click on the READ command. A dialog box appears so that you can choose a database and a view. Click the button called CHANGE PROJECT and then use the button with the three dots next to DATA SOURCE to find the MDB or Project that you created earlier, probably with your own initials. A view called viewMother should be present. Select this view and click OK. Note that the READ command appears in the program editor in the proper syntax. You are creating a program by responding to questions in the dialog boxes.

Seeing the Records

Click on LIST in the command tree. Select * for "ALL" and click OK to see the data you have entered. Note that the names, ages, and immunization status of the children is not shown, since it was entered in a Grid and has a separate data table.

READing viewOswego

Click on the READ command once more and than on CHANGE PROJECT. Find SAMPLE.MDB in the Epi_Info directory, and then choose viewOSWEGO. It should have 75 records.

Lists

Click on the LIST command. In the dialog that appears, choose one or more variables or click on "ALL" to choose all. Choose GRID as the output format and click OK. The variables are displayed in columns in a scrolling window.

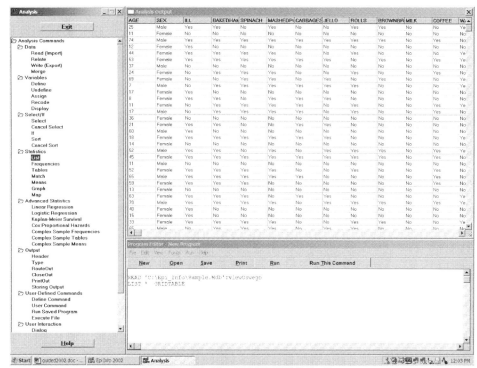

A LIST with the GRIDTABLE Option

Try the LIST command again, but choose HTML as the output format. This time the results appear in the form of an Internet web page in the Output windows.

Frequencies

Choose the FREQuencies command. In the dialog box, use the dropdown menu to select one or more variables, and then click OK. After a short wait, the results should appear in the browser window. Scroll up and down and note that each table is accompanied by yellow bars to the right that indicate the frequencies. Statistics will be displayed below the table if the value of the variable is numeric, as in AGE, but not for Yes/No fields like ILL.

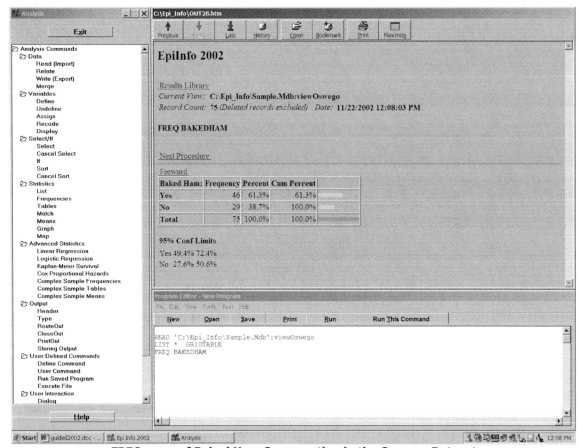

FREQuency of Baked Ham Consumption in the Oswego Dataset

Tables

Click the TABLES command. In the EXPOSURE VARIABLE field, choose VANILLA and for the OUTCOME VARIABLE, choose ILL. This will perform a cross-tabulation of VANILLA by ILL. Note that stratified analyses can be done by inserting the name of the stratifying variable(s). Summary data can be processed by setting WEIGHT equal to the name of a COUNT field. Click OK.

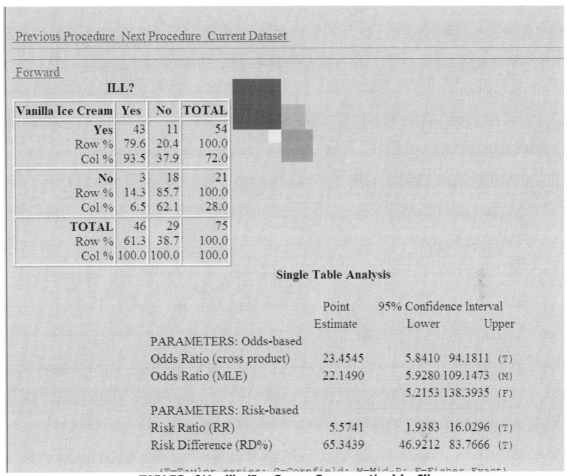

Previous Procedure Next Procedure Current Dataset

Forward

ILL?

Vanilla Ice Cream	Yes	No	TOTAL
Yes	43	11	54
Row %	79.6	20.4	100.0
Col %	93.5	37.9	72.0
No	3	18	21
Row %	14.3	85.7	100.0
Col %	6.5	62.1	28.0
TOTAL	46	29	75
Row %	61.3	38.7	100.0
Col %	100.0	100.0	100.0

Single Table Analysis

	Point Estimate	95% Confidence Interval Lower	Upper	
PARAMETERS: Odds-based				
Odds Ratio (cross product)	23.4545	5.8410	94.1811	(T)
Odds Ratio (MLE)	22.1490	5.9280	109.1473	(M)
		5.2153	138.3935	(F)
PARAMETERS: Risk-based				
Risk Ratio (RR)	5.5741	1.9383	16.0296	(T)
Risk Difference (RD%)	65.3439	46.9212	83.7666	(T)

(T=Taylor series; C=Cornfield; M=Mid-P; F=Fisher Exact)

TABLES of Vanilla (Ice Cream Consumption) by Ill

Note that the output in the browser includes a table and a graphic representation of the table values in each cell. Statistics are displayed below the table. If you have a printer connected, try printing the table by clicking on the PRINTOUT command and then OK without entering a file name. Information on the statistics in Epi Info is available in the Statistics section under HELP on the main menu.

Concept	Statistics in Analysis are produced in response to simple commands like Tables and Means. Tables yields the Odds Ratio with several kinds of confidence limits, 3 chi squares, and the Fisher exact test, as well as the Mantel Haenzel summary statistics for stratified tables. Means provides the 1-way Anova, student t, and Kruskal-Wallis tests.

Logistic Regression

Click on Logistic Regression and fill in values as follows:

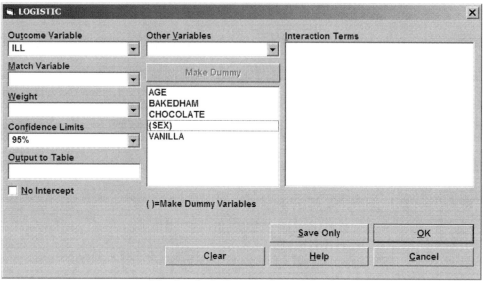

The Logistic Regression Dialog

Click OK and study the results, paying particular attention to the Odds Ratios and p values. Again Vanilla ice cream comes to the fore.

Term	Odds Ratio	95%	C.I.	Coefficient	S. E.	Z-Statistic	P-Value
AGE	1.0050	0.9760	1.0349	0.0050	0.0149	0.3326	0.7394
BAKEDHAM (Yes/No)	1.0033	0.2776	3.6261	0.0032	0.6556	0.0050	0.9960
CHOCOLATE (Yes/No)	0.9883	0.2587	3.7751	-0.0118	0.6838	-0.0172	0.9863
SEX (Male/Female)	0.2523	0.0684	0.9310	-1.3770	0.6660	-2.0674	0.0387
VANILLA (Yes/No)	30.7686	6.2714	150.9570	3.4265	0.8115	4.2225	0.0000
CONSTANT	*	*	*	-1.5644	1.0882	-1.4376	0.1505

Logistic Regression Output

Graphing

Epi Info can graph more than one variable at a time and also place more than one graph on a page. To illustrate this, choose the GRAPH command and enter the following values (the title is optional):

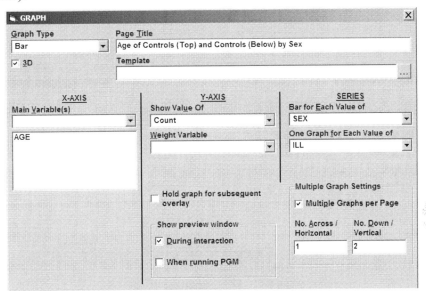

The GRAPH Dialog in Analysis

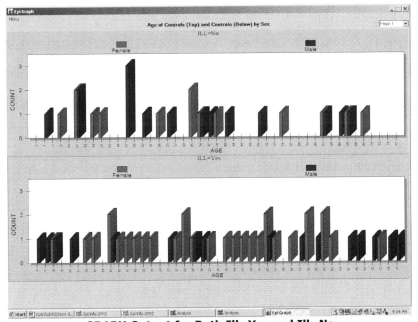

GRAPH Output for Both Ill=Yes and Ill=No

Note that we chose 3D and grouped bars to show off the capabilities of the GRAPH command, but that four separate graphs might have been clearer, and epidemiologists who care more about numbers than entertainment may advise against 3-dimensional graphs.

Viewing Previous Results

Click on CLOSEOUT to close the document you just created and then, click on the hyperlink called RESULTS LIBRARY at the top or bottom of the TABLES output in the browser. An index page appears, showing previous commands that have produced output files. Click on any of the entries to display it. An archiving system is provided so that important results can be selected and saved for future reference. You can learn more about storage of results by choosing the OUTPUT tab and examining the choices under STORING OUTPUT.

Setting the Display Values for Yes/No Fields

Click on SET under OPTIONS in the command tree on the left side of the screen. Note the options for customizing output. Change the values to be displayed for Yes/No fields, choosing from those available or typing your own, such as "Si" and "No" in Spanish. Choose LIST again and check the values displayed.

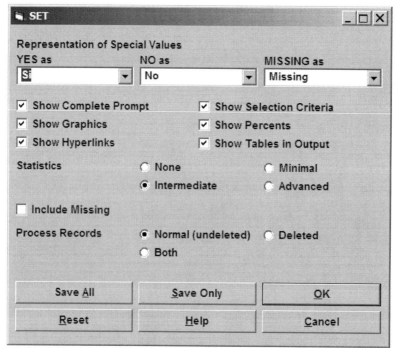

The SET Command. Choosing Spanish Values for Yes and No.

Defining a New Variable

Under Variables, choose the DEFINE command. Type STATUS as the name of a new variable. We want to set this variable to "Case" if the person was ILL and "Control" otherwise. A Standard variable, with the value reset for each record as the program passes through a table, is the best choice for this purpose. Click OK, and the necessary statement will appear in the program editor.

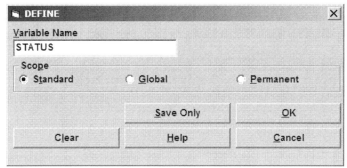

Defining a New Variable

An IF Statement

We can use an IF statement to set the value of the new STATUS variable. Choose the SELECT/IF tab and click on IF. The first item in the dialog is the condition under which the following statements should or should not be executed. The final format of the necessary IF statement is:

```
IF  ILL = (+)  THEN
     STATUS = "CASE"
ELSE
     STATUS = "CONTROL"
END
```

You will not have to remember the format, however, since filling in the blanks in the dialog will allow Epi Info to write the necessary command in the program editor. In the first blank, fill in the Condition as ILL=(+). To do so, you can choose the variable ILL from the list of variables in the second window and choose the equal sign and condition "Yes" (or "Si") by clicking on buttons with these labels. The button will display whatever label is specified for "Yes" in the SET dialog—"Yes", "Si", etc., but will convert the statement to the international symbol (+).

Regardless of the setting for Yes/No fields, "Yes" is always represented in the database as 1, No as 0, and Unknown as a blank or null value. These values can also be used, as in:

IF ILL = 1 THEN   (Note that numbers do not have quotation marks)
Etc.

If you are familiar with commands in Epi Info 6, you can type your own command in the box located under the then button. On the other hand, if you are experimenting for the first time with programming languages, you may want to use the aid available for IF statements. In the first case type STATUS="CASE" in the THEN box and STATUS="CONTROL" in the ELSE box.. Click OK to finish the command.

You can also click the THEN button to gain access to the command tree and insert one or several commands.

When the IF statement is completed, click on the OK button. The complete IFstatement will appear in the program editor.

Use the LIST command to verify that STATUS is indeed properly set, and that records where ILL = "Yes" have "CASE" as the value of STATUS.

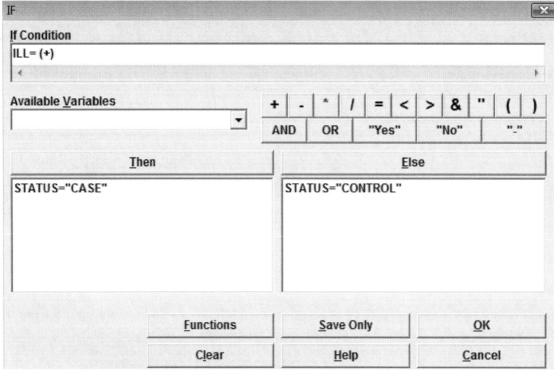

The IF Command Dialog

The SELECT Command

The SELECT statement limits subsequent analysis to particular records based on criteria that you specify. To work with cases only, for example, choose the SELECT statement and enter the condition STATUS = "CASE".

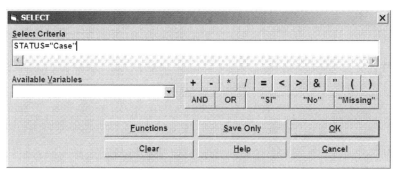

The SELECT Command

Use LIST or FREQ STATUS to show that cases only are included in the analysis.

To return to working with <u>all</u> the records, choose CANCEL SELECT and note that it places the word SELECT, without conditions, in the program.

The RECODE Command

To Group the values of AGE, first DEFINE a new variable called AGEGROUP, using the DEFINE command. Then Choose RECODE and specify that you will recode from AGE to AGEGROUP, using the drop down list. Click the FILE RANGES button and enter the range 0 for START and 80 for END, with 10 for BY. Click OK, and then do a FREQuency of AGEGROUP to see the results.

C:\Epi_Info\OUT30.htm

FREQ AgeGroup

Next Procedure

Forward

AgeGroup	Frequency	Percent	Cum Percent
>1 – 11	5	10.9%	10.9%
>11 – 21	10	21.7%	32.6%
>21 – 31	1	2.2%	34.8%
>31 – 41	8	17.4%	52.2%
>41 – 51	4	8.7%	60.9%
>51 – 61	9	19.6%	80.4%
>61 – 71	6	13.0%	93.5%
>71 – 80	3	6.5%	100.0%
Total	46	100.0%	100.0%

FREQuency of Age as Recoded by 10 Year Intervals

Creating a New File with the WRITE Command

At this point, we have made several improvements in the dataset, and might want to create a file containing the new variables. The new file can be either an Epi Info (Microsoft Access) file or one of many other file types. Choose the WRITE command, and then, from the list of Output Formats, choose "dBASE IV". Specify "All" variables and "Replace" so that an existing file by the same name will be overwritten. Give your Initials for the file name. Click on OK to write the file.

When writing a file other than an MDB, the box that asks for the "MDB" should be taken to mean the Folder or Directory, and the "Table" as the name of the file.

Concept	A program in ***Analysis*** is the collection of commands in the program editor that are generated by interaction with the command tree and dialog boxes. You can edit or type the commands yourself if you are familiar with the syntax. Programs can be saved, retrieved, and run again in ***Analysis***, or invoked from a menu (MNU) file.

Saving a Program (PGM)

To save the current program, click the SAVE button in the program editor (not in the command tree). In the dialog that appears, give a name for your program, such as your own initials, and click OK. Now delete the program from the program editor by clicking the NEW button in the editor. Retrieve the program by clicking on OPEN in the program editor and choosing the program name from the dropdown list. The editor will reload the program, ready to edit or run. By default, programs are saved in the current project or MDB, but, if you prefer, you can save or retrieve text file versions using the TEXT FILE button in the save dialog. By constructing an Epi Info menu to run an *Analysis* program (PGM) automatically, you can construct a convenient and permanent application to be used again repeatedly and execute any of the actions of which *Analysis* is capable.

READing a dBASE File

Now that you have produced a dBASE IV file, it is time to test the flexibility of *Analysis* in READing a variety of file types. Choose READ from the DATA tab, specify dBASE IV format, and read the .DBF file you have just produced. Use LIST and/or FREQ to verify that the variables you created and their values are contained in the new file.

CHAPTER 8: UTILITIES

Comparing Data Tables to Validate Data Entry

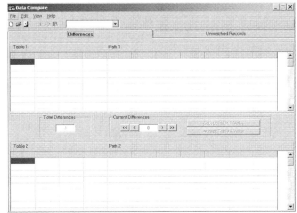

The TableDiff Program

To reach the TableDiff program for comparing two Epi Info data sets or Views, choose Data Compare from the UTILITIES menu. The program that appears is designed to compare two data tables entered by different people from the same set of paper documents. This method is often used for quality control in data entry shops, such as those supporting epidemiologic surveys.

To try out the program, you would first make a copy of the SAMPLE.MDB database, then edit the data in a few records in the Oswego View using Enter. Using the FILE menu in TableDiff to make a NEW script, you would choose the Oswego views in the two MDBs. The key to identify records (in case they are not entered in the same order) should be CODE. Differences in the tables will appear in the top and bottom so that you can make corrections until the two tables are identical or edit the one to be kept. Further details are given in the Help file.

File Encryption and Compression With EpiLock

Run EpiLock from the UTILITIES section of the Epi Info menu. It can be used to ZIP (compress) or encrypt files for transmission elsewhere or for storage.

Encryption scrambles data so that it cannot be recovered without the correct password. It is useful to protect sensitive data being sent over the Internet or by email, and also to protect data on a local computer or laptop if it is stolen or otherwise accessed improperly. Zipping or compression reduces the size of data files (sometimes up to 20-fold for MDBs), and is done automatically during encryption or can be selected without encryption.

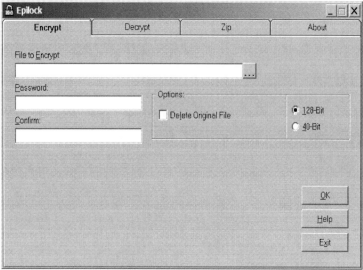

The EpiLock Encryption Screen

As with any good security procedure, a lost password is the same as lost data; hence be sure to keep a properly secured record of the password or backup copy of the data for any file encrypted with the instruction DELETE ORIGINAL FILE checked. To encrypt a file for transmission and keep the original file, do not check this box. It is useful, however, for protecting data on a laptop that could be stolen, or a desktop open to nighttime janitorial staff.

The level of encryption can be 40-bit or 128-bit. Generally, 128-bit is the right choice. In countries where US regulations do not allow versions of Microsoft Windows to do strong encryption, 40-bit may be chosen. If possible, use 128-bit encryption (.ELH) unless a file you are decrypting has been encrypted at 40 bits(ELS). The HELP feature in EpiLock gives more information..

Unfortunately some email systems do not allow zipped or encrypted file attachments. There are other services on the Internet that specialize in transmission of large or encrypted files. Try searching for "Send Encrypted Files" in Google to find these services, some of which are free or inexpensive. Since security resides in the encryption (and your management of the password), you do not have to worry too much about the details of the provider.

CHAPTER 9: VARIABLES, ASSIGNING VALUES, AND IF CONDITIONS

Variables

You have so far encountered variables in Epi Info as fields in a View or Column names in Analysis. As the name implies, the value of a variable can be different for each record in a database, AGE being 32 for one patient, 12 for another, and unknown or missing for a third. Variables can be subjected to mathematical or logical operations, and new variables can be created to hold the results. The latter are called "Defined" variables in contrast to "Table" or database variables. A defined variable can be given a value with the ASSIGN command. This chapter describes how to define and assign values to new variables, and how to determine the types of variables with the DISPLAY command.

DEFINE a New Variable

New variables may be a categorization of an existing variable (e.g., converting blood pressure information into hypertensive vs. not hypertensive), or a calculated field, such as calculating body mass index from weight and height.

You can think of the DEFINE command as creating a new column in a spreadsheet – there is a column heading (the variable name) and the column beneath it is blank. To place values in the column, you can use the ASSIGN, RECODE, or IF commands described later.

The dialog box for the DEFINE command is shown above. All it takes to create a new variable is to fill in a name and press OK. There are some rules concerning variable names: no spaces in the

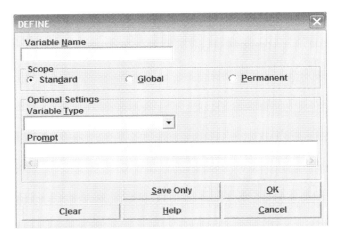

name; do not use a variable name that already exists in the data file; and do not use a name that is the same as any of the commands, operators, or functions (e.g., not names like AND, OR, LIST, etc.).

In most situations, the Scope of the variable should be Standard. Standard variables can assume a new value each time a record is processed, but only last until the next READ. If you want to make the newly DEFINEd Standard variable(s) a permanent part of the data file, you can use the WRITE command to create a new table containing the original data plus newly DEFINEd variables and their values.

Global variables persist until you EXIT from ANALYSIS.. They can therefore pass information from one PGM to another if the PGMs are run in the same session. Permanent variables are stored in the EpiInfo.INI file, and retain their values even when the computer is turned off. Their values are available to other Epi Info programs, such as ENTER and the Menu. Global and Permanent variables cannot be ASSIGNed values from database variables. They are not useful, for example, in calculating totals for a numeric field. Use the SUMMARIZE command for this purpose instead.

In recent versions of Epi Info, you have the option of specifying a data type, and also a Prompt that can be displayed in LISTs and TABLES when Display Prompts is SET to On. Here is the dialog for DEFINE in Version 3.4. If you do not specify a data type, it will be set automatically the first time you assign a value to the variable.

Variables, once defined, can be removed with UNDEFINE. This is not necessary for Standard scope variables, which are removed by the next READ command, but can be helpful in cleaning up after using Permanent variables, or in combating the error messages that are given about reDEFINing a Global variable when rerunning a program.

DISPLAY Variables

To view variable names and types, use the DISPLAY command which will present a dialog box as shown in the figure. If you have not done so, READ the EvansCounty data in Sample.MDB. Then click DISPLAY in the left command window, and then click on the OK button to see the available variables. The variable name, the field type (in this example, either a number, Yes/No, or text field), and the format are presented.

DISPLAY DBVARIABLES

Variable	Table	Field Type	Format/Value	Special Info	Prompt
AGE	EvansCounty	NUMBER	##		AGEC
AGEG1	EvansCounty	YES/NO			AGEG1
AGEG2	EvansCounty	NUMBER	#		AGEG2
CAT	EvansCounty	YES/NO			CAT
CHD	EvansCounty	YES/NO			CHD
Etc.........					
SMK	EvansCounty	YES/NO			SMK
Language	Defined	Text	ENGLISH	Predefined	

Output of the DISPLAY command, viewEvansCounty data, Epi Info

ASSIGN

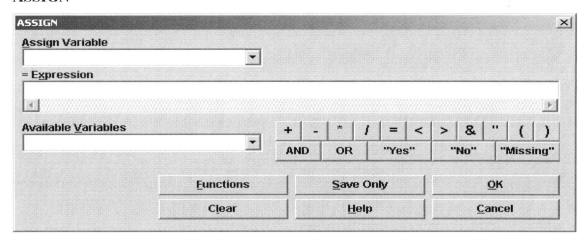

Simple Assignments

The ASSIGN command is way to give a value to a variable. In its simplest form, you can ASSIGN a variable the value of another variable or a new literal value, as follows:

```
DEFINE Cholesterol
ASSIGN Cholesterol=CHL
ASSIGN ReferenceDate=
```

The variable on the left can be a database variable or a DEFINEd variable. The word ASSIGN is not necessary, and can be omitted. If the variable on the left is a database or standard DEFINEd variable, you can expect it to assume its new value <u>for each record</u> during processing (in a LIST, FREQ, TABLE, etc.).

If the variable on the left is a Permanent or Global DEFINEd variable, it cannot be set equal to a database or standard DEFINEd variable, but it assumes the assigned value immediately and retains it as long as it is in Scope. For example, you might set a global or permanent variable for the starting date of a study.

```
DEFINE StartDate PERMANENT
StartDate=04/19/2008
```

There are a several predefined variables that are useful. These are SYSTEMTIME and SYSTEMDATE which give the current date and time, equivalent to the ones often displayed in the lower right hand corner of the screen in Windows. If you use these, be sure to check that the computer has the correct values, as it is fairly common to find users whose time is set for the time zone where the computer was first sold, or the wrong date. There is also a RECORDCOUNT variable that gives the number of records in the currently READ table or file. It is useful for avoiding errors if the RECORDCOUNT is zero and also as a denominator. ENVIRON and FILEDATE are other predefined variables that are sometimes useful.

Operators

ASSIGN basically sets up an equation, with a single variable on the left and a simple or complex expression on the right. The more interesting expressions require Operators, such as +,-,*, / ,MOD, and ^for addition, subtraction, multiplication, and division, modulus, and raising to a power. All but the last two are easily inserted in the ASSIGN statement with the buttons in the ASSIGN dialog.

The text (string) concatenation operator, &, joins two text variables or values into a single text item. "Mary" & "Beth" becomes "MaryBeth". "Mary " & "Beth" or "Mary"& " " & "Beth" becomes "Mary Beth.

MOD divides by a specified number and gives you the remainder (only). For example 365 mod 7 returns   1, there being 52 weeks and 1 extra day in a non-leap year. X^Y raises X to the Power Y, an expression often found in statistical calculations. X^0.5 takes the square root of X, a handy trick, since there is no square-root function available.

Functions

Functions are much like operators, since they accept values and return other values, but Functions require that the incoming values be placed in parentheses. Many Epi Info functions are also fussy about having no space before the initial parenthesis. The Help files available via the ASSIGN dialog FUNCTIONS button give the details for each function, but since you have to seach a bit to find them, here are the functions listed and a brief idea of their actions.

- Num is a variable or value that is numeric

- Txt is a text variable or text value. If it is a literal value, it must be in quotes.

- Date is a Date or DateTime variable or literal value

- Time is a DateTime or Date variable literal value

For Numbers	**For Text**	**For Dates and Times**
		Extract a value from a Date or Time
ABS(Num)—absolute value; removes a minus sign if there is one	FINDTEXT(Txt,TxttoFind)— returns numeric position if found, 0 if not	DAY(Date)
EXP(Num)--Raises e to the power Num	SUBSTRING(Txt,Start, how many chrs)	MONTH(Date)
LN(Num) –natural log		YEAR(Date)
LOG(Num)-log base 10		HOUR(Time)
NUMTODATE(Num)	TXTTODATE(Txt)	MINUTE(Time)
NUMTOTIME(Num)	TXTTONUM(Txt)	SECOND(Time)
RND(Num)	UPPERCASE(Txt)	Calculate duration between in different units
ROUND(Num)—rounds to nearest integer. Tends to put a strain on SQL.		DAYS(Date1, Date2)
SIN(Num), COS(Num), TAN(Num)		MONTHS(Date1, Date2)
TRUNC(Num)—rounds down to integer		YEARS(Date1, Date2)
		HOURS(Time1, Time2)
		MINUTES(Time1, Time2)
		SECONDS(Time1, Time2)

The FORMAT function always returns a text value, but the value can be in many "formats" depending on the starting variable and the Pattern given. The general idea is:

FORMAT(Variable or Literal, Pattern)

Patterns For Numbers	Patterns For Text	Patterns For Dates and Times
"General Number"	">"	"General Date"
"Currency"	converts to lowercase	"Long Date"
"Fixed"	"<"	"Medium Date"
"Standard"	to uppercase	"Short Date"
"Percent"		"Long Time"
"Scientific"		"Medium Time"
"Yes/No"		"Short Time"
"True/False"		MyStr = Format(Datevar,"Long Date")
MyStr = Format(23)		MyStr= Format(MyTime,"hh:mm:ssAMPM")
Returns "23".		Returns "05:04:23 PM"
MyStr = Format(5459.4, "##,##0.00")		MyStr = Format(MyDate,"dddd, mmm yyyy")
Returns "5,459.40"		
MyStr = Format(334.9, "###0.00")		
Returns "334.90"		
MyStr = Format(5, "0.00%")		
Returns "500.00%"		

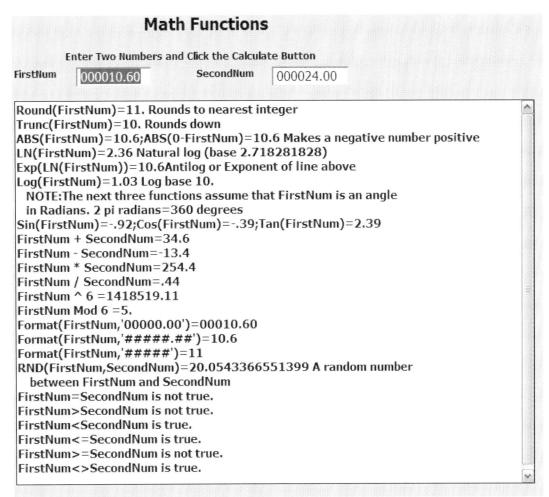

Data Entry Form Demonstrating Math Functions In EpiBookDemos.MDB

Data entry forms that allow experimenting with functions are provided in an MDB called EpiBookDemos in the exMISC folder of the Examples. Use the Enter program to open this MDB and see the three demos pictured here:

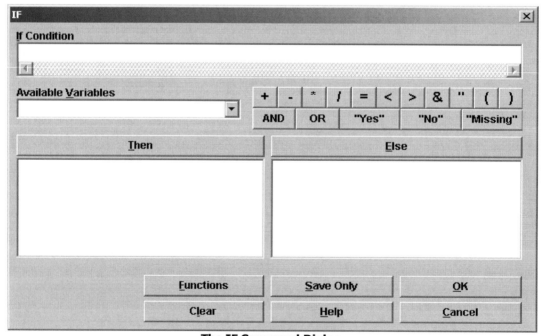

Date and Time Functions

First Date (and optional time) `2-07-1941 T: 08-00-00 AM`   Second Date (time optional) `D:05-25-2009 T: 12-00-00 A`

Insert SystemDate   Add SystemTime

Or, if you prefer separate fields, enter below and click a NUMTO button:

| Year | | Month | | Day | | NumToDate |
| Hour | | Minute | | Second | | NumToTime |

Results

```
____CALCULATING INTERVALS OR DURATIONS, e.g. age or incubation period____
YEARS(FirstDate,SecondDate)=67
MONTHS(FirstDate,SecondDate)=809
DAYS(FirstDate,SecondDate)=24641
HOURS(FirstDate,SecondDate)=591376
MINUTES(FirstDate,SecondDate)=35482560
SECONDS(FirstDate,SecondDate)=2128953600

____EXTRACTING A SINGLE ITEM FROM A DATE____
YEAR(FirstDate)=1941;  MONTH(FirstDate)=12;  DAY(FirstDate)=7
HOUR(FirstDate)=8;  MINUTE(FirstDate)=0;  SECOND(FirstDate)=0
```

Functions for Calculating Durations, and Converting Numbers to Dates and Times

The IF Command

The IF Command Dialog

The IF command is like a fork in the road. You specify conditions under which it should execute one set of commands or another, and then insert the necessary commands. The dialog box for the IF command is shown above. At the top is a condition, or multiple conditions joined by AND or OR. The two forks to be taken are in the larger boxes below, where you insert commands to be executed if the condition is true and if it is false.

Conditions

To specify conditions we will need some more operators, those specifying equality, less than, greater than, etc. Here they are:

>	greater than
<	less than
>=	greater than or equal to
<=	less than or equal to
=	equal to
<>	not equal to (If x<>y doesn't work, try not (x=y))

If you want to describe a condition that has more than one requirement, or that requires at least one of your specifications, you will need AND and OR. To specify the opposite of your condition, you need NOT. Finally, there is a seldom used conjunction called XOR that specifies that one and only one of two conditions is true, but it doesn't care which one. If you want to solidify and possibly show off your new knowledge, you should know that these are called Boolean Operators. George Boole, from Lincoln, England, was the no-nonsense mathematician to the right, who more or less invented the logic of zero and one, yes and no, true and false, but died in 1864 before he could see it transform the world as the basis of computer science.

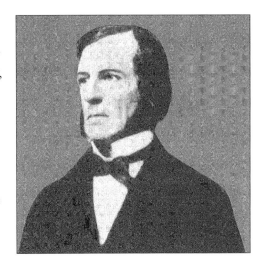

Here's an exercise in interpreting conditions. In most cases at least one of the values would be received as a variable, but literal numbers will work for illustration. Cover up the right hand column before you answer the following quiz.

Condition	Circle your Answer		Correct Answer
1=1	True(1)	False(0)	True
2>1	True(1)	False(0)	True
2=1	True(1)	False(0)	False
2>1 OR 2=1	True(1)	False(0)	True
2>=1	True(1)	False(0)	True
2<>3	True(1)	False(0)	True
2>1 AND 2=1	True(1)	False(0)	False
1<2 AND (5*20>=120)	True(1)	False(0)	True

In the viewEvansCounty, there is a variable CHL representing serum cholesterol, often considered to be elevated when over 200. . We can use the IF command box to make a Yes/No decision on

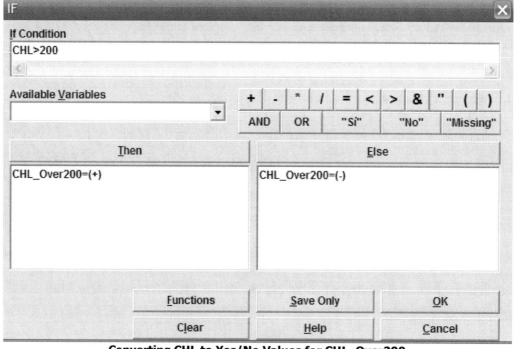

Converting CHL to Yes/No Values for CHL_Over200

CHL_Over200 and set the value of the variable accordingly. First, DEFINE a variable called CHL_Over200, click on the IF command, and fill in its dialog box as shown.:

The ASSIGNment statements that are the consequence of the IF decision are so simple here that we have just typed them in without the optional ASSIGN word, but the IF dialog also lets you use all the resources of the Analysis command tree to construct them if you click on the THEN or ELSE buttons. The first time is a little scary, but you will find that this mechanism works well.

Click OK, and you should have the following code in the program editor, assuming that you previously READ the View and defined CHL_Over200. .

```
READ 'C:\Epi_Info\Sample.mdb':viewEvansCounty
DEFINE CHL_Over200
IF CHL>200 THEN
    CHL_Over200=(+)
ELSE
    CHL_Over200=(-)
END
```

If you do a FREQuency of CHL_Over200, you will find that 57.8% of the study population had this level and the others did not. Note that we have not provided for subjects with missing values for CHL. Here we are dealing with final data from a study, and eveyone has a CHL value, but another IF statement could have been used to deal with missing values, as follows:

```
IF CHL=(.) THEN
    CHL_Over200=(.)
END
```

This one must come after the IF-THEN-ELSE statement, as the ELSE in the first statement would capture the missing values for CHL as "No"for CHL_Over200, and the second IF statement is needed to set them back to the missing value.

Once you have made an IF statement using the IF dialog, it is easy to copy and paste in the program editor to construct additional IF statements, editing the variable names and values as needed.

Note to Epi Info DOS users: In the DOS version of Epi Info, in Analysis, IF/Else commands were on a single line. In the Windows version of Epi Info, in the Program editor window the command is three or more lines with the last line having the command END.

The IF command can make more complex decisions by combining specifications For example, when using hemoglobin to define anemia status, adult females have a different cutoff value than males. Let's DEFINE a variable called Anemic (with apologies to our colleagues in the UK). An example of the code is shown below where HB is the variable name for hemoglobin value:

```
DEFINE Anemic
ASSIGN Anemic= (-)
IF SEX="F" AND HB<12 THEN
        anemic= (+)
END
```

> **IF SEX="M" AND HB<13 THEN**
>> **Anemic= (+)**
> **END**

The first line in the above code defines a new variable called "Anemic"; the second line assigns everyone a value of (-) or "No", meaning they are not anemic. The first and second IF commands set "Anemic" to (+) or "Yes" using if they meet the specified criteria for hemoglobin level by sex.

It is recommended that you LIST the original variable(s) and newly defined variables to make sure the coding worked as you expected. You can also use the TABLES and MEANS command for double-checking the accuracy of the new coding.

Logic
Often used with IF or SELECT commands
Enter Two Yes, No, or Blank Answers and Click the Go Button

FirstCondition (perhaps a symptom) `Yes`

SecondCondition (perhaps another symptom) `No`

```
_____Using AND, we check to see if BOTH conditions are true
IF FirstCondition=(+) AND SecondCondition=(+) then
   Conclusion='Both are TRUE'
else
   Conclusion='At least one is NOT TRUE
end...>>>In this example, the conclusion is : At least one is NOT TRUE
_____Using OR, we check to see if AT LEAST ONE condition is true
IF FirstCondition=(+) OR SecondCondition=(+) then
   Conclusion='AT LEAST ONE is True'
else
   Conclusion='NEITHER ONE is True
end...>>>In this example, the conclusion is : AT LEAST ONE is True.
_____Using XOR, we check to see if ONE and ONLY ONE condition is true
IF FirstCondition=(+) XOR SecondCondition=(+) then
   Conclusion='ONLY ONE is True'
else
   Conclusion='Both or Neither are true, but not one by itself.'
end...>>>In this example, the conclusion is : ONLY ONE is True
_____Using NOT, we check to see if a statement is NOT true.
IF NOT (FirstCondition=(+)) then
   Conclusion='FirstCondition is NOT true.'
else
   Conclusion='FirstCondition IS true
end...>>>In this example, the conclusion is : FirstCondition IS True
Logical statements can be combined to handle more complex cases,
and the conditions do not have to be Yes/No fields or equalities.
```

Summary of Logical Operators

Nested IF Statements

An IF statement can be placed inside another. IF statement. If it is in the ELSE clause, then it must begin on the line following the ELSE. Let's go back to our first IF example:

```
READ 'C:\Epi_Info\Sample.mdb':viewEvansCounty
DEFINE CHL_Over200
IF  CHL > 0  THEN
     IF  CHL>200  THEN
          CHL_Over200=(+)
     ELSE
          CHL_Over200=(-)
     END
END
```

Now we have protected our new variable from being set unless CHL is more than 0. Hence if CHL has a missing value, CHL_Over200 will also be missing. The result is the same as with the two IF statements we originally proposed, but this forms a neater package, and may be easier to understand.

Use of Parentheses ( )

For the ASSIGN and IF/Else commands, for multiple mathematical signs, you may need to use parentheses. Try evaluating this expression without the computer:

14 * 10 / 2 + 20

You would be tempted to do things in the order in which they occur. First, the multiplication is performed ($14 * 10 = 140$), followed by the division ($140 / 2 = 70$), and then the addition ($70 + 20 = 90$).producing a result of 90.

However, the 20 may have been intended to be under the division sign, as in 14 times 10 divided by 22 First $2 + 20$ equals 22; then $14 * 10 = 140$, which would then be divided by $22 = 6.3636$.

Even a mathematician would have trouble interpreting your expression, although he/she (and the computer) would use something called the "precedence of operators" which nobody wants to remember. The simple answer for humans and the computer is to place parentheses around the parts that are to be calculated first (or kept together), as in:

14 * 10 / (2+20) which everybody can agree is 6.3636

Whenever you have situations where it is not clear what belongs with what, it is a good idea to surround the separate parts with parentheses for clarity. This holds for expressions with both AND and OR as well as for equations with several types of operators.Leaving out the parentheses can lead to unexpected results; inserting them will do no harm, (unless they are unpaired.).

RECODE

Recode is used to assign new values to data that already exists. It can be used to recode 1 and 2 to "Male" and "Female", or to categorize numeric values like AgeInYears into age groups. Usually it is a good idea to DEFINE a new variable to receive the values before you use RECODE, although both RECODE and ASSIGN statements can put results into the same variable with which they began. The dialog box for RECODE is shown below.

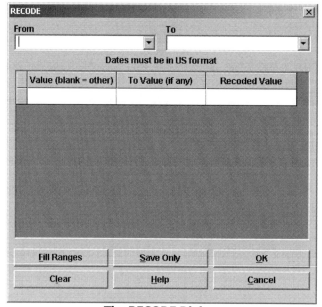

The RECODE Dialog

The RECODE command can be thought of as a shorthand version of a number of IF statements.

As an example, let's recode age into age groups using the viewEvansCounty file. First, DEFINE a variable called agegroup. Next, click on the RECODE command in the Analysis Command Window. The dialog box shown above will be displayed. In the From box, select the variable Age; in the To box, select the variable agegroup. Then click the button called FILL RANGES. The three boxes below the From/To section are, from left to right, the lowest category value, the highest category value, and the new category name. One way to complete these boxes automatically is to click on the Fill Ranges button near the bottom left of the dialog box; clicking on this button will present another dialog box

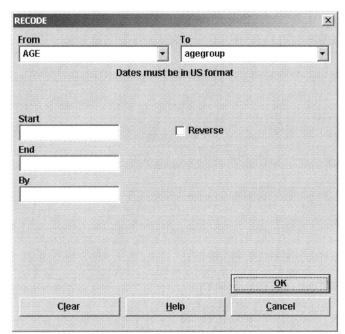

The FILL RANGES Dialog in the RECODE Command

The From variable is Age, the To variable is the recently defined variable called agegroup. There are three boxes below with the words Start, End, and By. For the Age to agegroup recode, Start would be the youngest age you want to categorize, End is the oldest age, and By and the interval, which in this example could be 5 or 10 or any year interval you desire. Try not to exceed 10 or 12 categories, as RECODE has a tendency to reject more complex requests.

In the viewEvansCounty data, the youngest person was 40 and the oldest 76, so the Start could be 39, the End 80, and the By 10. Pressing the OK button will result in the completed dialog box shown below. Why was 39 entered as the starting number? : The Start value is treated as >39, which in this example, would be 40-49 years of age. If you enter 40, the first age group would be 41-50, the second 51-60, etc. By entering 39 as the Start value, the first age group is 40-49, the second is 50-59, etc. You can double click in the boxes in the dialog to change values in the categories or the RECODEd Value (i.e., the label for the category).

Some notes on the use of the RECODE command. Text must be enclosed in quotation marks. Numeric ranges are separated by a space, hyphen, and space, as in 1 - 5. Negative values are permitted, as in -9 – -8. The words LOVALUE and HIVALUE may be used to indicate the smallest and largest values for the variable (see Figure 40). The word ELSE may be used to indicate all values not falling in the preceding ranges. RECODEs take place in the order stated; if two ranges overlap, the first in order will apply. In general, you cannot have more than 12 levels, although sometimes the command will work with more than 12 levels, even after receiving a warning message. Whenever using RECODE, it is recommended that you list the From and To variable from the RECODE dialog box and make sure that the recoding worked as expected.

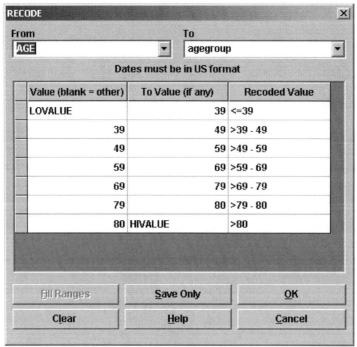

**RECODE Dialog with FILL RANGES for Age by Ten-Year
Intervals**

Practicing with the SELECT, DEFINE, ASSIGN, RECODE, and IF Commands

The following questions are based on the viewEvansCounty data.

You are interested in performing some analyses only on those with hypertension. In this data file, the variable name is HPT, and those who are hypertensive have the code "Yes." Use the SELECT command and answer the following questions:

1. What is the mean cholesterol (variable CHL) for the hypertensive group?

2. What is the risk ratio for the CAT-CHD relationship among those with hypertension?

At this point, please CANCEL SELECT.

An investigator has developed a new index for predicting coronary heart disease. This index is based on the measure of body size called QTI and cholesterol level (CHL). The index is calculated as:

CHD_index = 100 x QTI squared /Cholesterol level

1. Create this variable in the dataset. What is the mean CHD_index value?

2. Do those who developed CHD have a significantly higher mean CHD_index than those who did not develop CHD?

Using the RECODE command, RECODE age to agegroup using by 20-year age intervals: 40-59 and 50-79 years of age.

1. How many individuals are there in the 40-59 year age group and how many in the 60-79 year age group?

Let's use the hematocrit information to classify the men as anemic or not anemic. The cutoff for anemia is a hematocrit <39 for nonsmokers and hematocrit <40 for smokers. The variable name for hematocrit is HEM and the variable name for smoking is SMK, coded as "Yes"/"No".

1. DEFINE a new variable Anemic and use IF statements to give a value of 1 if anemic, a value of 0 if not anemic. What is the prevalence of anemia?

2. Save the DEFINE and IF statements into a program file called Anemic in the Sample.mdb file. ReREAD viewEvansCounty and Run the program.

Complexity

Sometimes after a series of IF statements or a multilevel recode, you may receive an error message like, "Statement too complex" with a display of SQL code that is full of "iif"s and parentheses. This means that the combination of commands that Epi Info makes into a SQL query for the Microsoft database module is rejected as being "too complex" or complicated.

The solution to this problem to examine your code for complex areas and, instead of letting all the Ifs, RECODES, and ASSIGNs accumulate automatically, use the WRITE command to capture the results part way through the process, and then READ the resulting file back in and add more code to continue with the logic or calculations. Here's the idea:

```
Define AA
ASSIGN AA=a+b+c+d+e+f+g+h+i+j+k+l+m+n+o+p+q+r+s+t+u+v+w+x+y+z
IF AA>3 then
  do something
END
```

If you had all these as numeric fields in a View, it is possible (although not likely) that this code might result in the "too complex" error. In order to evaluate the IF statement as each record is processed, the database engine must perform all 25 additions in the ASSIGN statement for each record.

The solution is to WRITE out the results of ASSIGN as a single field AA, READ the results back in, and continue with the logic that is based on AA—now a simple number in a field. Usually it is most convenient to include all the fields, both database and temporary, in the WRITE. When you READ this table back in, the fields that were formerly temporary are database fields (in the new file, not the original database) and no processing is needed to give them values.

```
Define AA
ASSIGN AA=a+b+c+d+e+f+g+h+i+j+k+l+m+n+o+p+q+r+s+t+u+v+w+x+y+z
WRITE REPLACE "Epi 2000"  tempsum *
LIST *  GRIDTABLE
* This writes all the database and DEFINEd variable values to a new table
* We READ the new table back in
READ TempSum
*Note that AA is now a database field with a numeric value in each record
*We have cleared the slate of complexity and can go on from here
IF AA>3 then
   do something
END
```

The SET Command

The user can specify many aspects of how information is presented using the SET command. Settings other than the default values are placed in the program editor when you click OK.

REPRESENTATION OF SPECIAL VALUES—These can be set to English or non-English representations of "Yes", "No", and "Missing", which are actually 1, 0, and blank or null in the database. The same settings can be made in the menu of the ENTER program as OPTIONS| YES/NO FIELDS. If you would like values not offered in the dialog, you can edit the SET commands that are inserted in the program editor, for example, to

SET (+) = "Si"
SET (.) = "--"

SET Command Dialog Box, Analysis, Epi Info.

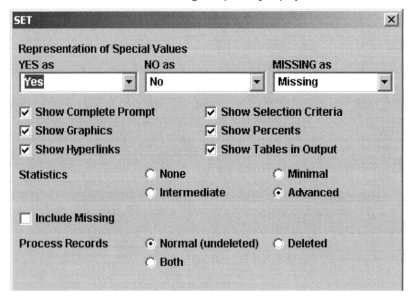

SHOW HYPERLINKS – when checked, hyperlinks for navigation are inserted in the web page output.

SHOW SELECTION CRITERIA – when checked, the SELECT settings are are shown in the output

SHOW PERCENTS – when checked, shows row and column percentages for the TABLES and MEANS commands. Uncheck this item to show only the numbers.

SHOW TABLES IN OUTPUT – when checked, shows tables for FREQuencies, MEANS, TABLES, or MATCH commands; when not checked, tables are not shown.

STATISTICS output can be turned off or set at various levels. NONE is good for large tables where only the counts and percentages matter. ADVANCED is needed to see all the available statistical results. The other levels are designed to prevent confusion if only minimal results are needed.

INCLUDE MISSING determines whether to include missing records in FREQuencies and TABLES. If missing values are included, and your dataset has such values, extra columns or rows will be added to the ouput, and missing value records will count as part of denominators. This can be part of a complete analysis, but it also turns two-by-two tables into three-by-three or three-by-two, and severely limits the kinds of statistics available. Odds ratios and risk ratios, for example are only available in two-by-two tables.

PROCESS RECORDS – Use this to process only UNDELETED records (the normal setting), to process only DELETED records or BOTH. This is handy in conjunction with LIST for seeing which records have been DELETED.

The RECODE Command

To Group the values of AGE, first DEFINE a new variable called AGEGROUP, using the DEFINE command. Then Choose RECODE and specify that you will recode from AGE to AGEGROUP, using the drop down list. Click the FILE RANGES button and enter the range 0 for START and 80 for END, with 10 for BY. Click OK, and then do a FREQuency of AGEGROUP to see the results.

Next Steps

You are now familiar with the main features of Epi Info. We suggest that you try working with your own data, either by designing a View and then entering data or by READing an existing dataset in the Analysis program. The Help files provide more detail on the programs, and the How To chapters sections have instructions for solving specific problems. Reference material is in the Commands chapter and is also available from the programs via the Help buttons in particular dialogs.

We hope that you will send your impressions and suggestions to the Development Team at the contact addresses in the front of the manual. The Epi Info Web Site is available at all times to provide information, updates of programs, and access to vendors, trainers, and the Epi Info Technical Support staff. One of this book's authors (AD) maintains a web site with additional materials relating to Epi Info at WWW.EpiInformatics.Com .

CHAPTER 10: STATISTICAL ANALYSIS WITH EPI INFO

Previous chapters have described the Analysis commands needed to gain access to data, define and manipulate variables, and do lists and tabulations of data values. In this chapter, we focus on the commands necessary to count, sum, cross tabulate, and graph the values in a given dataset.

Simple Analytic Commands and Graphics

The analytic commands, FREQuencies, MEANS, TABLES, and MATCH, are simple to use, but they provide a large number of statistical analyses that would otherwise have to be requested by name. The TABLES command, for example, given data from two Yes/No ("dichotomous") variables, produces not only a table of counts with percentages, but a graphic display of the size of the table cells, and the following statistics:

- Cross product Odds Ratio with confidence limits

- Maximum Likelihood Estimate of the Odds Ratio with exact confidence limits

- Risk Ratio(RR)

- Risk Difference(RD%)

- Chi-square—uncorrected and p value

- Chi-square—Mantel-Haenszel and p value

- Chi-square—Yates corrected and p value

- Mid-p exact

- Fisher exact

Adding one or more variables to the Stratify By choice, does a stratified analysis, making a separate table for each value of the new variable, with adjusted summary summary statistics that remove the confounding effect of the stratifying variable.

Which command to use depends on the type of data, and the purpose of the analysis. Rather than worry about the details, it is easier to try your best guess. Error messages will come up that provide guidance. Generally, FREQuencies and TABLES are used for COUNTING records. MEANS is used to SUM and AVERAGE the values in the records. For one variable, use FREQuencies for text values or MEANS for numbers. For more than one variable, use TABLES for text or Yes/No values and MEANS with two variables for numbers.

The Evans County Data in SAMPLE.MDB

In 1958, the National Institutes of Health began a long-term study of cardiovascular disease and its risk factors in a rural county of Southeast Georgia. Initially 3102 adults were examined and given laboratory tests.

The data in viewData are based on the Evans County heart disease cohort study on the seven-year incidence of coronary heart disease in 609 white males. The variable CAT (endogenous catecholamine level) was *fabricated* for illustrative purposes and dichotomized into categories "high" (top quintile of cohort values) and "low." There are no missing values in this dataset. Thanks to Dr. David Kleinbaum for making the data available[5].

For the examples that follow, use the READ Command to access the EvansCounty dataset in the project called Sample.MDB in the Epi_Info directory.

FREQuencies – Counting the Values

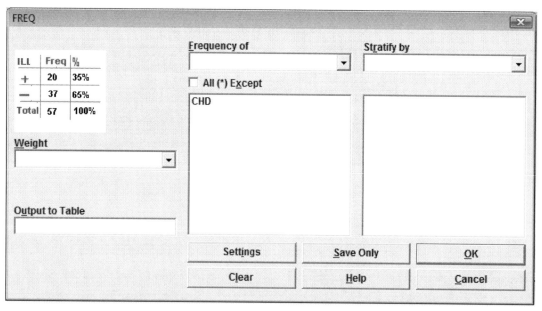

The FREQuencies command provides a table of the values and frequency of each of the values of a single variable. The dialog to do a frequency of the CHD (Coronary Heart Disease) variable in the Evans County dataset and the results are shown below. The Evans County data has been cleaned up so that it has no missing values, but otherwise, the exclusion or inclusion of missing values is controlled by a check box in the SET command.

---

5 Kleinbaum DG, Kupper LL, Morgenstern H. Epidemiologic Research: Principles and quantitative methods. Lifetime Learning Publications, Belmont, California, 1982.

CHD	Frequency	Percent	Cum Percent
Yes	71	11.7%	11.7%
No	538	88.3%	100.0%
Total	609	100.0%	100.0%

95% Conf Limits		
Yes	9.3%	14.5%
No	85.5%	90.7%

FREQuency of Coronary Heart Disease(CHD)

In the table above, the frequency or number of observations of each level of the CHD variable is presented, the percent at each level, and a cumulative percent. There is a small horizontal bar graph of the frequencies, and 95% confidence intervals are provided for each level. In the example above, 11.7% (71/609) of the men developed CHD during the study period with a 95% confidence interval of (9.3%, 14.5%).

Since there are no missing values, the "Cum Percent" or "Cumulative Percent" is 100% after both Yes and No have been tabulated.

You can suppress both the graphics and the statistics by making choices in the dialog box of the SET command.

The FREQuencies command will produce a count for each value of any of the common types of fields (except images), although doing a FREQ of, for example, DateOfBirth, in a large dataset will produce a very large list of counts, those on the same line having exactly the same birthday.

You can specify one or several variables to be tabulated in the FREQ dialog box, and the frequencies will be done automatically, one after the other. You can also choose to FREQ all of the fields in the dataset with a single command by choosing the * (asterisk) value at the top of the choice box. Since this often includes variables with a lot of values (dates, ages, laboratory values, names, or addresses), you can use the ALL EXCEPT check box to exclude these fields from the FREQuencies.

Stratification (i.e., Stratify by) in the FREQuencies command provides a separate table of the frequency for each level of the STRATIFY BY variable(s). If more than one STRATIFY BY variable is given, separate tables are made for each combination of values of the stratifying variables. The STRATIFY BY feature is useful if you want separate frequencies for records having different values of, say, COUNTY or SEX. Specifying one of these variables in STRATIFY BY will produce a separate frequency table for each value. Usually, it is better to produce a single table with both variables, as in TABLES SEX CHD rather than using FREQ CHD stratified by SEX, but the choice is available, especially if you are not interested in statistics for the comparison.

The OUTPUT TO TABLE option sends the results of the frequency to a data table in the current MDB. This allows you to READ the resulting table and perform additional operations on it--for example, SORTing it by frequency. This would be a good way to find the "Top 10" (or top 100) diagnoses in a clinical dataset with a field called Diagnosis. You might do a FREQ of Diagnosis, with OUTPUT TO TABLE specified as DiagFreq. Then READ the table called DiagFreq (check ALL rather than VIEWS in the READ command), SORT on the COUNT field, and LIST the results to produce a list ordered by frequency.

Working with Summary Data: the WEIGHT Field

In all Epi Info analyses except complex sample analysis, the Weight option in the dialog boxes may represent either the frequency of records which have similar characteristics for the given variables or they may represent a sample weight.

The View called Lasum (for Los Angeles summary) in Sample.MDB contains summary data from a study in Los Angeles to determine whether the effect of exogenous estrogen relates to endometrial cancer among 315 participants. The study had a matched case-control design in which each of 63 cases with endometrial cancer, is matched to four control women who were born within one year of the case, had the same marital status, and lived in the same retirement community for the same length of time. The dataset is in summary file format where individual records with similar characteristics are summarized into 25 groups with a COUNT variable to indicate the number persons represented by the record. A LIST of the data is shown below. OB=OBesity, DOS is the dose level of conjugated estrogen, and the OUTCOME is endometrial cancer.

Reference: Breslow and Day. Statistical methods in cancer research: Volume 1 – The analysis of case-control studies. Lyon : International Agency for Research on Cancer, 1980.

OB	DOS	OUTCOME	COUNT
Missing	Missing	1	2
Missing	0	0	41
Missing	0	1	3
Missing	1	0	2
Missing	2	1	1
Missing	3	0	2
0	Missing	0	2
0	Missing	1	2
0	0	0	41
0	0	1	3

Partial LIST of viewLasum Data

In the first row of the data shown the COUNT of 2, in this dataset, means there were 2 individuals with similar values for all other variables in the dataset. In the second data line, there are 41 individuals who were similar for the other variables. First, let's determine a frequency of outcome (a disease variable) using the Weight option. Fill in the variable names in the dialog box as shown in the figure below

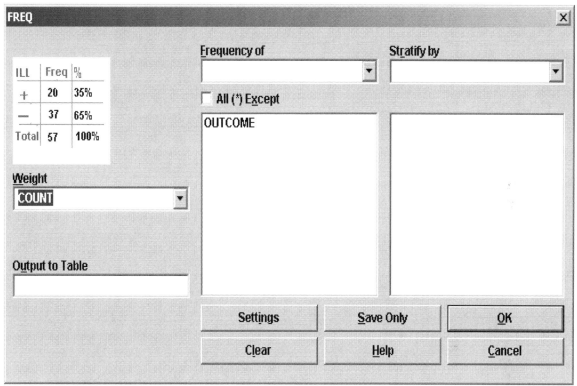

Dialog box for FREQuencies Command Using a Weight Variable, viewLasum Data

The output below shows that 63 individuals had disease and 252 did not, for a total of 315 observations. Without the Weight option, the result would have been 12 with disease out of 25. The latter would occur because each *record* would have been treated as an observation.

FREQ OUTCOME WEIGHTVAR=COUNT			
OUTCOME	**Frequency**	**Percent**	**Cum Percent**
0	252	80.0%	80.0%
1	63	20.0%	100.0%
Total	315	100.0%	100.0%

MEANS – Summing and Averaging

If you want the Sum, Total, and/or the average of values in a variable, the MEANS command is the tool you need.. Since it only works with numbers, the variable must be numeric, date, or time.

The dialog box for the MEANS command is shown below. An abbreviated example of the MEANS command for the variable CHL (cholesterol) follows. The results include the total number of observations ("Obs"); the sum of all observations ("Total"); the mean, variance, and standard deviation ("Std Dev") of the observations; minimum and maximum values; 25th, 50th ("median"), and 75th percentiles; and the mode. If the variable has two or more values (a tie) for the mode ("most frequent") value, the smallest will be presented in the Epi Info output.

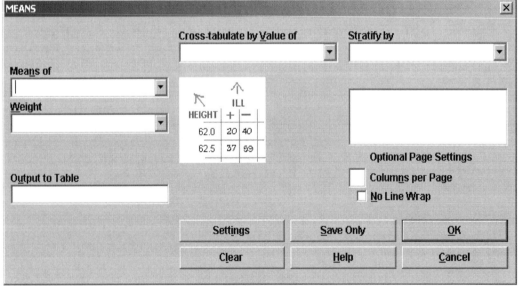

The MEANS Command Dialog

CHL	Frequency	Percent	Cum Percent
94	1	0.2%	0.2%
113	2	0.3%	0.5%
...	...	...	... ...
336	2	0.3%	99.8%
357	1	0.2%	100.0%
Total	609	100.0%	100.0%

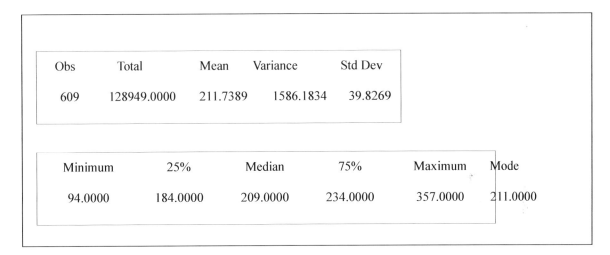

Obs	Total	Mean	Variance	Std Dev
609	128949.0000	211.7389	1586.1834	39.8269

Minimum	25%	Median	75%	Maximum	Mode
94.0000	184.0000	209.0000	234.0000	357.0000	211.0000

Output from MEANS command for a single variable, viewEvansCounty

Note that the cholesterol levels between 113 and 336 are omitted to save space

MEANS CHL CHD

CHD

CHL	Yes	No	TOTAL
94	0	1	1
Row %	0.0	100.0	100.0
Col %	0.0	0.2	0.2
113	0	2	2
Row %	0.0	100.0	100.0
Col %	0.0	0.4	0.3

...

Descriptive Statistics for Each Value of Crosstab Variable

	Yes	No	TOTAL
336	0	2	2
Row %	0.0	100.0	100.0
Col %	0.0	0.4	0.3
357	1	0	1
Row %	100.0	0.0	100.0
Col %	1.4	0.0	0.2
TOTAL	71	538	609
Row %	11.7	88.3	100.0
Col %	100.0	100.0	100.0

	Obs	Total	Mean	Variance	Std Dev
Yes	71	15758.0000	221.9437	1580.1111	39.7506
No	538	113191.0000	210.3922	1574.3431	39.6780

	Minimum	25%	Median	75%	Maximum	Mode
Yes	145.0000	195.0000	216.0000	242.0000	357.0000	228.0000
No	94.0000	182.0000	206.5000	232.0000	336.0000	211.0000

ANOVA, a Parametric Test for Inequality of Population Means (For normally distributed data only)

Variation	SS	df	MS	F statistic
Between	8369.4658	1	8369.4658	5.3139
Within	956030.0219	607	1575.0083	
Total	964399.4877	608		

T Statistic =2.3052
P-value =0.0215
Bartlett's Test for Inequality of Population Variances

Bartlett's chi square=	0.0004	df=1	P value=0.9838

A small p-value (e.g., less than 0.05) suggests that the variances are not homogeneous and that the ANOVA may not be appropriate.
Mann-Whitney/Wilcoxon Two-Sample Test (Kruskal-Wallis test for two groups)

Kruskal-Wallis H (equivalent to Chi square) =	5.4504
Degrees of freedom =	1
P value =	0.0196

Comparing Two MEANS, viewEvansCounty Data

Note that the cholesterol levels between 113 and 336 are omitted to save space

The MEANS command can also compare two or more means. When comparing two means an independent t-test is performed, and for comparing more than two means, a one-way analysis of variance (ANOVA) is performed. The independent t-test and ANOVA can be used if the following assumptions are met:

- The outcome variable is normally distributed in each group

- The underlying variances are the same in each group

Epi Info does not provide a statistical test to determine if the data are normally distributed; the data could be graphed to see if the data visually seem to be normally distributed. Epi Info does perform a test to determine if the second assumption above is met called "Bartlett's Test"; if the p-value is large (say >0.05) this would suggest the variances are approximately equal; if the p-value from Bartlett's test is small (say <0.05), this would suggest that the underlying variances are *not* the same and therefore the t-test and ANOVA results may not be appropriate for the data.

In the example shown, the cholesterol levels (CHL) of those who develop coronary heart disease (CHD) are compared to those without disease. The variances in Figure 13 can be assumed to be similar because the Bartlett's test p-value is 0.9838. What should you do if the variances are not equal? One option is to use the nonparametric test that does not require an assumption of normality. In this case the non-parametric p-value (p=0.0196) is similar in value to the t-test p-value. Another option is to transform the data, such as taking the log of the outcome variable. An independent t-test assuming unequal variances can be found in other programs such as SAS, SPSS, and OpenEpi.

In the example, since the variances can be assumed equal, we may wish to see if the mean cholesterol differs between those who developed CHD and those who did not. In this example, the mean cholesterol level in those who developed CHD was 222 mg/100mL compared to 210 mg/100mL in those who did not develop CHD. The t-test has a p-value of 0.0215 suggesting that those who developed CHD had a significantly higher mean cholesterol level.

If more than two means are compared, a p-value for this comparison will be presented based on the F-test for a one-way ANOVA. ANOVA, or Analysis of Variance, is the appropriate test to use for more than two columns of data, since there is not a "3-column t-test." Epi Info does not perform multiple comparison tests for one-way ANOVA tests.

Tests that depend on the assumption that the variable being assessed (the mean) has a known distribution pattern, in this case, Dr. Gauss's "normal" distribution. are called "Parametric". If this assumption cannot be made, there are "non-parametric" tests that do not require distribution assumptions. For data in two columns, the non-parametric test is called "Mann-Whitney/Wilcoxon two-sample test " If there are three or more columns, the test is called the Kruskal-Wallis test. Luckily, after that, the number of columns exceeds the number of statistician's names attached to the tests, and Kruskal and Wallis can still be relied upon.

Frequently, the non-parametric tests produce p-values quite similar to those from the parametric tests. In this case, if the results are "significant" with both, you can report the non-parametric results and not worry about whether the conditions for the ANOVA or t-test are met.

Occasionally, you may have trouble doing MEANS with a variable that appears numeric, but is a text variable, perhaps because the data were imported. If AGE, for example, is of text type, you can define a new variable, ASSIGN NumAge=TxtToNum(AGE), and then do the MEANS on NumAge.

Testing Associations with the TABLES Command

The TABLES command is used to compare two categorical variables, such as an exposure variable (exposed vs. unexposed) and an outcome variable (disease vs. no disease). To have the odds ratio (OR), risk ratio (RR), and risk difference (RD) calculated correctly, it is important the table be set up as shown in Table 1. Table setup for Epi Info to calculate the odds ratio, risk/prevalence ratio, and risk/prevalence difference.

	Disease	No Disease	Total
Exposed	a	b	a + b
Not Exposed	c	d	c + d
Total	a + c	b + d	n

The OR, RR, and RD are calculated as:

OR = (a x d) / (b x c)

RR = [a / (a + b)] / [c / (c + d)]   RD = [a / (a + b)] - [c / (c + d)]

The dialog box for the TABLES command is shown below. For an example using dichotomous (yes/no) exposure and disease variables, in the viewEvansCountry data, select CAT (catecholamine) as the Exposure variable and CHD (coronary heart disease) as the Outcome variable.

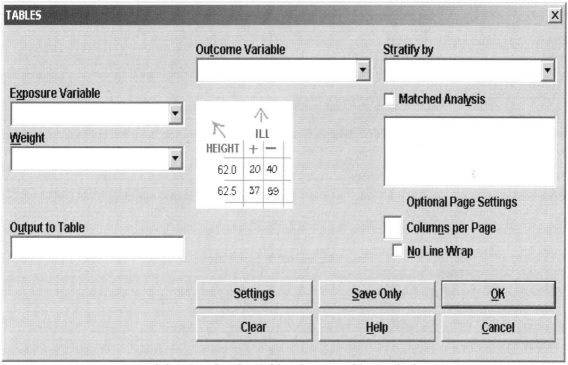

Dialog Box for the Tables Command in Analysis

If you observe the Exposure and Outcome suggestions, the tables will automatically be oriented for easy interpretation. In some cases, particularly for larger tables, Exposure and Outcome are not really relevant, and the variable inserted in the left blank will be shown vertically down the left side of pages, and the other will be horizontal across the top.

The output for two Yes/No variables, shown below, is a 2-by-2 table that contains: the number of observations in each cell, the row percent ("Row %"), and the column percent ("Col %"). Row and Column percents can be turned on or off from the SETTINGS command, the last one in the command list.

CORONARY HEART DISEASE (CHD)			
Catecholamine Level (CAT)	Yes	No	TOTAL
Yes	27	95	122
Row %	22.1	77.9	100.0
Col %	38.0	17.7	20.0
No	44	443	487
Row %	9.0	91.0	100.0
Col %	62.0	82.3	80.0
TOTAL	71	538	609
Row %	11.7	88.3	100.0
Col %	100.0	100.0	100.0

TABLES for Two Yes/No Variables, viewEvansCounty Data.

A graphic provided to the right of the table depicts how the observations are distributed within the table – the larger the box, the larger the number of observations.

The small red box represents the upper left cell of the table, the ill persons with with exposure to the risk factor. The large green box on the lower right represents the persons who were not ill and did not have the specified exposure. Both of these boxes are in favor of the hypothesis that there is an association between exposure and illness. The other two boxes in the upper right and lower left are discordant with the hypothesis.

The odds ratio, one of the measures of association, can be thought of as red x green divided by brown x yellow, or the product of boxes in favor divided by the product of boxes against the association. If the boxes against predominate, then the exposure may be protective (odds ratio less than 1.0). If the red and green boxes (upper left and lower right) win the day, the odds ratio exceeds 1.0, and there is a positive association. If all the boxes are the same size or the two cross-products are equal, the odds ratio is 1.0, suggesting no association.

Single Table Analysis

	Point	95% Confidence Interval	
	Estimate	Lower	Upper
PARAMETERS: Odds-based			
Odds Ratio (cross product)	2.8615	1.6878	4.8514 (T)
Odds Ratio (MLE)	2.8554	1.6690	4.8350 (M)
		1.6148	4.9853 (F)
PARAMETERS: Risk-based			
Risk Ratio (RR)	2.4495	1.5837	3.7887 (T)
Risk Difference (RD%)	13.0962	5.3021	20.8903 (T)

(T=Taylor series; C=Cornfield; M=Mid-P; F=Fisher Exact)

STATISTICAL TESTS	Chi-square	1-tailed p	2-tailed p
Chi square - uncorrected	16.2465		0.0000567826
Chi square - Mantel-Haenszel	16.2198		0.0000575712
Chi square - corrected (Yates)	14.9998		0.0001086935
Mid-p exact		0.0000911051	
Fisher exact		0.0001374257	

Remainder of Ouput from Tables with Two Yes/No Variables

Beneath the table is the Single Table Analysis that provides parameter estimates with confidence intervals and statistical tests. The first set of parameter estimates are based on the odds, with an odds ratio based on the cross product [i.e., (a x d) / (b x c)], and one based on the maximum likelihood estimation approach (MLE). Three different confidence intervals are provided, the Taylor series, mid-P exact, and the Fisher exact. Which one should you use? Our preference is the mid-P exact method. Note that the odds ratio calculated is an unmatched odds ratio – if the study used a matched case-control design, the MATCH command should be used.

Next are the Risk-based estimates - the risk ratio and the risk difference with their confidence intervals. Note that if the outcome variable is based on prevalent disease, then substitute the terms "prevalence ratio" and "prevalence difference" for "risk ratio" and "risk difference", respectively.

Finally, a number of statistical test results are provided: three different chi square tests and two exact tests. The chi square tests are presented as two-tailed p-values (although you could divide the two-tailed p-value by 2 to calculate a one-tailed p-value), and the exact tests are presented as one-tailed p-values (you could multiply the one-tailed p-values by 2 to get a two-tailed p-value).

In the example shown, we conclude that there is a statistically significant association between exposure and disease (p<.001), with individuals with high catecholamine (CAT=Yes) levels having a significantly higher risk of disease compared to those with "normal" catecholamine levels (CAT=No), 22.1% and 9.0%, respectively.

Stratified Analysis

To perform a stratified analysis, provide an exposure variable, an outcome variable, and at least one stratifying variable. For example, using the CAT and CHD variables from the previous example, stratify on cholesterol group (CHLG) to perform a stratified analysis. The risk ratio for CAT → CHD relationship was 12.1 in those in the high cholesterol group vs. 1.8 in those in the low cholesterol group (results not shown). The summary information indicates a much stronger exposure-disease relationship in the high-cholesterol group. This large difference in odds ratios between tables in two different strata is called "effect modification" or "interaction". If it is present, it is not legitimate to adjust the odds ratios over the strata and thus control for confounding.

Note: This particular file was fictiounally altered for teaching purposes; do not rush out to have your CATecholamine level measured or adjusted, no matter which CHLG stratum you may inhabit.

Parameters	Point Estimate	95%Confidence Interval Lower	Upper
Odds Ratio Estimates			
Crude OR (cross product)	2.8615	1.6878,	4.8514 (T)
Crude OR (MLE)	2.8554	1.6690,	4.8350 (M)
		1.6148,	4.9853 (F)
Adjusted OR (MH)	2.8716	1.6994,	4.8524 (R)
Adjusted OR (MLE)	3.0375	1.7551,	5.2156 (M)
		1.6962,	5.3868 (F)
Risk Ratios (RR)			
Crude Risk Ratio (RR)	2.4495	1.5837,	3.7887
Adjusted RR (MH)	2.4648	1.6173,	3.7564

`(T=Taylor series; R=RGB; M=Exact mid-P; F=Fisher exact)`

STATISTICAL TESTS (overall assoc)	Chi-square	1-tailed p	2-tailed p
MH Chi square - uncorrected	17.4807		0.0000
MH Chi square - corrected	16.1659		0.0001
Mid-p exact		0.0001	
Fisher exact		0.0001	
In the following two tests, low p values suggest that ratios differ by stratum			
Chi-square for differing Odds Ratios by stratum (interaction)	10.3638		0.0013
Chi-square for differing Risk Ratios by stratum	16.3645		0

(Above) Example of Output from TABLES Command for a Stratified 2x2 table, Summary Information Only, viewEvansCounty data, CAT x CHD, Stratified by Cholesterol Group(CHLG)

Epi Info presents both the crude odds ratio (which combines the strata into a single 2x2 table) and two different adjusted odds ratios (which "adjust" or "control" for the stratifying variable), one based on the Mantel-Haenszel method (MH) and one based on the maximum likelihood estimation method (MLE). Crude and adjusted risk ratios are also presented. Note that in this example the test-for-interaction for the risk ratio has a p-value of .0001, indicating that there is statistically significant interaction; therefore, the stratum-specific measures should be presented separately when describing the CAT → CHD association rather than the crude or adjusted risk ratio estimates. An example of confounding, not presented here, can be seen stratifying by the CAT → CHD example by age groups (AGEG1).

The general approach to stratified analyses is to determine if a variable modifies an exposure-disease relationship (i.e., assess for interaction). The statistical test for effect modification or interaction is shown at the bottom of the results. If it is determined that a stratifying variable does not modify the exposure-disease relationship, then the next question is whether the variable confounds the relationship. See the section on Logistic Regression for an example of how to assess confounding. If interest is in the risk difference, attributable fraction, or prevented fraction, these analyses can be performed using OpenEpi.

The MATCH Command

The MATCH command is for use with matched case-control studies. Each case is allowed to have one or more matched controls, and the number of controls can vary from case to case. The dialog box for the MATCH command is shown in Figure 17. To use the MATCH command, you need to specify an Exposure Variable, the Outcome Variable (i.e., case vs. control), and a MATCH Variable that links each case to their one or more controls. An example matched case-control dataset in the Sample.mdb file is called viewRely; please READ this dataset. These data are from a matched case-control study of toxic shock syndrome in which each case had three controls matched on potential confounders, such as age (see Appendix 1 for more details on this file). The primary exposure was the use of Rely tampons. After READing the data, view the data layout using the LIST command (see Figure 18). The name of the first variable (i.e., first column) is ID which is an identification number that links each case with her three controls; note the second variable/column in the dataset is CASE which has the values as either Yes (a case) or No (a control). The third variable/column reflects use of Rely tampons (Yes or No).

To run the MATCH command for the viewRely data, first READ viewRELY, then click the MATCH command and make the following entries in the dialog:

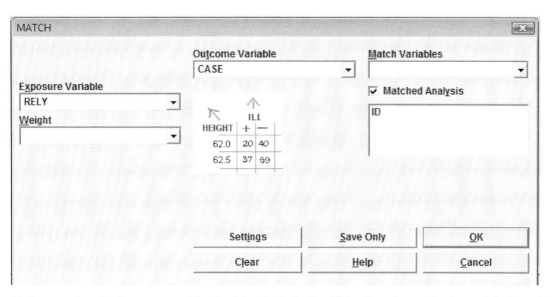

Make sure that the box next to Matched Analysis in the dialog box has a check mark in it, and then press the OK button. The output is shown on the next page.

RELY : CASE MATCH variables: ID

Matched Analysis of TABLES with Non-Zero Marginals
Matched Sets:12 Observations:48

Cases:1 Controls:3

	Exposed Controls			
Exposed Cases	3	2	1	0
1	1	1	5	4
0	0	1	1	1

	Point	95%Confidence Interval	
Parameters	Estimate	Lower	Upper
Odds Ratio Estimates			
Crude OR (cross product)	13.0000	2.4125,	70.0530 (T)
Crude OR (MLE)	12.2196	2.4762,	94.3799 (M)
		2.0935,	133.9356 (F)
Adjusted OR (MH)	7.6667	1.6061,	36.5973 (R)
Adjusted OR (MLE)	8.3589	1.9281,	58.2541 (M)
		1.6672,	81.7998 (F)
Risk Ratios (RR)			
Crude Risk Ratio (RR)	7.0000	1.7166,	28.5455
Adjusted RR (MH)	7.6667	1.6615,	35.3767

(T=Taylor series; R=RGB; M=Exact mid-P; F=Fisher exact)

In the output, one or more tables are presented to show the relationship between whether or not a case was exposed and the number of controls that were exposed. Next, odds ratio and risk ratio information is presented. In general, the only useful information from this part of the output is the adjusted odds ratios and their confidence intervals. In this example, the adjusted MH odds ratio is 7.7 indicating a strong association between toxic shock syndrome and use of Rely tampons. A number of statistical tests are provided at the bottom of the output, which, in this example, indicates a statistically significant association.

A common question is "what would happen if the matching aspects of the study design were ignored in the analysis?" To ignore the matching of controls to cases, use the TABLES command and provide Rely as the exposure variable and Case as the outcome variable. The odds ratio from the TABLES command, ignoring the match, is 8.2 (results not shown), compared to a matched odds ratio of 7.7. In this particular example, ignoring the matching of cases and controls overestimates the odds ratio (i.e., a bias away from the null).

SUMMARIZE Command

The SUMMARIZE command creates a new Data table (i.e., a dataset) containing descriptive statistics from the current dataset (Figure 20). Available Aggregate functions are COUNT, MIN, MAX, SUM, FIRST, LAST, AVG, VARIANCE and STANDARD DEVIATION. The basic principle is the same as that of Output To Table option in the TABLES, FREQ, and MEANS commands, but Aggregate functions are more powerful. The SUMMARIZE command can create a table that contains results from more than one function (e.g., COUNT, MIN, MAX, ...) specific to a single variable of interest or multiple functions for more than one variable.

Let's do an example. Using the viewEvansCounty data, if we wish to create a table that includes only mean values and standard deviations of AGE and diastolic blood pressure (DBP) along with total number of records, we can insert the following information into the fields un the upper left corner of the SUMMARIZE command dialog:

Aggregate: Average (choose 'average' from the available choices)

Variable: AGE (choose AGE from the list of available variables)

Into Variable: average_age (Name of a variable to be automatically created)

Then, click the Apply button. You can use the same technique for standard deviation (SD) of AGE, and means and SD of DBP (Diastolic Blood Pressure) as shown in the screen image below. The Aggregate function Count was applied to the AGE variable to get the overall number of records in the dataset.

In the Output to Table field, specify a name for the Data table that you want to create, in this example, summary_table (spaces not allowed). The table will be created and saved in the currently project, in this example, "C:\Epi_Info\Sample.mdb". Click OK to create the new Data table.

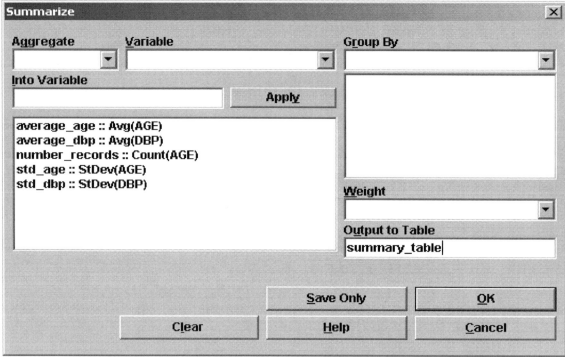

Dialog Box for the SUMMARIZE Command, viewEvansCounty Data, Epi Info.

Now use the READ command to READ the summary_table [note that you will need to click on ALL in READ dialog box. Have a look at the new table using the LIST command.

Example showing the effect of the SUMMARIZE command using LIST, Epi Info.

average_age	average_dbp	number_recs	std_age	std_dbp
53.70607553366	91.18062397372	609	9.25838769076145	14.4988731051949

These results are not particularly exciting, and could have been obtained with Frequencies and Means of the original dataset. Hang on, however, we are just getting started with the Summarize command.

To create a table that summarizes the number of records and mean values of age and DBP stratifying on CAT (catecholamine) and coronary heart disease CHD (present/absent), we can follow the same procedure as above, and then place the variables CAT and CHD in the Group By box. Group By, in this case, means "create a separate record of results for each combination of CAT and CHD values."

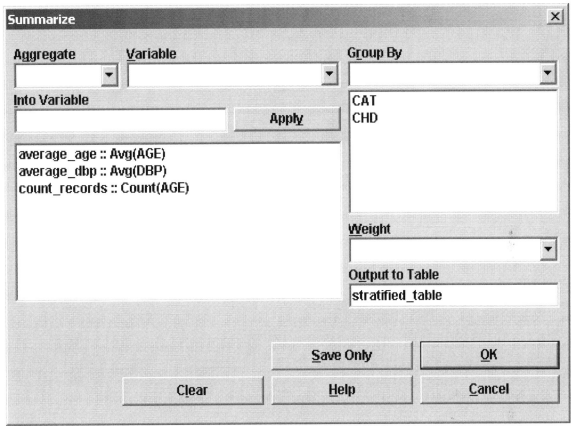

Dialog box for the SUMMARIZE Command Using the Group By Option, viewEvansCounty data

After clicking OK, use the READ command to read the file "stratified_table" from the current project "C:\Epi_Info\Sample.mdb" and look at the table by using the LIST command as in the previous SUMMARY example.

CAT	CHD	average_age	average_dbp	number_records
No	No	51.6433408577878	88.2121896162528	443
No	Yes	54.0909090909091	93.7272727272727	44
Yes	No	60.6736842105263	101.621052631579	95
Yes	Yes	62.4074074074074	99	27

The Output Table of the SUMMARIZE Command with the GROUP BY Option Using LIST

Please note that Aggregate functions 'FIRST' and 'LAST' are based on the current sort order of the dataset. (Warning; in case there is a tie for first—a duplicate—BOTH values are discarded.) For a variable with numeric value, 'Minimum' and 'Maximum' Aggregate function finds the minimum or maximum value of that variable. For date variables, Minimum value denotes earliest date and Maximum the latest date.

The really exciting use for SUMMARIZE, however, is its ability to find the latest or the earliest record in a series, for example, of visits by the same patient on different dates. This is nearly impossible in a relational database with other commands. Suppose that you have a database containing patient visits with PatientID, VisitDate, and Hematocrit. You would like to find the difference in hematocrit values between the first visit and the last visit.

Patient ID	Visit Date	Hemotocrit	UniqueKey	RecStatus
555	09-19-1995	44	7	1
555	08-08-2000	44	8	1
1	03-03-2002	13	1	1
1	04-04-2002	21	2	1
1	10-10-2002	25	3	1
222	02-02-2007	42	5	1
1	09-09-2008	42	4	1
222	10-10-2008	35	6	1
555	02-02-2009	22	9	1

Here's the strategy...First SORT the records by VisitDate, then use SUMMARIZE to create a new file in which the FIRST and LAST Hematocrit for each patient are in the same record. After that, it is a simple matter to define a variable Hct2MinusHct1 for the difference between the first and last hematocrits and assign it the value of the difference. The program and the dataset are in ..\Examples\exMisc.

```
*The following program , FirstLastHct.pgm does the work:
ROUTEOUT 'HctDifference.htm' REPLACE
READ 'Summarize.mdb':viewVisitsHct
SORT VisitDate
LIST *
SUMMARIZE FirstHct :: First(Hemotocrit) LastHct :: Last(Hemotocrit) TO FirstLastHct
STRATAVAR=PatientID
READ 'Summarize.mdb':FirstLastHct
LIST * GRIDTABLE
DEFINE Hct2MinusHct1 NUMERIC
ASSIGN Hct2MinusHct1=TxtToNum(LastHct)-TxtToNum(FirstHct)
LIST *
```

Here is the final result:

PatientID	FirstHct	LastHct	Hct2MinusHct1
1	13	42	29
222	42	35	-7
555	44	22	-22

We conclude that Patient #1 had a dramatic increase in Hematocrit over the course of treatment. Perhaps he/she was first seen for a serious bleeding episode due to trauma, and the hematocrit had returned to normal by the last visit. Patients #222 and #555 both had decreases in Hematocrit, perhaps due to malignancies and/or chemotherapy.

In a later chapter, we will use the RELATE command to link a SUMMARIZE output table to a dataset and make information from the first visit, or an average of all visits, available in each record of patient data.

CHAPTER 11: THE GRAPH COMMAND

The Graph module is one of the hidden gems of Epi Info. You can choose from 18 different graph types, put up to 9 graphs on a page, overlay one graph on another, and produce a whole collection of graphs with a single command. After producing a graph, you can change colors, axes, symbols, and many other features by editing the graph itself. The edits can be saved as a "template" to use with future data sets. Graph types include:

- Area
- Bar
- Box-Whisker
- Hi-Low
- Histogram
- Line

- Moving Average
- Pareto
- Pie
- Points
- Polar
- Pyramid

- Rotated Bar
- Scatter 3D
- Scatter XY
- Spline
- Stacked Histogram
- Step

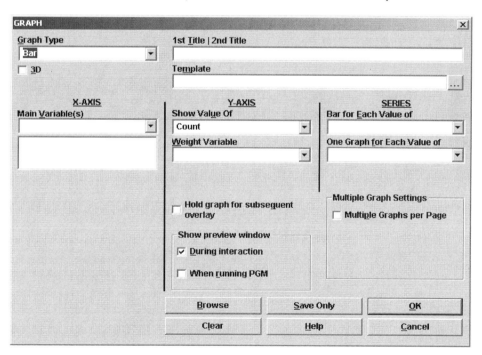

Graphing One Variable

By choosing the name of a single main variable for the X-axis, you can produce graphs that give information similar to that of the FREQ command. Here are examples, using the EVENTNAME field from ..\exSurveillance\Surveillance.mdb:viewCaseReports, a sample of surveillance data from a US state.

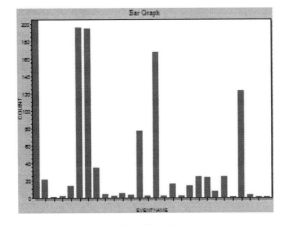

Bar Graph

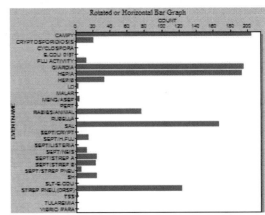

Horizontal Bar Graph

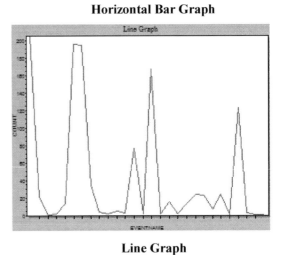

Area Graph

Line Graph

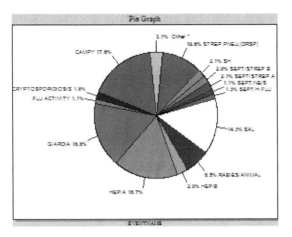

Pie Graph

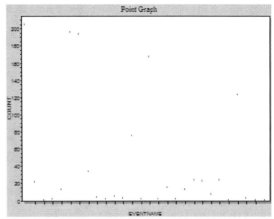

Point Graph

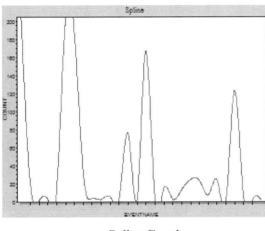

Spline Graph

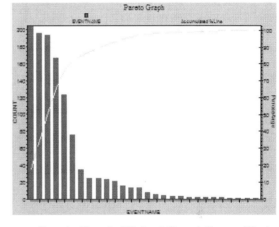

Pareto Graph. Highest Count Comes First

Graphing Time Data

In the classical epidemiologic descriptors of Person, Place, and Time, the time course of events is often best shown as a graph, also known as the Epidemic Curve. Although a bar, line, or point graph can be used with a Time variable like Date or Date/Hour, they give a false impression when there are missing dates, since no values are plotted when there are no values in the dataset. Note that there are no gaps in the following bar graph of the DateOnset field in our favorite dataset, Sample.mdb:viewOswego.

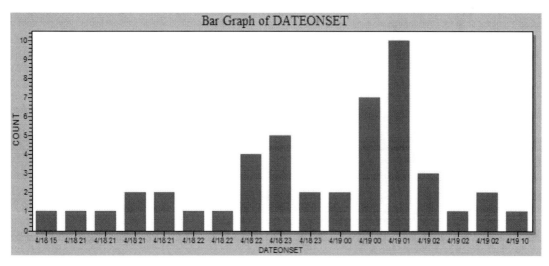

There is another Graph type that is smarter about dates and other numeric series, however. A HISTOGRAM can depict dates or times with zero cases, as illustrated by the graph below

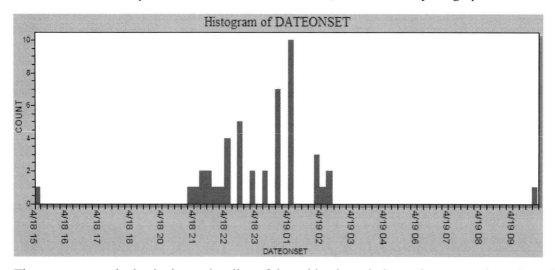

The two cases at the beginning and ending of the epidemic period gave important clues about the etiology of the epidemic, as they had eaten the contaminated ice cream at times other than the main supper hour. The histogram makes these cases and the intervals before and after much clearer than the bar graph.

When you choose HISTOGRAM in the Graph command dialog and the variable is a Date or Date/Time variable, you can choose the DISPLAY FORMAT, e.g., DD/MM/YYYY. If you choose an interval, such as "WEEK," the data are automatically grouped, in this case, by 7-day intervals, as shown in the second graph below.

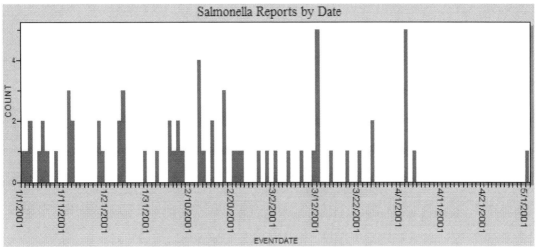

Reports By Date, In Other Words, By Day

Here is the one with the Interval set to weeks. Note that a recode statement could have accomplished the same thing, but less conveniently.

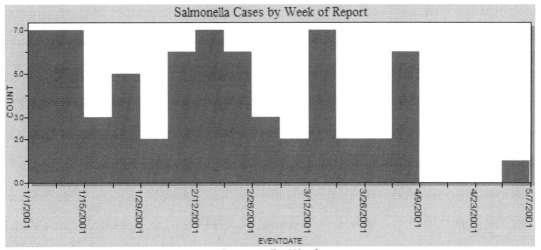

Reports By Week

Multiple Graphs

The Graph command can make a number of graphs with a single command, using the ONE GRAPH FOR EACH VALUE OF feature. In the following example, the request for a separate graph for each COUNTY produces 22 separate graphs.

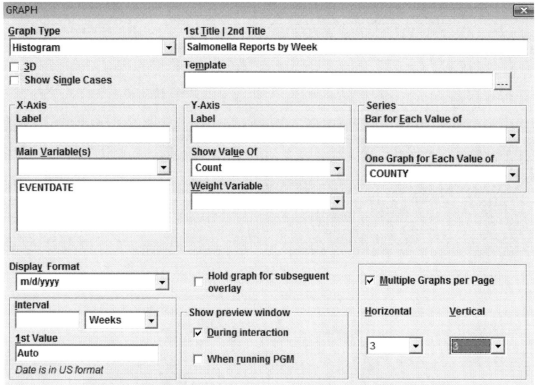

Graphing EVENTDATE with a Separate Graph for Each COUNTY

Here's the output:

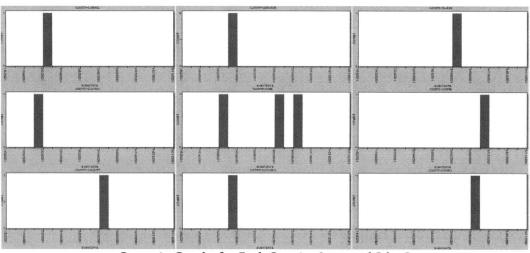

Separate Graphs for Each County, Arranged 3 by 3

Graphing Two or More Variables

The ScatterXY graph takes two numeric variables and plots them in XY configuration with the addition of a linear regression line.

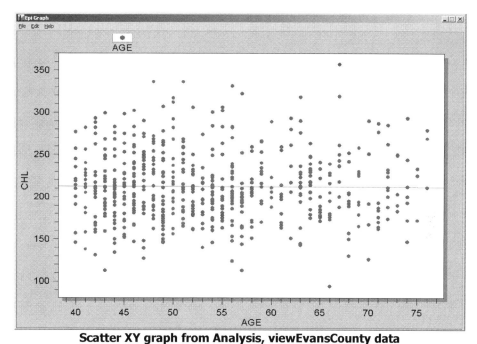

Scatter XY graph from Analysis, viewEvansCounty data

Epi Info can place more than one graph on a page. To illustrate this, enter the following values.:

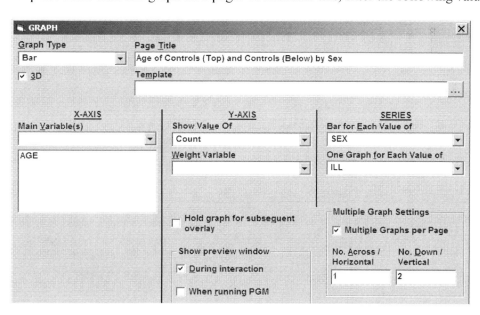

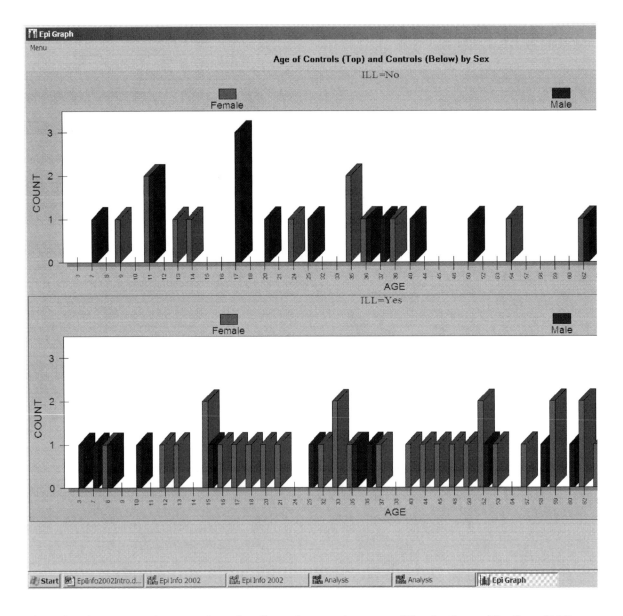

Note that the two graphs are reshaped to fit on the page because of the 1 x 2 specification. BAR FOR EACH VALUE of SEX produced separate bars for males and females. Here we chose 3D and grouped bars to show off the capabilities of the GRAPH command, but four separate graphs might have been clearer, and epidemiologists who care more about numbers than entertainment may advise against 3-dimensional graphs.

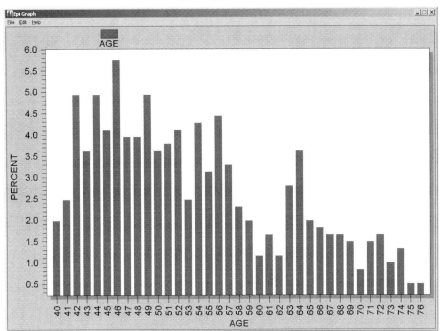

Bar Graph from viewEvansCounty Data

To change an axis label, left click on the label and a dialog box will appear which allows the user to specify the label text. A similar approach can be used to change data point labels. To alter features such as the font style, font size, numeric precision, right click on the item. The image files created by the graphing command are automatically included in the HTML output (discussed later).

Templates

Graphs can be customized after they are produced, and the properties saved as a Template that can be invoked again, as long as the graph type (e.g., bar) remains the same.

To "customize" a graph, first produce it with the Graph command, and then double-click anywhere on the graph without closing the graph view. The Customization dialog box will appear on the screen. (Note: other ways to view the Customization... dialog box are through the pull-down menu system (Edit→Launch Dialog Box) or by right clicking on the on the screen and then selecting the option Customize Dialog).

The customization dialog provides a host of options to modify the graph, in a series of tabs. Probably the best way to learn about them is to experiment.

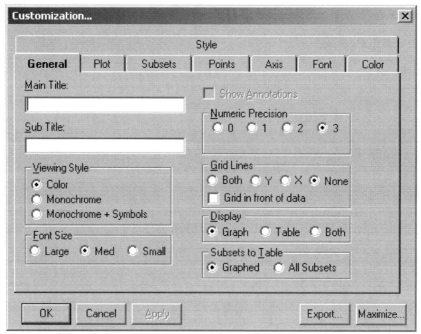

Right Click on a Graph to See this Customization Dialog

After customizing a graph, you can save the properties in a template so that they are applied by specifying the template in the GRAPH dialog in Analysis. To save the properties, use the SAVE TEMPLATE entry on the FILE menu at the top left corner of the graph window.:

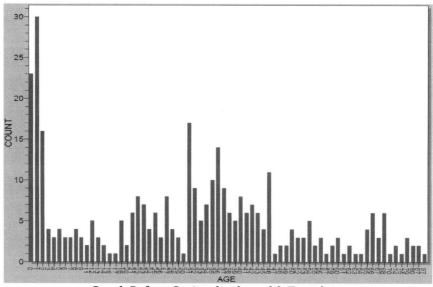

Graph Before Customization with Template

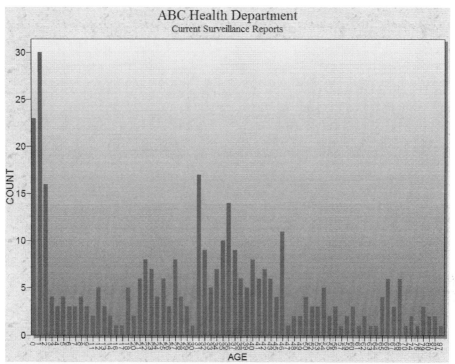

Same Data As Previous Graph, Customized with Template

After customization, the properties were saved from the menu at the top of the Graph page with the Save Template feature, as BarChartTemplate.CHT. They can be imposed on any new dataset using the Graph command with BAR and the template, BarChartTemplate.CHT. Although the properties of charts are good for esthetics and for hours of fun, they also can be quite useful, for example, in adjusting the maximum and minimum values on the Y axis to facilitate comparison among data sets with different numbers of records, or adjusting fonts and sizes to improve legibility.

Practice with the MEANS, TABLES, and GRAPH Commands

Using the viewEvansCounty file, answer the following questions:

1. What is the mean hematocrit (HEM)?

2. Does hematocrit (HEM) appear to be normally distributed? (Note: use a graph to display the distribution of the values.)

3. Does the mean hematocrit (HEM) differ between younger individuals (<55 years of age, variable AGEG1=No) and older individuals (>55 years of age, variable AGEG1=Yes)?

4. What is the mean socioeconomic status score (SES)?

5. Does SES appear to be normally distributed? (Note: use a graph to display the distribution of the values.)

6. Does SES vary by the seven age group categories (variable AGEG2)?

7. What is the odds ratio and risk ratio when assessing the relationship between the cholesterol group variable (CHLG) and CHD? Is there a statistically significant association?

8. Assess whether the variables in the table below modify or confound the CAT-CHD relationship based on the odds ratio. "Modify" (also referred to as effect modification or interaction) is considered present for the odds ratio when the Chi-square for differing Odds Ratios by stratum (interaction) p-value is < 0.05. If there is no interaction, the assessment of confounding will be a 10% or greater difference between the crude and adjusted odds ratio:

$$\frac{\left| \hat{OR}_{crude} - \hat{OR}_{adjusted} \right|}{\hat{OR}_{adjusted}} x100$$

Third Variable	Interaction p-value	Crude OR[1]	Adjusted OR[2]	Interaction, and/or Confounding?
ECG				
MAR				
SMK				
AGEG1				
QTIG				
HPT				

Resources

Sample and exercise files for this chapter are found in **exGRAPH** in the **Examples** folder. The "answers" to the exercises are found in a file in the **..\Examples\exMisc** folder.

CHAPTER 12: ADVANCED STATISTICS

This chapter covers Linear Regression, Logistic Regression, Kaplan-Meier Survival, Cox Proportional Hazards, and the commands for analyzing complex sample designs (Complex Sample FREQuencies, Complex Sample TABLES, and Complex Sample MEANS).

Linear Regression

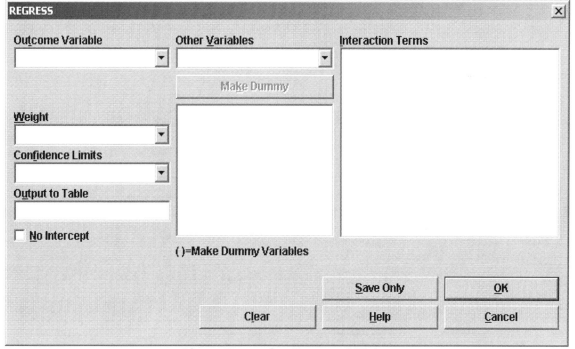

Linear Regression Command Dialog

Linear regression is used when the outcome variable is continuous, as with blood pressure, hemoglobin, or cholesterol. The Linear Regression command can be used for simple linear-regression and simple correlation (only one independent variable), or for multiple linear regression (more than one independent variable). The primary interest is to predict one dependent (outcome) variable (y) from one or more independent (predictor) variables (x,x1,..).

Simple Linear Regression

As an example of simple linear regression, we will use the viewEstriolandBirthweight data which can be found in the Sample.mdb file. In this example, the Outcome Variable is Birthweight and the Other Variable is Estriol. Estriol is the mother's estriol level measured near the end of pregnancy. Both are continuous variables, similar to those we would use for a ScatterXY graph.

Linear Regression

Variable	Coefficient	Std Error	F-test	P-Value
Estriol	0.608	0.147	17.1616	0.000286
CONSTANT	21.523	2.620	67.4656	0.000000

Source	df	Sum of Squares	Mean Square	F-statistic
Regression	1	250.574	250.574	17.162
Residuals	29	423.426	14.601	
Total	30	674.000		

Linear Regression Results, viewEstriolAndBirthweight data

Note: The Correlation Coefficient, frequently referred to as "r", is **not** the same as r^2 or r^2

Coefficient, Std Error, F-test, and P-value: For the predictor variable, the Regression COEFFICIENT is the slope of the line. In this example, 0.608 tells us that, for every one-unit increase in estriol (1 mg/24 hr), there is a 0.608 increase in birth weight units (g/100). A line with a positive coefficient slopes upward, one with a negative coefficient slopes downward, and a coefficient of 0 means the line is straight across (no relationship). The standard error ("Std Error") of the slope here is 0.147. The F-test is the same as the F-Statistic presented later in the output for simple linear regression, and the P-value, in this example, is 0.000286. For the CONSTANT, the coefficient is the y intercept, i.e., that when the the birthweight is 0, the Mom's estriol level should be 21.523, a good illustration of the need to consider biology and common sense when using linear regression.

F-Statistic: The F-statistic is the Regression mean square / Residual mean square. In the example, 250.574 / 14.601 = 17.162. In a simple linear regression, the F-statistic is calculated to determine if the slope of the regression line is significantly different from 0. For a simple linear regression, note that the F-Statistic in the lower half of the output is the same as the F-Test for the predictor variable in the upper half of the output which has a p-value = 0.000286.

The equation of the simple linear regression line is:

$$y = a + bx$$

where y is the dependent variable, a is the intercept, b is the slope, and x is the independent variable.

In the above example, the regression line is:

Birthweight = a + b(estriol)

Birthweight = 21.523 + 0.608(estriol)

For any given value of estriol, a Birthweight value can be predicted. For example, using the mean estriol level of 17.226:

Birthweight = 21.523 + 0.608(17.226) = 31.996

An example of a Scatter XY graph for the data with the regression line is shown on the next. page

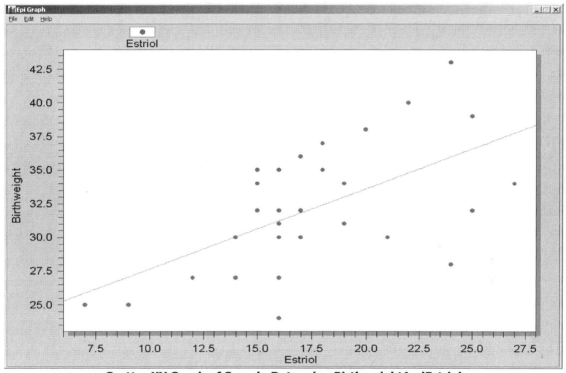

Scatter XY Graph of Sample Data, viewBirthweightAndEstriol

Within Epi Info, the predicted values and the residuals could be added to the file. For example, the following commands could be used for the data presented above:

```
DEFINE PREDICTED
ASSIGN PREDICTED = 21.523 + 0.608 * ESTRIOL
DEFINE RESIDUAL
ASSIGN RESIDUAL = BIRTHWEIGHT - PREDICTED
```

Multiple Linear Regression

An example of multiple linear regression is presented using viewBabyBloodPressure which can be found in Sample.mdb. The outcome (dependent) variable is systolic blood pressure (SystolicBlood), and the other (independent) variables are birth weight (Birthweight) in ounces and age in days (AgeInDays). .

Linear Regression

Variable	Coefficient	Std Error	F-test	P-Value
AgeInDays	5.888	0.680	74.9229	0.000002
Birthweight	0.126	0.034	13.3770	0.003281
CONSTANT	53.450	4.532	139.1042	0.000000

Correlation Coefficient: r^2=   0.88

Source	df	Sum of Squares	Mean Square	F-statistic
Regression	2	591.036	295.518	48.081
Residuals	13	79.902	6.146	
Total	15	670.938		

Linear Regression with More than One Variable, viewBabyBloodPressure

For each independent variable the following information is provided: the coefficient (i.e., slope), its standard error ("Std Error"), and the F-test value and associated p-value. The interpretation would be that both birth weight and age have statistically significant associations with systolic blood pressure even after controlling for the other variable. The CONSTANT coefficient term is the y intercept.

The regression line is: SBP = 53.450 + 0.126*BWT + 5.888*AGE

A Scatter 3D graph is shown below. We give the graphing engine "A" for effort.

To predict the SBP in an infant who weighs 128 oz and is 3 days old:

> SBP = 53.450 + 0.126*(128) + 5.888*(3)

> SBP = 87.242 mm Hg

r^2 As in the simple linear regression, this is Regression Sum of Squares / Total Sums of Squares. In this example, 591.036/670.938 = 0.88.

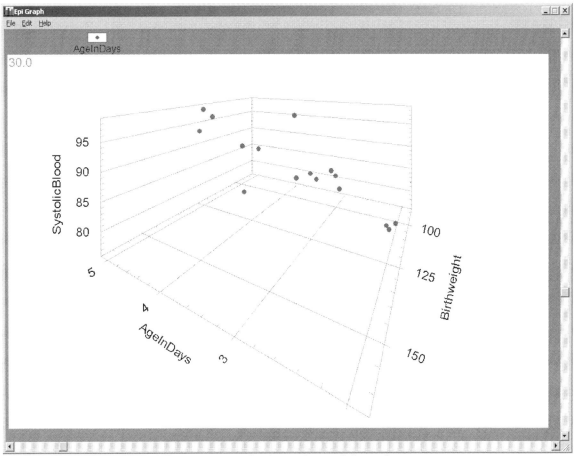

Scatter3D Graph of SBP for Weight and Age

The linear regression dialog box also provides the ability to create dummy variables and interaction terms. Dummy variables are usually used with variables that are ordered categories (such as mild, moderate, and severe) or nominal (such as race/ethnicity). Using the MAKE DUMMY option will create c-1 new variables, where c is the number of categories. Epi Info uses the 1/0 coding approach to creating dummy variables, where the smallest (XXXX Kevin and Minn—Do you mean the FIRST value??) value in the categorical variable will be treated as the comparison group. For additional details on coding dummy variables, please consult a statistical text such as *Applied Regression Analysis and Other Multivariable Models* by Kleinbaum et al.

Logistic Regression

In using Linear Regression above, we quickly ran into unlikely situations by moving too far along the straight line of the regression, babies of zero or negative weight and mothers with crystals of estriol in their veins delivering babies heavier than elephants. Logistic Regression is frequently used in biology, medicine, and public health because it provides an "S" shaped curve that, at the extremes, describes reality better.

When should you use Logistic Regression? First, there must be an Outcome variable with only two values, typically Ill=Y/N, Coronary Heart Disease=Y/N, Deceased=Y/N, etc. If this is not the case, it may be possible to split a study into manageable pieces with binary outcomes, as required for logistic regression. The predictor and/or confounder ("Other") variables can be of various types--text, numeric, or yes/no.

The usual reason for using Logistic Regression is that several predictor variables contribute to the outcome, as is true for age, sex, hypertension, smoking, and cholesterol level as predictors of coronary heart disease risk. It can also produce answers (odds ratios) for systems with only one or two significant predictor variables, such as the Oswego outbreak, where Vanilla ice cream consumption was highly associated with illness, and Chocolate ice cream was somewhat "protective," but the TABLES command is adequate to deal with such situations.

In order to use Logistic Regression, many experts recommend that you first analyze the dataset with simple cross-tabulation (TABLES), stratifying if necessary to control for confounding, and to detect effect modification (interaction) as a difference in odds ratios between strata.

Epi Info can perform either <u>un</u>conditional logistic regression for <u>un</u>matched case-control, cross-sectional, cohort, and randomized clinical trial study designs, or <u>conditional</u> logistic regression for matched case-control study designs (the <u>condition</u> being the match). The outcome variable must be a Yes/No variable or a numeric variable coded as 1/0 where 1 is for those with the outcome of interest and 0 for those not having the outcome of interest. Predictor variables can be Yes/No, have many categories, or be numeric. Hence, logistic regression requires a vary clearly defined binary outcome, but the other variables can be of various types.

Unconditional Logistic Regression

First, let's perform an unconditional logistic regression using the cohort study data viewEvansCounty, the outcome variable is CHD and the primary exposure variable is CAT. Complete the logistic regression dialog box as follows and click on the OK button:

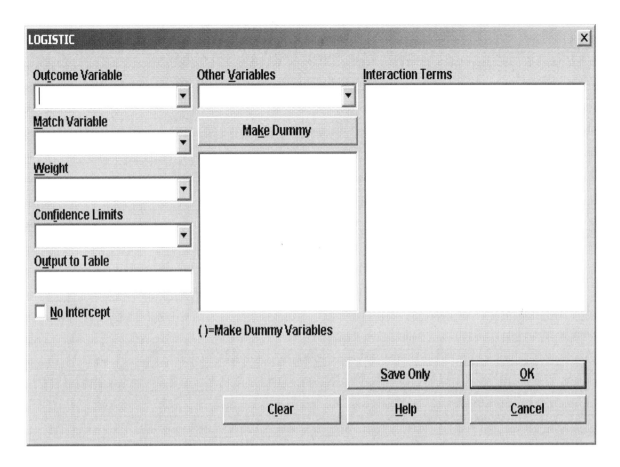

The results for this simple unconditional logistic regression analysis are presented in the next table. The odds ratio could be described as a "crude" odds ratio because the model does not control for any other variables. The crude odds ratio for the CAT→CHD relationship is 2.86 with a 95% CI (1.69, 4.85) and this is a statistically significant association (p<0.001). Note that the odds ratio, confidence interval, and p-values are similar to those calculated using the TABLES command in Figure 15.

Say the investigator wants to assess whether another variable (i.e., a "third" variable) modifies or confounds the CAT→CHD relationship. As an example, use the ECG variable (electrocardiogram results). To determine if ECG modifies the CAT→CHD relationship, we need to create an interaction term which can be done using the dialog box. Using the Logistic Regression dialog box, do the following:

Outcome Variable:	CHD
Other Variables:	CAT
Other Variables:	ECG

Unconditional Logistic Regression

Term	Odds Ratio	95%	C.I.	Coefficient	S. E.	Z-Statistic	P-Value
CAT (Yes/No)	2.8615	1.6878	4.8513	1.0513	0.2693	3.9033	0.0001
CONSTANT	*	*	*	-2.3094	0.1581	-14.6103	0.0000

Convergence:	Converged
Iterations:	5
Final -2*Log-Likelihood:	424.4271
Cases included:	609

Test	Statistic	D.F.	P-Value
Score	16.2465	1	0.0001
Likelihood Ratio	14.1312	1	0.0002

Sample Output for Unconditional Logistic Regression, viewEvansCounty Data,

The variables CAT and ECG should appear in the middle of the dialog box; click on each variable to highlight them. Note that after highlighting the two variables, the button above these two variables will change from Make Dummy to Make Interaction. Click on this button and in the right side of the dialog box, below where it says Interaction Terms, you should see CAT*ECG, the interaction term. Click on the OK button and the results are shown in Figure 51. To determine whether or not there is a statistically significant interaction between CAT and ECG, use the P-value for the CAT*ECG interaction term, in this example, p=0.4196, which would lead to the conclusion that there is no statistically significant interaction.

Unconditional Logistic Regression

Term	Odds Ratio	95%	C.I.	Coefficient	S. E.	Z-Statistic	P-Value
CAT (Yes/No)	3.0743	1.4002	6.7502	1.1231	0.4013	2.7988	0.0051
ECG (Yes/No)	1.7278	0.8523	3.5027	0.5469	0.3605	1.5168	0.1293
CAT (Yes/No) * ECG (Yes/No)	0.6276	0.2025	1.9452	-0.4658	0.5771	-0.8071	**0.4196**
CONSTANT	*	*	*	-2.4314	0.1844	-13.1868	0.0000

Convergence:	Converged
Iterations:	5
Final -2*Log-Likelihood:	422.2477
Cases included:	609

Test	Statistic	D.F.	P-Value
Score	18.1738	3	0.0004
Likelihood Ratio	16.3106	3	0.0010

Unconditional Logistic Regression with an Interaction Term, viewEvansCounty data

With no statistically significant interaction, the next question would be whether ECG confounds the CAT→CHD relationship. To determine this, run another model with:

Outcome Variable:	CHD
Other Variables:	CAT
Other Variables:	ECG

This time, do not create an interaction term; press the OK button to run the model. The output from this model is shown below. The odds ratio for CAT is 2.4483; this would be interpreted as the odds ratio for the CAT→CHD association controlling for ECG. The crude odds ratio for the CAT→CHD association was 2.8615 (as presented in Figure 50), and, controlling for ECG, the adjusted OR is 2.4483. Are these values different enough to say that ECG confounds the CAT→CHD association? One approach is to use the following formula; if the crude and adjusted estimates differ by more than some amount, say 5% or 10%, we could conclude that there is important confounding:

$$\frac{\left| \hat{OR}_{crude} - \hat{OR}_{adjusted} \right|}{\hat{OR}_{adjusted}} x100$$

In this example, by applying the formula, we find a value of 18%, and therefore conclude that ECG is an important confounder of the CAT→CHD association in this population.

For predictor variables with more than two levels or categories, by clicking the variable and then the Make Dummy button, Epi Info will create n-1 dummy variables using a 1/0 coding scheme. For example, in the viewEvansCounty data, there is the variable AGE2 which has seven age group levels coded from 1 to 7. To create n-1 (i.e., in this example six) dummy variables, click on the Make Dummy button and age group level 1 will be the comparison category for levels 2-7.

Unconditional Logistic Regression

Term	Odds Ratio	95%	C.I.	Coefficient	S. E.	Z-Statistic	P-Value
CAT (Yes/No)	2.4483	1.3677	4.3828	0.8954	0.2971	3.0139	0.0026
ECG (Yes/No)	1.4393	0.8147	2.5427	0.3641	0.2904	1.2540	0.2098
CONSTANT	*	*	*	-2.3860	0.1723	-13.8455	0.0000

Sample Output for Unconditional Logistic Regression to Assess for Confounding, viewEvansCounty

Conditional (Matched) Logistic Regression

As an example of a conditional logistic regression, which is most frequently used with matched case-control data, READ the viewRely data file in the Sample.mdb project – a description of this data is presented for the MATCH command described earlier in this document. To analyze this data using logistic regression, using the dialog box, enter the following:

Outcome Variable: CASE

MATCH Variables: ID

Other Variables: RELY

The output from this conditional logistic regression model is shown below. The odds ratio, taking into account the matching, is 8.4, indicating a strong association between the use of rely tampons and development of Toxic Shock syndrome. The odds ratio from the conditional logistic regression is similar to those calculated using the MATCH command described previously.

The conditional logistic regression model is useful in that it is possible to assess for interaction and confounding which are not possible using the MATCH command. In conditional logistic regression, you can also have continuous predictor variables, like AGE in years.

LOGISTIC CASE = RELY MATCHVAR = ID

Conditional Logistic Regression

Term	Odds Ratio	95%	C.I.	Coefficient	S. E.	Z-Statistic	P-Value
RELY (Yes/No)	8.3589	1.7589	39.7237	2.1233	0.7952	2.6701	0.0076

Convergence:	Converged
Iterations:	5
Final -2*Log-Likelihood:	29.0544
Cases included:	56

Test	Statistic	D.F.	P-Value
Score	9.5238	1	0.0020
Likelihood Ratio	9.7618	1	0.0018

Conditional (Matched) Logistic Regression, viewRely Data

Logistic Regression with Summary Data using WEIGHT

To show the use of WEIGHT with Logistic Regression, READ viewLASUM in Sample.MDB, choose Logistic Regression, and fill in the dialog as shown.

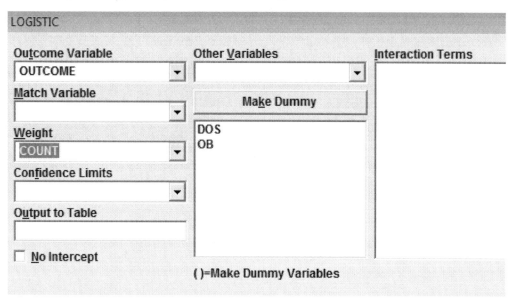

Unconditional Logistic Regression

Term	Odds Ratio	95%	C.I.	Coefficient	S. E.	Z-Statistic	P-Value
DOS	1.9710	1.4763	2.6315	0.6786	0.1475	4.6018	0.0000
OB	1.7396	0.8643	3.5013	0.5537	0.3569	1.5515	0.1208
CONSTANT	*	*	*	-2.5373	0.3697	-6.8622	0.0000

The output shows that the odds ratio is 1.9710 with a very small p-value, suggesting a significant association between OB (Obesity) and disease (endometerial cancer) regardless of Oebesity. If the WEIGHT option had not been used, only 19 observations would have been analyzed, with an incorrect odds ratio and p-value.

The WEIGHT option allows analysis of data that is already in Summary form, with a count variable present. If you begin with data that is in the form of one record per individual, you can produce summary data with a COUNT variable, such as we see in LASUM, by doing a FREQuency and specifying OUTPUT TO TABLE. Hence Epi Info can transform individual data into summary data with OUTPUT TO TABLE, and then treat it as individual data again, using the WEIGHT feature.

WEIGHT variables are also used to adjust records according to their importance in the analysis, for example, if a record represents a large population rather than a small one in a complex or stratified sample. The mechanism is the same--a weight of 2 means that the record has the same effect in the analysis as 2 records of the same type—but weights do not necessarily have to be integers unless they are counts.

References

Kleinbaum DG, Klein M. Logistic Regression: A Self-Learning Text, 2nd Ed. Springer Verlag Publishers, 2002.

Kleinbaum DG, Kupper LL, Morgenstern H. Epidemiologic Research: Principles and Quantitative Methods. John Wiley and Sons Publishers, New York, 1982.

Kleinbaum DG, Kupper LL, Muller KE, Nizam A. Applied Regression Analysis and Multivariable Methods, 3rd Ed. Duxbury Press, 1998.

Kleinbaum DG, Sullivan KM, Barker N. ActivEpi Companion Textbook. Springer Verlag Publishers, 2003.

Rosner B. Fundamentals of Biostatistics, 5th Ed. Duxbury, Pacific Grove, 2000.

An on-line source is: http://faculty.chass.ncsu.edu/garson/PA765/logistic.htm

CHAPTER 13: ANALYSIS OF FOLLOW UP STUDIES

Kaplan-Meier Survival Analysis

The Kaplan-Meier (KM) method is used to analyze studies in which defined events are recorded over time in a series of followup encounters. The event of interest may be "death," but it could also be recurrence of a disease, abandoning medication, or another end point expected of the cohort being followed.

KM methodology estimates the probability of "survival" over a given time period. "Survival" means that the event of interest has not occurred. KM provides an estimate of the probability of being free of the event at time *t*. Conversely, 1.0 *minus* the probability of being free of the event at time *t*" is the probability of *having* the event at time *t*.

What distinguishes survival analysis from most other statistical methods is the presence of "censoring" for incomplete observations. In a study of survival following two different treatment regimens, for example, analysis of the trial typically occurs well before all the patients have died. For those still alive at the time of analysis, the true survival time is known only to be greater than the time observed to date. Such an observation is said to be "censored," a rather odd way to describe ones inability to see into the future.

There are two other sorts of incomplete observation: the "lost to follow-up" (patient missing during the study duration) or the appearance of an event other than the event being studied. These observations are also considered censored. For survival analysis, the censored variable, the time variable, the units of time (day, month, year), and the group of patients (if studying the effect of a treatment) must be specified. The time variable is numeric. The censored variable is coded: "1" if the patient experiences the event (uncensored data), "0" if the event is not known to occur (censored data). (Don't ask about the coding; just do it as Kaplan and Meier specify.)

Survival data is often presented using a "+" for the censored observation, so that a set of times might be 8, 11+, 14, 2, 36+, etc.

Coding of Censored Variable for 6 Patients with Bladder Cancer

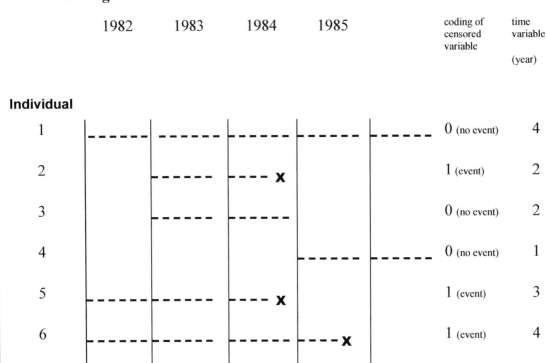

The censored variable has the value of "0" for individuals 1, 3, and 4, and "1" for individuals 2, 5, and 6, who experienced event X.

Dialog box for Kaplan-Meier Survival

The Censored Variable is the variable that contains information as to whether or not an individual developed an event during the study, and Value for Uncensored is the code identifying those who developed the event (think of Value for Uncensored as Value for Event Occurred). The Time Variable is the follow-up time for each individual until an event (success/failure) occurred or, for subjects who did not develop the outcome, i.e., "censored", the amount of follow-up time.

The Time Unit is optional and allows the user to specify the unit of follow-up time, such as hours, days, weeks, months, or years. A Group Variable must be provided and must be categorical (1 or more categories). Graph Type is optional with a default setting of a Survival Probability plot – the other two graph options are None and Log-Log Survival.

As an example, let's perform a Kaplan-Meier Survival analysis using a dataset from a clinical trial of leukemia patients, named Anderson (for MD Anderson Cancer Hospital) in Sample.mdb. Note that there is no View for this data table—you must click ALL under File Type in the READ dialog to see it.

Fill in the Kaplan-Meier dialog box as follows and click the OK button.

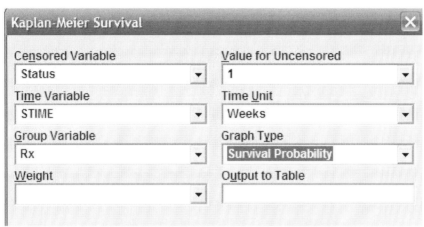

Kaplan Meier Survival Command Dialog

(For the treatment group Rx=0 for the placebo group, Rx=1.)

The results are shown below. The Kaplan-Meier Survival curves are a visual comparison between treatment (Rx=0, for reasons known only to the Anderson group) and placebo Rx=1) groups. A small table at the bottom provides information on two statistical tests for comparing the survival curves: the Log-Rank test and Wilcoxon test. Based on the small p-values in this example, we would conclude that the treatment and placebo groups have statistically significant different survival curves with the treated group (Rx = 0) having a significantly longer survival.

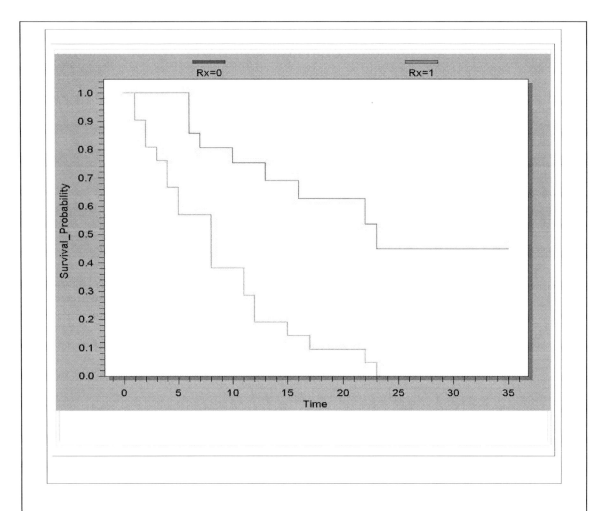

Test	Statistic	D.F.	P-Value
Log-Rank	16.7929	1	0.0
Wilcoxon	13.4579	1	0.0002

Cox Proportional Hazards

The Cox Proportional Hazards model is used with the assumption that predictor variables are time-independent, that is, the values of a given individual do not change during the study (e.g., race, sex, country of origin). The Cox Proportional Hazards model is more powerful than Kaplan-Meier Survival approach in the sense that the Cox Proportional Hazards model not only compares the groups in terms of hazard ratio, but can also assess whether other variables modify or confound the relationship between the main predictor variable and time to event. The dialog box for the Cox Proportional Hazards model is shown below.

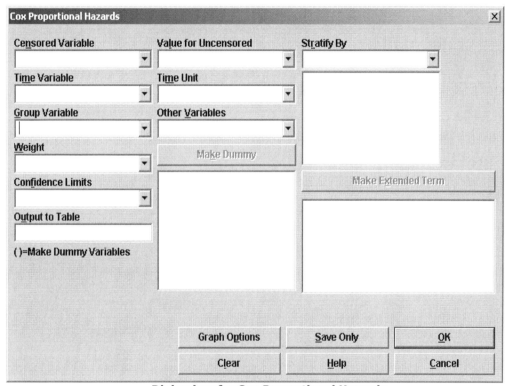

Dialog box for Cox Proportional Hazards

The variable options are more or less the same as the Kaplan-Meier Survival procedure: Censored Variable, Value for Uncensored, Time Variable, Time Unit, and Group Variable. The Graph Options button can be used to hide or display different forms of unadjusted Kaplan-Meier Survival curves in the output screen. The default setting is to plot the survival probability.

Let's perform a simple Cox Proportional Hazards model, again using the Anderson dataset from a clinical trial of leukemia patients to compare the treatment and placebo group survival. Complete the Cox Proportional Hazards dialog box as follows and click on OK button.

Censored Variable	STATUS		Value for Uncensored	1
Time Variable	Stime		Time Unit	Weeks
Group variable	Rx			

The results are shown below. The hazard ratio for placebo vs. treatment group is 4.5231, which is a crude ratio that describes the relationship between the treatment variable (Rx) and time to event without taking into account other variables. The p-value from the Z-statistics is 0.0002, which denotes a significant treatment effect. In conclusion, we can say that the hazard for the placebo group is 4.5 times the hazard for the treatment group. When using the Group variable with a 1/0 coding, the value of 1 is treated as a "Yes" response and a value of 0 is treated as a "No" response. In this example, because the placebo group (Rx = 1) had a poorer survival, it makes sense to code the placebo group as a 1 and the treatment group as a 0 to have a hazard ratio > 1.

Sample output for Cox proportional hazards,.

Cox Proportional Hazards

Term	Hazard Ratio	95%	C.I.	Coefficient	S. E.	Z-Statistic	P-Value
Rx(Yes/No)	4.5231	2.0269	10.0932	1.5092	0.4095	3.6851	0.0002

Convergence:	Converged
Iterations:	4
-2 * Log-Likelihood:	172.7592

Test	Statistic	D.F.	P-Value
Score	15.9305	1	0.0001
Likelihood Ratio	15.2109	1	0.0001

Note: Coding for Rx was 0 for the treatment group and 1 for placebo group; the program treats "0" for the grouping variable as "No" and "1" as "Yes"

Say the investigator wants to assess whether another variable (e.g., a "third" variable) modifies or confounds the relationship between the Group variable and time to event. As an example, let's use the log_wbc (log-value of white blood cell counts) as a third variable. To determine if log_wbc modifies the treatment effect (Rx), we need to create an interaction term (Rx_logwbc) by using the DEFINE and ASSIGN commands. First, DEFINE the Rx_logwbc variable, then ASSIGN it the following value: Rx_logwbc=Rx*log_wbc. This is a little more tedious than creating an interaction term in logistic regression where one can get it directly from the Logistic Regression dialog box.

Complete the Cox proportional hazards dialog box as follows and click on OK button.

Censored Variable	**STATUS**	**Value for Uncensored 1**	
Time Variable	**Stime**	**Time Unit**	**Weeks**
Group Variable	**Rx**	**Other Variables Log_wbc, Rx_logwbc**	

The results are shown the figure below To determine whether or not there is a statistically significant interaction between Rx and Log_wbc, use the p-value for the Rx_logwbc interaction term. In this example, p=0.5103, and thus, it can be concluded that there is no statistically significant interaction.

Sample output for Cox Proportional Hazards model with an interaction term.

Cox Proportional Hazards

Term	Hazard Ratio	95%	C.I.	Coefficient	S. E.	Z-Statistic	P-Value
Rx(Yes/No)	10.5375	0.3907	284.1802	2.3549	1.681	1.4009	0.1612
log_wbc	6.0665	2.5277	14.56	1.8028	0.4467	4.0359	0.0001
rx_logwbc	0.7102	0.2565	1.9668	-0.3422	0.5197	-0.6584	0.5103

Convergence:	Converged
Iterations:	6
-2 * Log-Likelihood:	144.1314

Test	Statistic	D.F.	P-Value
Score	45.9021	3	0.0
Likelihood Ratio	43.8387	3	0.0

Because the interaction term was not significant, we can ask whether Log_wbc confounds the relationship between Rx and time to event. To determine this, run another model without an interaction variable and complete the dialog box as follows:

Censored Variable: STATUS   **Value for Uncensored:1**
Time Variable: Stime   **Time Unit: Weeks**
Group Variable: Rx   **Other Variables: Log_wbc**

The output from this model is shown below.

Cox Proportional Hazards

Term	Hazard Ratio	95%	C.I.	Coefficient	S. E.	Z-Statistic	P-Value
Rx(Yes/No)	3.6476	1.5948	8.3426	1.2941	0.4221	3.0658	0.0022
log_wbc	4.9746	2.6088	9.4859	1.6043	0.3293	4.8716	0.0

Convergence:	Converged
Iterations:	5
-2 * Log-Likelihood:	144.5585

Test	Statistic	D.F.	P-Value
Score	42.9382	2	0.0
Likelihood Ratio	43.4116	2	0.0

Sample output for Cox proportional hazards model to assess for confounding.

The hazard for the placebo group is 3.65 times the hazard for the treatment group, adjusting for Log_wbc. This is 24% higher than the crude hazard ratio of 4.5231. It can be concluded that log_wbc is an important confounder of the treatment effect (Rx) in the study population.

Stratification in the Cox proportional hazards model

The Cox proportional hazards model is frequently used with the assumption that the predictor variable is time-independent, that is, that the values for a given individual do not change while under study. However, when the Cox proportional hazards (PH) assumption is not met because of changing values of predictor variables, one must perform either a stratified Cox PH analysis or extended Cox model approach. We will focus on the stratified Cox PH approach.

As a general rule, before performing a Cox PH analysis, one must check whether PH assumptions are met. ("Survival Analysis: A Self Learning Text" by Kleinbaum).

There are basically three approaches in checking the PH assumption:

1. The graphical approach (presence of nonparallelism of the log-log curves of the variable of interest)

2. Creating a time-dependent variable (converting a predictor variable into a time-dependent variable by means of creating a product term with a function of time).

3. A goodness of fit test (not available in Epi Info)

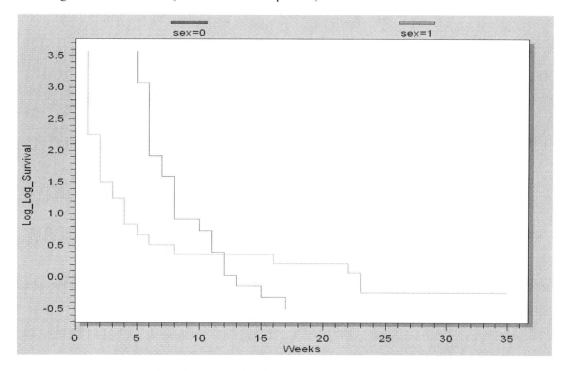

Log-log Kaplan-Meier Survival curves, Anderson Data

Here we will use the graphical approach using the Anderson dataset in Sample.mdb. As shown in the graph, the Log-Log KM curves of sex cross each other, a violation of the Cox PH assumption. Use the Kaplan-Meier Survival curves procedure described earlier and select the Log-Log KM curve. Note that Log-Log curves of Rx and log_wbc showed no strong evidence of non-parallelism (figures not shown), thus, these variables meet the proportional hazards model assumption.

The Cox PH assumption is not met for Sex in the above model because of strong evidence of nonparallelism. Therefore, in this example, stratified Cox PH analysis should be performed where the predictor variables Rx and/or Log_wbc (which meets the PH assumption) can be placed in the Cox PH model statement when stratified on the Sex variable.

Stratification in the Cox PH models is conceptually similar to stratification in the TABLES command where, when you stratify ing on a variable produces an adjusted summary estimate for the predictor variable, i.e., the adjusted hazard ratio, controlling for the stratified variable. This adjusted hazard ratio is compared to a Cox PH model without a stratification variable where the crude hazard ratio is estimated. If there is a significant difference between the adjusted and crude hazard ratios, then confounding may be present.

Dialog box for Cox Proportional Hazards, stratified by sex, Anderson data

Let's continue the stratified Cox PH analysis using the Anderson dataset. We must first assess whether sex confounds the relation between Rx and survival time. Complete the Cox PH dialog box as shown above and click the OK button.

The results are shown below. The adjusted hazard ratio of placebo against drug treatment is 3.5469, controlling for sex. The crude hazard ratio of placebo against drug (not controlling

for sex) is 4.5231 as seen in Figure 77. Using the same formula for assessing the confounding effect at 5-10% cut point as in logistic regression, the crude hazard ratio is 28% higher than the adjusted hazard ratio. Therefore, sex is an important confounder of the treatment effect (Rx) and should be included in the modeling strategy when describing a treatment outcome.

COXPH STIME = (Rx) * Status (1) TIMEUNIT="Weeks" STRATAVAR=sex							
Cox Proportional Hazards							
Term	**Hazard Ratio**	**95%**	**C.I.**	**Coefficient**	**S. E.**	**Z-Statistic**	**P-Value**
Rx(Yes/No)	3.5469	1.5085	8.3397	1.2661	0.4362	2.9024	0.0037

Convergence:	Converged
Iterations:	4
-2 * Log-Likelihood:	135.8371

Test	Statistic	D.F.	P-Value
Score	9.1471	1	0.0025
Likelihood Ratio	9.2823	1	0.0023

Output of Adjusted Hazard Ratio from Stratified Cox PH Model after Controlling for Sex,

	COXPH STIME = (Rx) * Status (1) TIMEUNIT="Weeks"						
		Cox Proportional Hazards					
Term	**Hazard Ratio**	**95%**	**C.I.**	**Coefficient**	**S. E.**	**Z-Statistic**	**P-Value**
Rx(Yes/No)	4.5231	2.0269	10.0932	1.5092	0.4095	3.6851	0.0002

Convergence:	Converged
Iterations:	4
-2 * Log-Likelihood:	172.7592

Test	**Statistic**	**D.F.**	**P-Value**
Score	15.9305	1	0.0001
Likelihood Ratio	15.2109	1	0.0001

Output of Crude Hazard Ratio from Cox PH Model

Note that the stratified Cox PH analysis assumes no interaction between the stratified variable and main predictor of interest, that is, it assumes the hazard ratios of the main predictor are the same across all covariate strata. You can assess interaction terms in the Cox model as well as perform an extended Cox model analysis that takes into account several time-dependent variables. These types of advanced analyses are beyond the scope of this module, and readers are encouraged to refer to textbooks, such as Survival Analysis: A Self-Learning Text by David Kleinbaum, Springer Verlag Publishers, 1996.

CHAPTER 14: ANALYZING COMPLEX SAMPLE SURVEYS

Adapted from Chapter 14 of the Epi Info for DOS Manual, written by William Kalsbeek, PhD, University of North Carolina at Chapel Hill, and Ralph Frerichs, DVM, DrPH, Department of Epidemiology, University of California, Los Angeles (UCLA)

The FREQ, TABLES, and MEANS commands in Epi Info perform statistical calculations assuming the data were collected using simple random sampling (SRS) or unbiased systematic sampling. In many surveys, more complicated sampling strategies, like stratification, cluster sampling, and the use of unequal sampling fractions, are used. Data from such complex sample designs should be analyzed with methods that account for the sampling design, and ANALYSIS provides three commands to analyze complex sample design data. These are Complex Sample Frequencies, Complex Sample TABLES, and Complex Sample MEANS.

Generally, in complex sample analysis, there is a variable for the primary sampling unit (PSU) or Cluster from which a sample subject was selected. If the PSUs were chosen from different Strata (e.g., states or counties), and there may be a stratification variable (Stratify by). The concept of sample stratification in complex sample designs differs from the concept of stratification during epidemiologic analysis using the TABLES command, as the Strata are chosen in the sampling process before analysis. If there are unequal selection probabilities, In addition, a weight variable (Weight) is used when sampling strategies result in unequal selection probabilities. The complex sample commands in Epi Info can compute proportions or means with standard errors and confidence limits. If a 2x2 table is requested, the odds ratio, risk ratio, and risk difference are provided.

Sampling Concepts and Terminology

Calculations for Complex Samples in Epi Info assume that the individual records are members of a sample in which random (or complete or unbiased systematic) sampling has been used in some part of the design. There are three other basic features of sample design that might be used and that must be accounted for in analysis: *cluster sampling, stratification,* and *unequal sampling rates.* When none of these features is used, methods for simple random samples (FREQ, TABLES, and MEANS in ANALYSIS) are appropriate.

Before discussing the three complicating features of sampling designs more fully, it is necessary to define a few basic concepts related to samples and sampling. A sample is chosen to represent a larger universe called the sample's *target population.* This population consists of individuals called *members* who are the object of study. The data items gathered for the study describe these population members, although data gathering may not involve them directly (e.g., when data is abstracted from medical records).

A sample of population members is chosen from one or more lists called the *sampling frame* whose individual entries are called *sampling units.* In list samples (e.g., a sample chosen for a physician survey from a list of physicians), the population members and sampling units are the same, but in other samples this is not necessarily the case (a list of households for a survey of individuals). Simple random sampling is a form of list sampling in which selections are made at random and with equal probability from a complete population frame. Simple random selection can be done *with replacement,* meaning that a member can be chosen again once it is selected the first time, or it can be done *without replacement,* in which case a selected member is not allowed to be chosen again. The calculations in CSAMPLE assume that random sampling has been done *with replacement.* If the sample is a small fraction of the population, the assumption of sampling with replacement may be made for practical purposes, as described below, even if this was not the original sampling method.

Stratification

Stratification is a common feature in sampling designs. In sampling terminology, stratification means that the frame is subdivided into mutually exclusive and complete (exhaustive) groups called strata and that samples are chosen separately from each stratum. This use of the word "stratum" should be clearly distinguished from "stratification" during data analysis--the process that occurs when you add a third dimension to a TABLES command in ANALYSIS and a separate table is made for each stratum. In sampling the strata are determined prior to data collection; in epidemiology, data are generally stratified after data collection.

Sample stratification is commonly used in list sampling, with simple random sampling being the selection method within each stratum. The result is what is called a stratified simple random sample. Stratification is also often used in conjunction with cluster sampling. In general stratification tends to reduce the variance (narrow the confidence limits), at least partially offsetting the opposite effect of cluster sampling. While, in principle, stratification can be used in each stage of a multi-stage cluster sample, it is most commonly used for the first stage of selection. Stratification for choosing Primary Sampling Units (PSUs) is called primary stratification, and is described below.

Cluster Sampling

A sampling design is said to involve *cluster sampling* if at some point in the selection process the sampling units consist of one or more mutually exclusive groups, called clusters. The clusters used for survey sampling are typically spatial (e.g., a sample of residential households that is obtained by selecting counties or villages), organizational (e.g., a sample of students that is identified by sampling schools), or temporal (e.g., a sample of patients visiting a health clinic chosen by sampling days the clinic is open).

The Expanded Program in Immunization (EPI) coverage surveys are cluster surveys. All villages and cities (i.e., clusters) are listed, and then a sample of villages and cities is selected for the survey.

The clusters in real populations rarely have the same number of members and may vary greatly in size. Cluster sampling is often done in more than one step or stage of selection. This type of design produces what is called a multi-stage cluster sample. To do so requires the existence of a hierarchical configuration of clusters, so that the clusters at any given stage consist of members or clusters in the subsequent stage(s). For example, a three-stage sample of households in the U.S. might be chosen by designating counties to be the sampling units in the first stage (called primary sampling units, or PSU's), by assigning block groups to be the second stage sampling units for sampling within each PSU, and by designating households to be chosen separately within selected block groups as the third stage.

Cluster sampling usually increases the variance (widens confidence intervals) of survey estimates. This happens because members of the same cluster tend to be more alike than the population as a whole. Members of a sample from the same cluster therefore tend to provide less information about the population than do members from different clusters. This reduction in information from a clustered sample translates into estimates that are likely to be less precise than estimates obtained using simple random sampling.

Primary sampling units (PSU's) are the units chosen from a list in the first (upper) stage of sampling that involves choosing clusters. For example:

Stage	List Used	Sampling Method
One	Regions	Stratification
Two	States	Random within region
Three	Counties	Random within state
Four	Census Tract	Random within county
Five	Block	Random within census tract
Six	Household	Random within block
Seven	Person	Random within household

Stage two contains the Primary Sampling Units--the "clusters" at the first stage where clusters are randomly chosen. Each record must contain an identifier for the state from which it came. The file may contain identifiers for each of the other levels as well, but those below stage two will not be used by the Complex Sample commands. They may be necessary for the calculation of weights prior to running the analysis, however.

Unequal Selection Probabilities

The third feature that complicates a sampling design is having unequal selection probabilities for population members. This happens when the ratio of sample to population size differs for different parts of the sample. In stratified sampling this can happen if the sample sizes are not proportional to the population of the strata. Unequal selection probabilities may be found in cluster samples in a variety of ways (e.g., sampling clusters with unequal probabilities in a one-stage sample, using simple random samples of the same size in both stages of a two-stage design where the clusters vary in size, etc). They also occur during the course of a survey through differing response rates in different areas, and other factors that may be ascertained through the survey itself, such as response rates or household size.

Unequal selection probabilities are accounted for in the analysis of data by computing sample weights for each member of the sample (i.e., record of the dataset). Producing these weights is usually done just prior to analysis. Determining selection probabilities requires that good records be kept for each selection step of the sampling process so that the selection sequence can be explicitly recreated. For multi-stage cluster samples this means knowing the first stage selection probability for the PSU of which the member is a part, the selection probability for the second stage cluster of which the member is a part, and so on up to the selection probability of the member in the final stage cluster. For designs with stratified sampling this implies having separate information for sampling in each stratum (e.g., sampling rates for stratified simple random sampling).

A sample weight for a sample member in its most basic form is simply 1 divided by the member's selection probability. More intuitively, it is the number of population members whom this member represents. The sample weights found in survey data sets are rarely seen in this form, however. They are often adjusted (i.e., multiplied by some appropriate adjustment factor) to compensate for such things as imbalance in the sample due to failure of the frame to fully cover the population (i.e., undercoverage), failure to secure participation from all sample members (i.e., nonresponse), and departures from the demographic composition of the population due to randomized sampling. Users who are interested in more details about weights and adjustments are referred to Lessler and Kalsbeek (1992, Section 8.1). The weights may also be normalized so that they sum to a designated value (e.g., the total sample size), although this is not required by CSAMPLE.

Complex Sample FREQuencies

The table viewEpi1 in Sample.mdb contains an Expanded Program for Immunization (EPI) cluster survey. Using the EPI method, a team selected 30 communities (i.e., clusters) from the chosen geographic area and visited each of the 30 communities. In each, they selected seven children in an appropriate age range and determined each child's immunization (VAC) status.

Choose ANALYZE DATA from the main Epi Info menu, then use the READ command to access the View called EPI1 in SAMPLE.MDB. Complete the dialog box as below and then click the OK button.

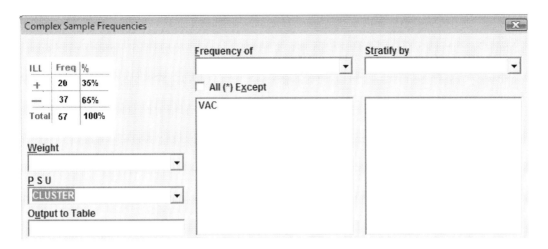

Click OK to receive the output on the next page. If it does not appear, check that the Statistics option in the SET command is set to Advanced, then try again.

	VAC	TOTAL
1		155
	Row %	100.000
	Col %	73.810
	SE %	4.599
	LCL %	64.795
	UCL %	82.824
2		55
	Row %	100.000
	Col %	26.190
	SE %	4.599
	LCL %	17.176

```
                    Sample Design Included:

                    Weight Variable: None
                    PSU Variable: CLUSTER
                    Stratification Variable: None
                    0 records with missing values
```

VAC denotes whether a child is vaccinated or not; 1=Yes and 2=No

Information provided in the output includes:

Row %	**For a frequency will always be 100%**
Col %	**The column percent; in the above example, 73.8% were vaccinated (VAC = 1)**
SE %	**The standard error, which takes into account the complex sample design**
LCL %	**Lower Confidence Limit**
UCL %	**Upper Confidence Limit**
Total	**Total number of individuals/elements surveyed**
Design Effect	**Ratio of variance assuming complex design divided by variance assuming a simple random sample**

Additional information is provided in the paragraph labeled Sample Design Included at the bottom of the output. In these results, 73.8% (155/210) of the children were VACcinated with 95% confidence limits of (64.8%, 82.8%) taking into account the cluster design. Note that had the FREQuencies command been used, ignoring cluster design, the proportion immunized would also be 73.8% but the confidence interval would be too narrow (67.3%, 79.6%).

As another example using the Complex Sample FREQuencies, READ the viewEpi10 file in Sample.mdb. These data are similar to viewEpi1 except that this is a stratified cluster survey with a separate 30-cluster survey completed in each of 10 strata . As in viewEpi1, there is a variable for whether or not a child is vaccinated (VAC,1=yes,2=no). To correctly analyze this dataset, we need to take into account the Stratum variable (LOCATION) where each child lives (LOCATION). The population sizes of the 10 LOCATIONS are different, meaning that each subjects in different LOCATIONS represent different numbers of people. To account for differences in population sizes between strata therefore, there is a Weight variable called POPW.

Complete the dialog box as follows to see the results are presented below.

Frequency of : VAC ; Stratify by: LOCATION ; Weight: POPW; PSU: CLUSTER

A second example of output from Complex Sample FREQuencies, viewEpi10 file, Epi Info.

VAC	TOTAL
1	1242
Row %	100.000
Col %	55.263
SE %	2.620
LCL %	50.128
UCL %	60.398
2	910
Row %	100.000
Col %	44.737
SE %	2.620
LCL %	39.602
UCL %	49.872
TOTAL	2152
Design Effect	5.98

Weight Variable: POPW
PSU Variable: CLUSTER
Stratification Variable: LOCATION

The overall estimate of the percentage of children vaccinated is 55.3% with 95% confidence limits (50.1%, 60.4%) taking into account stratification, the cluster design, and population weights.

Complex Sample TABLES

The Complex Sample TABLES command is similar to the TABLES command in that you specify an Exposure Variable and an Outcome Variable. Using the viewEpi10 data, let's analyze the data using whether or not the mother received prenatal care (PRENATAL) as the Exposure Variable and, for the Outcome Variable, the child's vaccination status (VAC). If the mother had received prenatal care, PRENATAL=1 else PRENATAL=2. The dialog box should be completed as follows:

- **Outcome Variable**   **VAC**
- **Stratify by**   **LOCATION**
- **Exposure Variable**   **PRENATAL**
- **Weight**   **POPW**
- **PSU**   **CLUSTER**

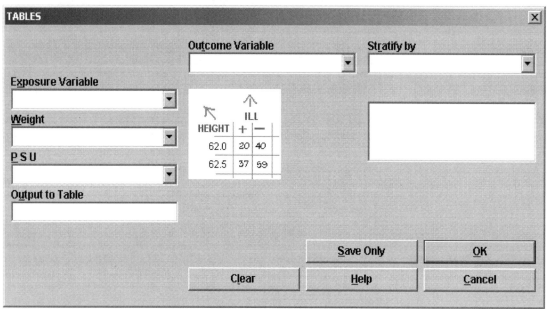

Dialog box for Complex Sample Table

Note the inconsistency between the command name Complex Sample Table and the dialog box name TABLES.

Here is the second part of the results:

CTABLES COMPLEX SAMPLE DESIGN ANALYSIS OF 2 X 2 TABLE

Odds Ratio (OR) 2.088
Standard Error (SE) 0.307
95% Conf. Limits (1.50, 2.901)

Risk Ratio (RR) 1.427
Standard Error (SE) 0.110
95% Conf. Limits (1.23, 1.660)
RR = (Risk of VAC=1 if PRENATAL=1) / (Risk of VAC=1 if PRENATAL=2)

Risk Difference (RD%) 18.174
Standard Error (SE%) 4.021

95% Conf. Limits (10.26, 26.089)
RD = (Risk of VAC=1 if PRENATAL=1) - (Risk of VAC=1 if PRENATAL=2)

Sample Design Included:

Weight Variable: POPW

PSU Variable: CLUSTER

Stratification Variable: LOCATION

records with missing values: 0

The results may appear similar to the output for the Complex Sample FREQuencies command, but there are some important differences. First, with the goal of assessing whether or not children whose mother had received prenatal care were more or less likely to be immunized compared to those with mothers who had not received prenatal care, the important proportions are the Row% in the first column. Among children whose mothers had received prenatal care, 60.7% were immunized compared to 42.3% among those whose mothers did not receive prenatal care. The confidence limits (LCL and UCL) are for the Row% values.

Estimates of the odds ratio, risk ratio, and risk difference are provided for 2x2 tables. In order to assure that these parameters are estimated correctly, the table setup must be the same as described for the TABLES command (i.e., exposure as the row variable and outcome as the column variable.). Note that complex sample designs are most frequently applied to cross-sectional data and that cross-sectional surveys usually estimate "prevalence" or "coverage", not risk. Therefore, in many situations the correct names for the epidemiologic parameters would be the prevalence odds ratio, the prevalence ratio, and the prevalence difference.

The prevalence odds ratio in the sample data below is 2.088, the prevalence ratio is 1.427, and the prevalence difference is 18.2%. The prevalence ratio says that 1.427 times as many children of women who received prenatal care were immunized (60.734% /42.560% = 1.427) compared to children born to women who had not received prenatal care, a 40% difference.

CTABLES COMPLEX SAMPLE DESIGN ANALYSIS OF 2 X 2 TABLE

Odds Ratio (OR) 2.088
Standard Error (SE) 0.307
95% Conf. Limits (1.50, 2.901)

Risk Ratio (RR) 1.427
Standard Error (SE) 0.110
95% Conf. Limits (1.23, 1.660)
RR = (Risk of VAC=1 if PRENATAL=1) / (Risk of VAC=1 if PRENATAL=2)

Risk Difference (RD%) 18.174

Standard Error (SE%) 4.021
95% Conf. Limits (10.26, 26.089)
RD = (Risk of VAC=1 if PRENATAL=1) - (Risk of VAC=1 if PRENATAL=2)

Sample Design Included:
Weight Variable: POPW
PSU Variable: CLUSTER
Stratification Variable: LOCATION

A random digit telephone sample might be selected as follows. Clusters of telephone numbers are defined, with each cluster consisting of numbers with the same first eight digits of a 10-digit telephone number. Separately for each county, a with-replacement sample of clusters is randomly chosen with probabilities that are proportional to the size (PPS) of (i.e., number of residential telephone numbers in) the cluster. Next, a random sample of three participating households is selected within each selected cluster. Finally, an interview is completed with one adult who is chosen at random within each participating households. This design produces a stratified three-stage sample, with clusters of telephone numbers as PSUs, primary stratification by county, residential telephone numbers as second stage clusters, and member adults as sampling units in the third stage. While this design would produce an equal-probability sample of residential telephone numbers, the final sample of adults would have unequal selection probabilities (and therefore require sample weights) since the number of adults and the number of telephone numbers that can be dialed to reach the households varies among households.

Stage	List Used	Sampling Method
One	8-digit clusters by county	Random PPS within 8-digit clusters, stratified by county
Two	Clusters from stage one	3-random households per cluster
Three	Households from stage two	One random adult per participating household

A record would be created for each adult interviewed in stage three. Primary sampling units in this case are identified as 8-digit clusters. Stratification is by COUNTY.

WEIGHTS would be determined by the number of adults in each household interviewed, the simplest method being to use the number of adults in the household as the weight. If one household contained 100 adults, the interview in that household would be weighted as 100 in comparison with an interview with a single-adult household (weight 1). If participation rates differed among counties, additional weighting would be done to compensate for this--a county with 90% participation would have a weight of 100/90 in comparison with a county with 70% participation having a weight of 100/70. A household with two telephones has twice the chance of being selected and would have a weight of 0.5 in comparison with a one-telephone household.

Complex Sample Means

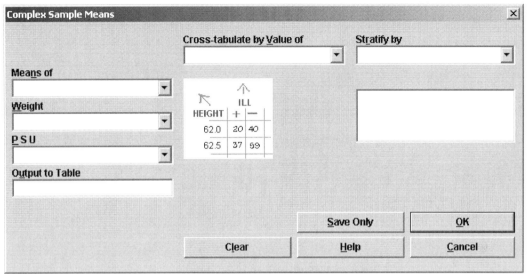

Dialog for Complex Sample Means

The Complex Sample Means command can be used when the outcome variable is continuous, such as age, cholesterol level, etc. You can either calculate an overall mean with it's measures of variation or compare means across a grouping variable.

As an example of computing an overall mean, use the viewSmoke data file located in Sample.mdb. This is a stratified three-stage cluster survey with the need to apply sample weights. To calculate the average number of cigarettes smoked among those who reported smoking, complete the dialog box with the following values:

- Means of   NUMCIGAR

- Stratify by   STRATA

- Weight   SAMPW

- PSU   PSUID

The result below is that among the 82 individuals who smoked cigarettes, the average number of cigarettes smoked per day was 17.3 with 95% confidence limits of 15.4 and 19.2 cigarettes per day. Note that the viewSmoke file has 337 individuals. However, the number of cigarettes smoked per day (NUMCIGAR) was asked only of the 82 smokers; for nonsmokers this variable was left blank and therefore is treated as missing data and excluded from analysis.

	Count	Mean	Std Error	Confidence Limits		Minimum	Maximum
				Lower	Upper		
TOTAL	82	17.256	0.972	15.391	19.193	2.000	40.000

Sample Design Included

Weight Variable: SAMPW
PSU Variable: PSUID
Stratification Variable: STRATA

records with missing values= 0

Complex Sample MEANS, Calculation of an Overall Mean, viewSmoke Data

As an example of calculating means with a grouping variable, again use the viewSmoke data file. In this example, the investigator is interested in determining if, among smokers, there is a difference in the average number of cigarettes smoked between males and females. In these data, the variable SEX is coded as 1=male and 2=female.

Complete the dialog box as follows:

Means of	NUMCIGAR
Cross-tabulate by Value of	SEX
Stratify by	STRATA
Weight	SAMPW
PSU	PSUID

The results of this analysis are shown below. Males smoked, on average, 18.7 cigarettes per day compared to 16.1 cigarettes in females. The difference is 2.6 cigarettes per day, with 95% confidence limits of −1.1 and 6.4. Because the confidence interval includes the null value of zero, one could reasonably conclude that there does not appear to be a statistically significant difference in the average number of cigarettes smoked per day between males and females in these data.

SEX	Count	Mean	Std Error	Confidence Limits		Minimum	Maximum
				Lower	Upper		
1	36	18.722	1.577	15.631	21.814	2.000	40.000
2	46	16.109	1.167	13.822	18.395	2.000	40.000
TOTAL	82	17.256	0.972	15.351	19.161	2.000	40.000
Difference		2.614	1.950	-1.208	6.435		

Sample Design Included

Weight Variable: SAMPW
PSU Variable: PSUID
Stratification Variable: STRATA
records with missing values: 0

Sample output for Complex Sample MEANS, Calculation of Means for Males and Females, viewSmoke Data

CHAPTER 15: OPENEPI—STATISTICS FOR SUMMARY DATA

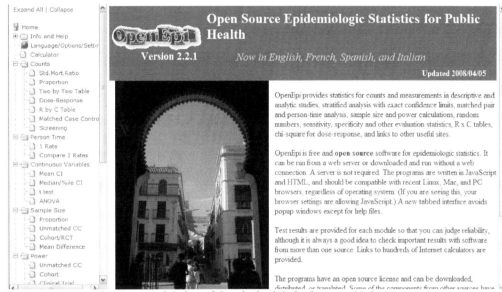

The OpenEpi Suite of Statistical Calculators--Main Menu

Introduction

Statcalc is a pre-Microsoft Windows utility that is still supplied with Epi Info on the UTILITIES menu. It provides interactive calculations for summary table data, dose-response and sample-size calculations. Although Statcalc is still useful, OpenEpi performs the same calculations and many more, comes with a complete set of exercises and documentation, and provides links to many more epidemiologic and statistical resources on the Internet. In this chapter we will focus on finding and using the resources in OpenEpi.

Let's assume that you are either using OpenEpi directly from its website (www.openepi.com) or that you have installed it on your computer using the instructions in the previous chapter on installing Epi Info and OpenEpi, and that you are looking at the OpenEpi main screen, shown above. We will hit some of the high points of resources available.

Information Resources

Click to expand the INFO AND HELP option on the menu and explore the resources available, including instructions for USING OPENEPI, a guide to types of statistical methods for different data and study types, and NEWS about the current version. Click on the METHODS guide to explore the many types of statistical methods, and their use. Not all are found in Epi Info or OpenEpi, but Internet searches can reveal software for many of the others. Near the bottom of the menu under NET LINKS, you can click on LOTS OF STAT PAGES to gain access to hundreds of other resources.

Near the center of the menu list under SEARCH are two very useful links to search sites for Google and to PubMed, a portal to the US National Library of Medicine's search engine. You may have your own favorite search sites; these are placed here for convenience, and can be replaced with others if you install OpenEpi on your computer and edit the OpenEpi.MNU file.

Exploring A Statistical Module

Click on the TWO BY TWO TABLE entry in the menu to show the Start page for this module. Then click the button called LOAD DEMO DATA to see a table populated with sample data. There are two strata that can be seen by choosing in the control box at the top of the page. To see results, click the CALCULATE button or the RESULTS tab at the top. Now return to the START tab (for OpenEpi, not Windows), and try the ENTER NEW DATA, entering you own numbers in the four cells of the table, and choosing CALCULATE to see results.

Return to the Start page again, and click on DOCUMENTATION at the top of the page. Here is the place to read about the statistical background of the module, and to see the equations behind the calculations. Each of the modules has a document of this kind.

Go back to top of the Start page for TWO BY TWO again and click EXERCISES to see several practice scenarios with data to enter in TWO BY TWO. These are useful both for learning the module, and also for classroom use in teaching others. Since the EXERCISES are automatically translated into the language chosen in LANGUAGE AND SETTINGS, they can be printed in English, Spanish, French, or Italian.

Saving Results

OpenEpi presents the results in the browser as HTML. You may want to copy the results window to a word processor, such as Microsoft Word or OpenOffice Writer, or print the contents of the window. Printing is relatively easy, just use the print function of the browser. To copy and paste results from the browser screen, first, "select" the data, that is, move the mouse to the top of the results that you want to copy, hold the left button and move the mouse to the bottom of the output you wish to copy. To copy the data, you can press the control key ("Ctrl") and the "c" key ("c") simultaneously, e.g., Ctrl+C. This will copy the data to the clipboard. (Note: an alternative method is after you have selected the data, from the Internet Explorer (or other browser) menu, click on Edit and then Copy, or right click in the highlighted area and a small menu should appear and click on Copy.) Next, open the word processor, place the cursor where you want to paste the data, and press Ctrl+V (or, alternatively, from the word processing menu Edit and then Paste). Once in the word processor you can change font sizes and make other modifications in the results.

For those who have installed OpenEpi onto their computer using OpenEpi.MSI (and are therefore using Windows), one of the icons labeled "OpenEpi SAVE". By clicking on this icon to run

OpenEpi all of the output will automatically be saved as HTM files in the folder …
OpenEpi\RESULTS.

Language and Settings

Click on the LANGUAGE AND SETTINGS entry in the OpenEpi menu.

Language: As of this writing, the languages supported by OpenEpi are English, French, Italian, and Spanish, with a Portuguese translation in progress. As languages are added, they will be added to the **Select Language** pull down menu on the LANGUAGE AND SETTINGS screen. To choose a language, first select it in the drop-down box and then place the cursor after the OpenEpi address in the browser address space and press Enter. The other option is to hold down the shift key and click the Refresh button at the top of the browser.

Settings for a 2 x 2 Input Table: This option allows the user to specify whether disease forms the columns and exposure the rows, or vice versa. It also allows the user to specify the order of those with the event, i.e. "(+)", or without the event, i.e. "(-). Different textbooks and different software programs may have different ways in which a 2 x 2 table is presented. Settings for couple of common textbooks can be chosen by clicking one of the choices, effectively rotating the table so that Disease and Exposed are exchanged. If you have another combination in mind, finer choices can be made for the columns and rows.

There are eight possible ways to orient a 2 x 2 table, and it seems probable that somewhere there is an epidemiologist who prefers each one. OpenEpi is ready for this rugged individualist. For a given definition of disease and exposure, only one of these tables will provide the correct risk ratio and risk different estimates.

Confidence level for confidence intervals: Ninety five percent confidence intervals are the default, but users can select from a list of levels. The output in the Results screen will specify the confidence level.

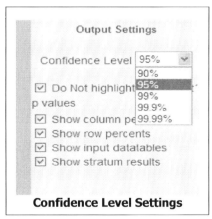

Confidence Level Settings

Do Not highlight "significant" p-values: If this box is checked, all p-values and confidence intervals are presented in a black font. If this box is ***not*** checked, p-values <0.05 and confidence intervals that do not capture the null value are presented in a blue font – all others will be in a black font. There will also be the following message in the output:

P-values < 0.05 and confidence limits excluding null values (0,1, or [n]) are highlighted.

Show column percents, row percents, input tables, stratum results: This option applies to the Two x Two Tables and Compare Two Rates modules. At this time it appears that the Show input datatables and Show stratum results are always on, that is, the data tables and stratum results are also presented in the results.

Note: The settings are saved in a browser cookie. This works with most browsers, but the Google Chrome browser refuses to save or read cookies when the OpenEpi files are on a local hard disk rather than on a server. Hence, we recommend that you use other browsers if OpenEpi has been dowloaded and installed. Perhaps this will change with future versions of the Chrome browser.

Using OpenEpi on PDA's and Cell Phones

OpenEpi works on some PDA's and cell phones, although OpenEpi was not developed with small screens in mind. Whether OpenEpi will work on a PDA or cell phone depends on the extent to which the browser can run JavaScript. We have been able to use OpenEpi on an iPhone. Open the browser and go the www.OpenEpi.com and determine whether you can see both the menu and the main screen. Some browsers seem to have problems showing both the menu and main screen. In this case,, it is possible to avoid the OpenEpi menu system and to go directly to each module. The web site address for each separate module can be found by moving the cursor to "hover"on a menu link. The address of the linked program should appear in the browser line at the bottom of the screen. There are also some similar modules and other programs at www.sph.emory.edu/~cdckms. A future version of OpenEpi will have a simpler menu more suitable for handheld devices.

Links to Other Sites

The menu offers some useful epidemiologic tools in the form of links to other sites. Both Google and MEDLARS searches are found here, althoug, of course, you may have your own search facility for MEDLARS. The other sites are a collection of those useful in epidemiology and computing, and they offer hundreds of links to other such sites.

The Calculator

The Calculator entry on the menu brings up a calculator with higher math functions. For statistics, this one is somewhat more useful than the simpler calculator that comes with Microsoft Windows.

CHAPTER 16: RELATING RECORDS IN A HIERARCHY—PATIENTS AND VISITS

In a questionnaire View, each set of entries—whether one page or many—creates one record in the data table. The record corresponds to one instance of whatever the questionnaire or form represents, whether it is a person, a visit, an interview, a health provider, a case report, a hospital or clinic record, a medication order, a laboratory test, a surgical instrument tray, or an entire hospital.

A data system often needs more than one View to represent different entities that are related to one another. Clinical records, whether paper based or electronic, usually contain a single "face sheet" record for each patient, giving name, address, date of birth, etc., but a patient may have multiple clinic visits, operations, medications, or laboratory tests. These in an Epi Info system are separate Views, with records related to the patient record by numeric (or text) keys.

Epi Info offers methods of creating and linking such different views so that they function as a single data system. In the system to be created here, a Mother record has two related views, for Children and Lab Tests. The views are linked by identifiers created automatically by Epi Info.

Relational file systems created by data managers often consist of many related files, and most public health professionals require the services of programmers to put the pieces back together for analysis. While Epi Info does not remove the need for careful design and understanding of such systems, the RELATE command in the Analysis program allows several Views to be Related (linked) for analysis with minimum difficulty if the automatic key structure of Epi Info is used. Keys that have been set up in other systems can also be used during analysis.

The examples in this chapter, found in the folder exRELATE, of the EXAMPLES, present a data system with mother, child, and laboratory records. Each "mother" has zero to several children and one or more laboratory tests.

Mother's Record

Mother Record Number   000555

Mother Birthdate   11-11-1985

Children   Lab Tests

The Mother View

In the Analysis program, the LIST command displays the following records. Note that the UniqueKey field has been generated automatically and given a unique value for each record.

Mother Record Number	Mother Birthdate	UniqueKey	RecStatus
1	11-11-1980	1	1
2	11-11-1982	2	1
3	11-11-1979	3	1
44	11-11-1990	4	1
555	11-11-1985	5	1

Clicking on the CHILDREN button shows the CHILD view.

Child's Record

Child Name   `Matilda`   Child Birthdate   `01-01-2004`

Child HIV Positive at 18 Months?   `No`

The Child View

During data entry, identification numbers ("keys") are generated automatically behind the scenes and stored in fields with the special names UniqueKey and FKey (for Foreign Key). LISTing the Children's records we have:

Child Name	Child Birthdate	Child HIV Positive at 18 Months?	UniqueKey	RecStatus	FKey
Tom	11-11-2000	No	1	1	1
Mary	11-11-2002	No	2	1	1
Ralph	01-01-2004	Yes	3	1	1
Rene	11-11-2001	No	4	1	2
Leila	01-01-2004	No	5	1	4
Jose	01-01-2003	No	6	1	5
Matilda	01-01-2004	No	7	1	5

As with every Epi Info View, UniqueKey is generated for each record. The important thing to notice here is Fkey, which is the UniqueKey of the corresponding MOTHER record. Tom, Mary, and Ralph all belong to the Mother with UniqueKey 1, and Jose and Matilda to the Mother whose UniqueKey is 5. Ignore the RecStatus field for now; it is used to identify records marked as deleted in the Enter program.

Clicking on the LAB TESTS button navigates to the Lab Test records for this Mother.

Lab Tests

Lab Test Date		Lab HIV Antibody Present?	
	01-01-2003		Yes

The Lab Test View

Again the Fkey field "points" or links back to the corresponding MOTHER UniqueKey. The

Lab Test Date	Lab HIV Antibody Present?	UniqueKey	RecStatus	FKey
11-11-2000	No	1	1	1
11-11-2002	No	2	1	1
11-11-2003	No	3	1	1
01-01-2004	Yes	4	1	1
11-11-2001	No	5	1	2
11-11-2001	No	6	1	3
01-01-2004	Yes	7	1	4
01-01-2003	Yes	8	1	5
02-02-2004	Yes	9	1	5

mother with UniqueKey 1 had four negative HIV tests before having a positive test on 01/01/2004. The mother with UniqueKey 5 had two positive HIV tests.

Epi Info takes care of linking the records so that the three Views behave as a single system, controlled by the Relate buttons CHILDREN and LAB TESTS and the BACK button on the left side of the data entry screen for navigation. The result is very similar to navigating from one linked page to another in an Internet browser.

When Epi Info views are used for related records, the UniqueKey and Fkey system illustrated here is employed during data entry. In many other software systems, however, Key fields are specified when the database is set up, and may consist of, for example, the Mother's Clinic ID number. Almost any unique identifier or combination of identifiers (mother's name and date of birth) could be used as a key to link Mothers and Children, although identifiers that will change (name) or contain mistakes (date of birth) are usually excluded in favor of unique numbers. Using Check Code, such explicit keys can be created during data entry as an alternative to the UniqueKey and FKey system. An optional section at the end of this chapter will show how to do this.

In Analysis, the RELATE command uses the UniqueKey and Fkey if the Views to be related are from Epi Info and no other keys are specified. It is possible, however, to use keys generated in other systems, including those involving more than one field (County, State, and CaseID, for example). Analyzing such data is done in Analysis by specifying the keys needed to RELATE two data tables or Views.

Creating Related Views and Entering Data

(Instructions for setting up Views and Data tables similar to those described above, and contained in RELATED.MDB in the exRelated folder of the book EXAMPLES.)

1. Using the MakeView program, from the FILE menu choose NEW and create a new MDB Project in the exRelated folder in the EXAMPLES for this book, using your initials for the file name--for example, ABC.MDB. Name the View MOTHER (in capital letters to indicate the main View) and create data entry fields for Mother Record Number (of type Number with pattern ######) and Mother Birthdate (a Date type). Of course, a working system would have other details like address and medical history, but we will keep this simple to illustrate principles. It is not necessary to include the word Mother in each field name, but it will make the rest of the exercise easier to follow.

2. Right click on the screen to create the next field and give the prompt as "Children". Then click on the button called RELATED VIEW. In the next dialog, leave the entries as they are, with the View accessible "any time", and click OK. Choose the default value in the next dialog, "Create a New Related View", and click OK. A button will appear on the form with the caption "Children."

3. Move the mouse cursor over the button to see instructions for accessing, moving, editing, and resizing the button. In this case we want to access the new blank View and add some fields. Hold down the control key and left click the button. You should see a blank View similar to the one on which you created the mother's View. Right click to create a field, and make a text field called Child Name. Create additional fields for "Child Birthdate" as a Date field, and "Child HIV Positive at 18 months?" as a Yes/No field. When the form is complete, click on BACK to return to the MOTHER form, agreeing to make the data table when asked.

4. Now repeat the same process to create a button called "Lab Tests" and develop a View that contains fields "Lab Test Date" as a Date and "Lab HIV Antibody Present?" (Yes/No). When you are satisfied with the new View, click the BACK button to return to the MOTHER View, again agreeing to make the data table. EXIT from MakeView (FILE menu| EXIT) to the main Epi Info menu. If asked, agree to make the data table.

5. Let's enter some data! Use the values shown in the paragraphs above, but ignore the field UniqueKey, Fkey, and RecStatus. Click ENTER DATA on the main Epi Info menu. Choose OPEN from the FILE menu and find the MDB with your initials, and within it, the View called MOTHER. Enter data for the first mother from the tables below, and then click the CHILD button. Now enter the data for her 3 children. After you enter the last field in each record, a new blank record appears. Click the BACK button on the left panel when you are ready to return to MOTHER record number 1. Click LAB TESTS in the first MOTHER's

record and use the same techniques to enter her 4 laboratory tests. Use the BACK button to return to the Mother's record. Click NEW to enter the second mother. Noting that mother number 3 has a LAB TEST, but no children, enter the rest of the data, using NEW to create new mother's as needed. (We have made it easy to enter the dates by using a lot of 1's for days and months.).

When you have finished, return to the MOTHER View and use the navigation keys on the lower left panel to check your data against the paper copy. (With a larger dataset, you could also use the LIST command in Analysis to display all the records for review.) Make changes if necessary. When you are satisfied, choose EXIT from the FILE menu or click the red X at the top of the screen to return to the Epi Info main menu.

Analyzing Relational Data

Analyzing a dataset of this size is most efficiently done with tick marks on a sheet of paper, but our purpose is to illustrate how it can be done for 10,000 or a million records, where the tick-mark approach becomes tedious.

Children of HIV positive mothers can have positive HIV serology after birth from passively transferred maternal antibody, but, if the child has negative serology at 18 months, transmission is assumed not to have occurred. Without antiretroviral medication to prevent transmission, about 25 to 40% of children born to HIV- positive mothers will be positive at 18 months—that is, HIV infected.

Let's set some goals for the analysis. Before consulting the detailed instructions, you might write down or discuss the steps that you think are necessary to accomplish each task. Use the spaces below to record your preliminary ideas. In a real situation, it may take considerable trial and error to arrive at a suitable series of steps.

Goal 1: For each child calculate the mother's age when the child was born, i.e., the difference between the mother's date of birth and the child's birthday.

Goal 2: For each mother, find the date of the first positive HIV Lab Test.

Goal 3: Calculate the rate of transmission of HIV infection from seropositive mothers to their children.

Goal 1: Relating Mother/Child Views and Calculating Mother's Age at Child's Birth

The two variables are in different Views (and Data tables), which requires that we RELATE the two views before doing the calculation. To illustrate how the tables are related, we will also LIST the data before and after using the RELATE command.

1. Run ANALYZE DATA from the main Epi Info menu and use READ and the Change Project button to read the RELATED.MDB project that is similar to the one you have just created and named. You can use your own MDB instead if your data entry went well. Use the CHANGEPROJECT button to navigate to the exRelated folder, choose RELATED.MDB or your own MDB, and then viewChildren within the MDB. LIST (choosing ALL) the data and confirm that the variable ChildBirthdate is present, but that the Mother's age or birthdate is not. There are 7 children. Note that the FKey field contains numbers that provide a link to the Mother's record for each child.

2. Now use the RELATE command to link the MOTHER View to the CHILD View. Simply click on RELATE, choose the MOTHER View, and click OK. Since you have not specified the keys on which to RELATE, Epi Info will automatically use UniqueKey in the parent file and FKey in the related file. If we wanted to include the MOTHER who has no children (perhaps because the first one is on the way), we would check the box USE UNMATCHED (ALL), but there is no reason to do so for the present exercise.

3. Use LIST again and note that there are still seven records, one for each child, but that now each row of the table contains both ChildBirthdate and MotherBirthdate. You can expand the column width in the grid by clicking and dragging the vertical line between two column headings.

4. The relationship will persist until we either READ another table or exit from Analysis. Use the DEFINE command to create a new standard variable called MOTHERAGE. Click on the ASSIGN command and then on the FUNCTIONS button. The syntax of the YEARS function that calculates the difference between two dates in years is YEARS(EarlierDate,LaterDate). Returning to the ASSIGN dialog, choose MOTHERAGE as the variable to which a value will be assigned. In the second blank, type YEARS(MotherBirthdate, ChildBirthdate) and then choose OK. (Since this is a function, the initial parenthesis must follow YEARS without a space.) Use LIST to see that each child now has a calculated MotherAge.

5. The result is satisfying, but not permanent, until we WRITE a new table to preserve the new calculations. Use the WRITE command to WRITE a new file in the Epi Info 2000 format, naming it NewRelated.MDB and writing a table called MotherChildAge with all the variables shown. Set the Output Mode to REPLACE, in case a table by this name already exists.

6. Confirm that the new data table exists. Click on READ, then Change Project and find NewRelated.MDB. Click the ALL choice to see data tables, choose MotherChildAge, and use LIST to see the records.

7. Save the program commands generated during this interaction by clicking the SAVE button in the program editor (lower right window) and then the TEXT FILE button in the dialog that appears. Name the program GoalOne and click OK.

Goal 2: Using SUMMARIZE to Find the First Positive HIV Test for Each Mother

Relational database tables are, strangely enough, not processed in any particular order, even after sorting, and the SUMMARIZE command in Analysis is required to do the work of picking out the first (minimum) date with a positive HIV test for each mother. Here we use SUMMARIZE to find the first date on which the Mother had a positive lab test and write it and the Mother's UniqueKey identifier to a new data table called FirstHIVPosDate, using the same name for the variable. Once having obtained the FirstHIVPosDate for each mother, the new information can be related to the Mother's record and written to a new table containing the enhanced records.

1. Run the Analysis program. If there are already program statements in the lower right window, click the NEW button and YES to remove them. Use READ with the ChangeProject button to READ viewMOTHER in Related.mdb. Then RELATE viewLabTests. It is not necessary to specify a key when doing so. Use LIST to see that there is now one record for each lab test, and that each of the 9 lab tests has the related Mother information.

2. Click on the SELECT command and insert the condition, LabHIVAntibody="Yes". Now only the records containing a Lab test positive for HIV antibody will be processed. There should be 4 records.

3. Click on the SUMMARIZE command, fill it in as in the image below, click the Apply button. (This dialog has one peculiar feature—after filling in all the information, you must click APPLY before clicking OK.)

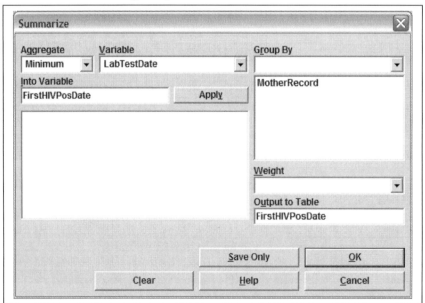

(We are telling SUMMARIZE to find the Minimum value of LabTestDate for each group of records with the same MotherRecord number, and write it to a new variable called FirstHIVPosDate in a new table called FirstHIVPOsDate. There will be one record for each MotherRecord number in the new table, and it will contain the FirstHIVPosDate value.)

4. The necessary text appears in the larger box as in the next picture. After clicking APPLY, the dialog should look like this:

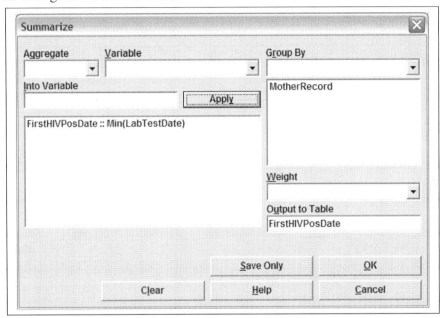

5. Click OK. Agree to replace the existing output table, if any. A new table will be written containing one record for each Mother and the value of her FirstHIVPosDate, if any.

6. Use the READ command to READ the viewMOTHER table without the Lab Test View. This also cancels the previous selection of HIV positive records.

7. Use LIST to see the currently active records, and ascertain that the new table is not yet connected with the original Mother records with which we started. We must use the RELATE command to link it by RecordNumber to these records.

8. To relate the new table to the other Views, click on the RELATE command, click the ALL choice in the middle of the dialog so that you can see data tables as well as Views, and highlight the table called FirstHIVPosDate, but do not click OK yet. We want to use the MotherRecordNumber key to guide the linking, so we have to tell RELATE what keys to use.

9. Click the BUILD KEY button. The dialog that appears is useful, but has some peculiar features that are not entirely intuitive. Note that Current Table is selected. In the Available Variables field, find MotherRecordNumber and select it. It appears in the field at the top,

but belongs in the larger field below Current Table. Now click on Related Table, and MotherRecordNumber appears under Current Table. Use Available Variables again to see the variables in the Related Table and choose MotherRecordNumber again. This is the copy of the Mother's RecordNumber that was written to the FirstHIVPosDate table. How do you get MotherRecordNumber to show up in the large field on the right under Related Table? Strangely enough, it is by clicking once again on Current Table, which will make the choice show up in Related Table!! Or you can simply type MotherRecordNumber in both of the large text fields in the BuildKey dialog. Click OK and you will see MotherRecordNumber::MotherRecordNumber at the bottom of the RELATE dialog. Again, after a little experience, you may decide just to type the key definition into this field rather than using Build Key. Now check the item Use Unmatched (ALL) and click OK in the RELATE dialog. Use LIST to see the results. What has been achieved?

10. Use the WRITE command to write the related table formed from Mother and FirstHIVPosDate tables to a new table called MotherPosDate1 in the file NewRelated.MDB. The achievement mentioned above is that each positive mother now has a date of her first HIV positive test attached to all of her records or virtual records.

11. Click the SAVE button in the program window and save the program as a TEXT FILE named GOALTwo.pgm

Goal 3:Finding the Rate of HIV Transmission from HIV-Positive Mothers

The strategy for this section is to use the newly enhanced mother's record containing the date of first HIV positive test, and RELATE the child records. To find the number of children born to seropositive mothers, we select children whose BirthDate is on or after the Mother's FirstHIVPosDate. Since we have selected only exposed children, a simple frequency of those who are HIV positive (at 18 months, which rules out passive antibody transfer from the mother) and the total number at risk gives the HIV transmission rate.

1. Click the NEW button in the Analysis program editor and then YES to remove the previous program.

2. Use READ and Change Project to READ the data table, MotherPosDate1 in NewRelated.MDB, containing the dates of first positive for each mother.

3. RELATE MotherChildAge, containing a record for each child, by using the key combination MOTHERRECORD::MOTHERRECORD in the KEY field at the bottom of the RELATE dialog.

4. SELECT records for which ChildBirthdate >= FirstHIVPosDate, in other words, the child was born on or after the mother's FirstHIVPosDate. There should be 4 records.

5. Do a Frequency of ChildHIVPositive to determine the rate of infection in children born on or after the date the mother was shown to have LabHIVAntibody. The result is a 25% rate of transmission, about what studies show occurs without antiretroviral preventive treatment.

6. Use the SAVE button in the program editor to save the program as GOALThree.pgm.

This was a lot of keystrokes and dialogs, but there are two principles to remember:

The RELATE command gives you the power to relate different types of tables, as long as they have key fields that can be used to make the link. UniqueKey must be unique (no duplicates) within the tables in which it resides, although several Fkeys can point to the same UniqueKey in the parent record.

The SUMMARIZE command makes up for not being able to process records sequentially and count on a particular order of processing. Writing the summary information to a new table and relating that table back to the original table is a very useful trick for making the information (e.g., date of first positive HIV test) accessible from any record in the original table.

One to Many and Many to One

In order to solidify your understanding of related Views and data tables, think about situations in your own work environment for which related file systems might be useful. We have so far related children and laboratory values to Mothers, using Epi Info's built-in and automatic keys (UniqueKey and Fkey). If you specify Keys for the RELATE command, however, a world of possibilities open up. Epi Info provides a hierarchical form of RELATE, to use terms you might find in a textbook on computer science and database design. This means that data records on one side of the relationship must have unique, non-duplicative keys. ONE record in a table can RELATE to MANY records in another table that have the same key. Conversely MANY records in a table can RELATE to ONE record in another table for which the keys match. Examples of useful relations might include:

Relating many VISITS to one patient RECORD (see below) using a unique patient ID or Epi Info's automatic keys.

Relating one population or other census record to many records in any other table containing City identifiers (assuming these are codes or spelled the same way).

Relating one environmental sensor to its many readings over time

Relating many students to one classroom or teacher

Relating many contacts to one case of sexually transmitted disease

Relating many different laboratory values with results and dates to a patient

(Database purists can break this down further as one patient/many specimens, one specimen/many tests, one test/many sources of payment, ...well, you see why database design takes some thought, and putting together someone else's relational database for analysis may not be an easy task)

These can be handled with one-to-many and many-to-one relationships, but one of the common problems is the human family, which appears to require many-to-many relationships between parents, step-parents, and children. It is likely that the problem can be solved by creating a new type of record, perhaps called a Marriage, or a ParentalRelationship, that would then RELATE to children's records and to records for the two partners in the relationship. Geneticists will of course have to think about how to handle different kinds of incest, but we leave that to the experts.

Using such intermediary records can theoretically solve the many-to-many problem, but, in practice, convenience dictates different locations for the various files involved, and perhaps different kinds of keys. We have not yet reached the day when everyone has his/her record in the Internet cloud, and other records merely consist of identifiers that point to it.

How Many Fields Is Too Many?

Epi Info does not impose a limit on the number of fields in a View. You can meander on for many pages in your questionnaire, but there are some details to consider. Since Microsoft Access Tables DO have a limit of 255 fields per table, Epi Info, behind the scenes, constructs additional related Views and manages the keys so that, hopefully, you do not need to know about them. According to the Epi Info help desk, however, deleting a field from one of the automatically created related Views will cause corruption of the database. Hence, it is best to avoid creating Views in which the *main* form contains more than about 200 fields. There should be no problem in creating a *main* form with *related* Views that each contain another 200 fields.

If you find that your questionnaire has an ungainly number of fields, you should also think whether they are all necessary and will be analyzed. Then decide how to divide them into logical Views that serve the same purpose through relational database structure. Avoid the situation where you construct twelve identical pages of questions, in case a family has up to twelve children, and also the disease surveillance system where the main form contains fields with specialized questions for each type of disease. Put the children in twelve records in a related View, accessed from a single RELATE button on the main form, and the specialized questions for each disease in related views.

Even if the cause of your questionnaire's obesity is legitimate, the View and its logic might be a lot neater with a main page that has a number of RELATE buttons connecting Views that are subsections of the questionnaire. Think of the buttons as tabs in a clinical record that mark the various parts, such as Clinical History, Social and Family History, Laboratory, etc. You can always relate the various parts in Analysis using, for example, Patient ID number, but you will not need large numbers of fields in any one section. We mentioned above that Epi Info divides huge questionnaires into sections automatically, but it makes more sense for you to do this yourself when setting up the Views to take advantage of better access and clarity. Some users have had trouble with very large related Views, and our suggestion is to keep related Views from much exceeding 200 fields by splitting them into several pieces, each with its own RELATE button.

Seeing Inside Groups of Records with SUMMARIZE

The database in the exRELATE folder called HEMATOLOGY.MDB contains a small clinical record system, with the following Views:

Patient Record

PatientID	3874	Name	Vidal
Date Of Birth	08-06-1944	Initial Diagnosis	Ca Prostate

Other details of patient's face sheet here... items that will not repeat or change over time

VISIT

Clicking on VISIT reveals a VISIT record. Each Patient has several VISITs.

VISIT Record

Date of Visit	12-03-2008	Hematocrit	30
Duration of Visit (Minutes)	023		

Fields for other details of visit and lab findings.....

Here's another practice exercise to solidify you knowledge of the Epi Info UniqueKey / Fkey automatic relational system. In Patient and Visit clinical record system above, how would you do the following in the Analysis program?

1. Find the hematocrit at the first visit for each patient, given that there is a field in VISIT called Hematocrit where the information is recorded and that each visit has a DateOfVisit.

2. Find the hematocrit at the last visit for each patient.

3. Find the difference between first and last visit hematocrit for each patient.

4. Find the average number of minutes spent per visit for each patient (assuming that VISIT records have a Duration field)

5. Find the date of first hematocrit above 35 for each patient (in an anemia clinic).

Here's the program that we developed in Analysis after several experiments and false starts. You can load it into Analysis by clicking OPEN in the program editor panel and finding the Text file program called Hematocrit.pgm within the ..\Examples\exRELATE folder. Once loaded into the program editor, you can run it line by line with RUN THIS COMMAND or all at once with the RUN button.

```
*The first part of this exercise requires finding the Hematocrit values"
* from the first and last visits of each patient and subtracting to find"
* the difference."
ROUTEOUT 'Hematocrit.htm'
READ Hematology.MDB:viewPatient
RELATE viewVISIT
SORT DateofVisit
* The SORT is necessary so that the records are in order by date
* for the First and Last functions in SUMMARIZE
```

•

Here's the dialog for SUMMARIZE, after filling in values and clicking APPLY twice.

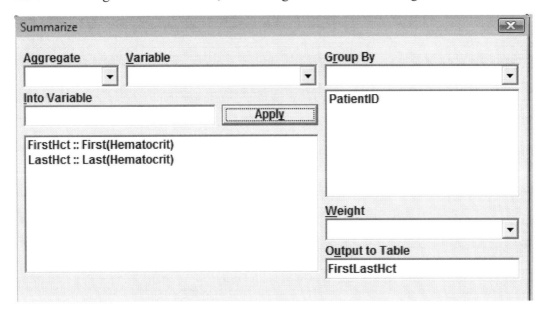

```
SUMMARIZE FirstHct :: First(Hematocrit) LastHct :: Last(Hematocrit) TO
FirstLastHct STRATAVAR=PatientID


* Now we READ viewPatient again to remove the relation  to viewVISIT
READ viewPatient
RELATE FirstLastHct PatientID::PatientID
```

```
DEFINE HctIncrease NUMERIC
ASSIGN HctIncrease=LastHct-FirstHct
LIST  PatientID Name FirstHct LastHct HctIncrease
```

*The next challenge is to find the AVERAGE duration of visits for each patient

```
*First we read the VISIT view
READ viewVISIT
*DURATION is in the VISIT view, but we RELATE the PATIENT view to have
* the patient name, ID, and Diagnosis available
RELATE viewPatient
SUMMARIZE NumberOfVisits :: Count(DurationofVisitMinutes) VisitDuration ::
Avg(DurationofVisitMinutes) TO VisitDuration STRATAVAR=PatientID
READ viewPatient
RELATE VisitDuration PatientID::PatientID
LIST  PatientID Name InitialDiagnosis NumberOfVisits VisitDuration
*VisitDuration has too many decimal places; let's fix it
Define Duration
*The FORMAT function can use a pattern, but produces text and not a number, so we
need a new variable
Duration = Format(VisitDuration,"##.#")
LIST  PatientID Name InitialDiagnosis NumberOfVisits Duration
```

```
READ 'C:\_EpiBook\Examples - Copy\exRelate\Hematology.MDB':viewPatient
RELATE viewVISIT
SELECT Hematocrit>35

SUMMARIZE DateFirstHctGT35 :: Min(DateofVisit) TO FirstHctGT35
STRATAVAR=PatientID
READ 'C:\_EpiBook\Examples - Copy\exRelate\Hematology.MDB':viewPatient
RELATE FirstHctGT35 PatientID::PatientID
LIST  PatientID Name InitialDiagnosis DateFirstHctGT35
```

In plain words rather than commands, here is what the program does:

1. Find the Hematocrit at the last visit for each patient.

    a. Use the same steps, but select Maximum rather than Minimum in step b.

2. Find the difference between first and last visit hematocrits for each patient.

    a. RELATE the table from 1. above to the main table by PatientID

    b. RELATE the table from 2. above to the main table by PatientID

    c. Define two new variables, FirstHCT and LastHCT

    d. Use IF statements to ASSIGN the variables

---

       i.   IF VisitDate=FirstVisit THEN ASSIGN FirstHCT=Hematocrit

      ii. IF VisitDate=LastVisit THEN ASSIGN LastHCT=Hematocrit

  e. Define another variable called LastMinusFirstHCT and assign it the value of LastHCT-FirstHCT

3. Find the average number of minutes spent per visit for each patient (assuming that VISIT records have a Duration field)

  a. Use SUMMARIZE with AVERAGE of the DURATION field for each PatientID, writing to a variable and table called AverageVisitDuration.

4. Find the date of first hematocrit above 35 for each patient (in an anemia clinic).

  a. Select Hematocrit>35

  b. Use SUMMARIZE to write the Minimum of VisitDate for each PatientID

Adding Alternative Keys in a Relational System (Optional)

By now, you should have an idea of how Epi Info creates UniqueKeys for each parent record and an FKey (for foreign key) in each child record that "points" back to the parent record (by being a copy of the UniqueKey of the parent).

Since keys are so important to data integrity, it is reasonable to use two key systems in a large dataset—the built-in, automatic mechanism, and a second set of visible keys. The latter are entered by the user for the master (Mother) record, but can be copied to the children automatically using Check Code.

For those who prefer to use the extra key system, here's how to install it in the database we have already constructed.

Installing an Alternate Key System

The objective is to insert new fields in the related Child and Lab Test views to match the MotherRecord number. In order to transmit the MotherRecord number to each record in the related Views, a global variable called MoGlobalID is created in Check Code and set to MotherRecord before each RECORD is accessed in the Mother View. MoGlobalID is then used to set the value of the Record Number in each related View before one of their RECORDs is accessed.

To preserve the work already done, use MyComputer from the Windows Start menu or Desktop to copy your own MDB or the sample provided as Related.mdb. Click once on the filename to select it and then do Ctrl-C to copy and Ctrl-V to paste. This will make a copy of the file called "Copy of…" Right click on its icon and use the RENAME feature to rename it to BetterRelated.MDB or another name that you prefer.

1. Return to Epi Info, run MakeView, and open BetterRelated.MDB and the MOTHER View.

2. To make sure that no record has a blank MotherRecord number, double click on the prompt words, Mother Record Number to bring up the field dialog and then click in the checkbox next to Required. Click the OK button. The user will now be required to enter a MotherRecord number before leaving each record.

3. With the MOTHER View visible, click the blue PROGRAM button in the left screen panel. This brings up the Check Code programming panel.

4. We want to transfer the MotherRecord value to a global variable so that it can be used to set the corresponding keys in the CHILD and LAB TEST Views. In the dropdown box under Choose field where action will occur, choose DEFINEDVARIABLES. Click the DEFINE command button, enter the name MoGlobalID, and check the variable type as GLOBAL. Click OK to create the global variable.

5. In order to cover both new records and existing records when a user browses back through the table, we must set the value of MoGlobalID in two places—immediately after a new MotherRecord number is entered, and also in the block called RECORD, which will set it before every record is displayed. A modifier called ALWAYS … END will make sure that it is set even when the user is paging through records and not entering a new record. In the space for FIELD WHERE ACTION WILL OCCUR, choose MotherRecord, then click on the Assign command and locate the MoGlobalID variable for the top blank and MotherRecord for the second one. Click on OK. This will set the global variable, MoGlobalID to MotherRecord immediately after the MotherRecord number is entered by the user.

6. Now choose RECORD as the location where action will occur, click BEFORE, and then make the same assignment, setting MoGlobalID equal to MotherRecordNumber. Note that the command appears before the marker ENDBEFORE, meaning that the assignment will occur before entering rather than after leaving the RECORD.

7. One more thing is necessary to make the assignment occur even when the user is scrolling back through records and making no entries. In the edit window, surround the assignment with the words ALWAYS and END. The code in the RECORD block should look like this:

```
ALWAYS
  Assign MoGlobalID=MotherRecord
END
ENDBEFORE
```

8. Click OK to return to Mother's main screen.

9. Hold the Ctrl key and click the CHILDREN button. In the child form, right click near the top to add a field. Name the field Mother's Number. Make it a NUMBER field with the pattern ###### (6 digits). This is important, as keys in one View must match by field type and pattern, or they cannot be used to RELATE the Views. Check the property called READ ONLY. Click the OK button. The user will not be able to enter data in this field, but we will use Check Code to do so automatically. The global variable MoGlobalID is visible

from the CHILD form--that's why we made it GLOBAL—and we can now use it to set the
value of MothersNumber in the CHILD View. Click the Program button and insert the
following Check Code in the RECORD block:

ALWAYS
   Assign MothersNumber=MoGlobalID
END
ENDBEFORE

10. Close the Check Code screen, and then click BACK to return to the MOTHER View.

11. Hold the Ctrl key and click on Lab Tests. Make the same changes in this View that you
made in the child View, except that the 6-digit field should be called Patient Number and
the ASSIGN should be adjusted accordingly.

12. Test your new code from the MOTHER View in Enter and make sure that the child forms
always contain the Mother's number. If not, look for errors in the Check Code and consult
with your colleagues or instructor. To insert the new keys in related records you will have
to visit each record.

13. A working version of the code is found in EnhancedRelated.MDB.

Grid Fields for Views

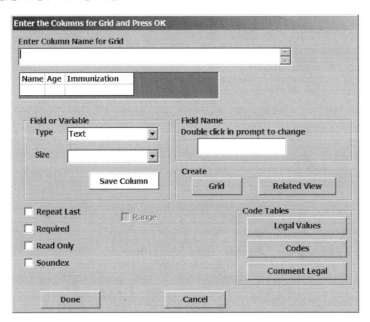

So far we have described the creation and analysis of related tables through the Create RELATED
VIEW option in MakeView. There is an alternative way to create related tables. If you choose
Create GRID in the field dialog, you will be able to create a table within the data entry View. In the

dialog above, we have already named the field CHILDREN and then clicked on Create GRID. This grid will allow recording the Name, Age, and Immunization status of a Mother's several children on the same page with the mother's data.

The result will be a table called recGridMotherChildren that is the equivalent of the CHILD table created in the main exercise for this chapter. In Analysis, after READing the MOTHER View, you can RELATE recGridMotherChildren and do analysis just as with the related Views. Although this is theoretically a neat idea, there is no way to add Check Code to fields in a grid, and grids are apt to be a bit flakey. We do not recommend that you use them with caution and careful testing until some future version of Epi Info makes them more stable.

Analyzing Data in a Grid

To see the children's data, use the RELATE command. Choose the view called RecGridMotherChildrenIn or something similar, and click OK. The number of records increases, if you entered more than one child per mother. There now is a "record" for each child, linked to the mother by an internal UniqueKey number maintained by Epi Info. To see the records, use LIST again with * for "ALL", and note that each child has data and that the mother's data items are duplicated for each child. You can now analyze the data to find out how many children there are, and the ages of their mothers, for example.

Concept

Relational or hierarchical tables are an important way of dealing with data for a person with repeated visits or episodes, a household or parent with many children, etc. The "parent" and "child" records are linked by a UniqueKey identifier that is created automatically by Epi Info. Related tables are created by inserting a grid or by creating a related View using the RELATED VIEW button in the field dialog of *MakeView*.

Resources

Sample and exercise files for this chapter are found in **exRelate** in the **Examples** folde r

CHAPTER 17: DATA MANAGEMENT WITH EPI INFO

Data management and statistics are, in some respects, separate topics. Database programs such as Microsoft Access, dBASE, and Foxpro focus on data management, and do not offer ready-made statistics. Many statistical programs such as Stata, SPSS, and SAS focus mainly on statistics and less so on database management.

In this chapter, we will explore the data management features in Epi Info that allow it to support disease reporting systems, clinical and research databases, and other activities where data management is at least as important as statistical processing.

Review of Data Storage

Epi Info's data access features are described in previous chapters. The native or default storage format is that used by Microsoft Access, the MDB file. MDB files can be considered as containers or bags containing up to 999 separate tables. Each table consists (conceptually) of rows and columns like a spreadsheet, with capacity for millions of rows. An MDB is a Windows file, and is stored in a Windows Folder or Directory on a hard disk, a removable memory device (memory stick), a ZIP drive, or in a network. An MDB can be copied to a CDROM for backup or distribution, but the the MDB cannot be used directly from a write-once CDROM. For use, you must copy the MDB to a hard disk or other medium with read/write access.

MDB's can be ZIPed for storage, and they often compress remarkably—10-fold or even 20-fold. After they have been used and a many changes have been made to the data, they contain a lot of empty space that can be reduced by the COMPACT DATABASE feature on the FILE menu in the ENTER program.

A VIEW in Epi Info is an MDB table, such as "viewOswego" that describes the appearance of the data-entry screen and its relationship to the data. It is used by Epi Info to construct the database table and display the form or questionnaire. The other table usually has a matching name, such as "Oswego" without the "view" prefix. There may be other tables with prefixes like "code" that provide Legal or Code values for fields in the View.

You can examine the tables in an MDB directly with the UTILITY called VISUALIZE DATA available from the Epi Info menu. It is good practice to make a copy of the MDB before using VISUALIZE DATA. An easy way to do this in Windows XP and Vista is to click once on the filename in Windows Explorer/MyComputer to select, then use Ctrl-C, Ctrl-V to make a new file called "Copy of ..." in Windows XP. You may have to scroll to the bottom of the list of files to see

it, as My Computer does not realize that it has a dual-processor, turbocharged, CPU mill underneath that could sort the list faster than you can think, "Where is it?"

To see the tables in SAMPLE.MDB, use VISUALIZE DATA to Open the MDB as an Epi Info Project, then expand the TABLES item and double-click on a table icon to see the rows and columns. Have a look at the inside of viewOswego and the corresponding Oswego data table. Any changes that you make are permanent; that's why you made an extra copy of the MDB.

Sending MDB Files

Unfortunately, some email security systems consider an MDB to be "an executable file" and will not permit it to be sent as an attachment, even if it is ZIPped (compressed) first, although if you change its name to something like MBB and ZIP it, it may sail through. The recipient has to unzip it and change the name back to MDB. Hopefully this note will be of only historical significance within a couple of Internet Years. Meanwhile, there are Internet services that allow sending large or executable files without using this trick, and you can also subscribe to an FTP (file transport protocol) site that will store or transport essentially any kind of file. The easy way to find them is to Google for "send file" (without the quotes) or something similar ("send file securely"). Be sure to try out the service you choose, and check to see if it is legal in your organization to send data this way. For extra security, you can encrypt files with EpiLock, and transmit the password to the recipient by some route other than email.

Using Epi Info on a Local Area Network

Computers connected by Ethernet cables and/or wireless connections at a single site are known as a Local Area Network or LAN. Epi Info can access MDB files located remotely on a LAN, and people on separate computers can enter data in the same MDB. Each computer must have a copy of Epi Info installed, but you can keep the Epi Info installation file(s) on a server to make installation easy.

Several users can access the same MDB, the same dataset, and even the same records in a server-based MDB. For example, people can enter data in a clinic database from the Pediatric and Adult medicine offices, both supported by the same file server, and adding to the same MDB and dataset. If both access the same record, a warning pops up with instructions so that one of the entries does not override the other without a decision being made by the operators.

There is a limitation with the Analysis program. It does not recognize network addresses like \\MyDiskServer\Somedata.mdb. You have to "Map" the address to a drive letter like R: to be able to READ the file in Analysis. To do this, open My Computer and click the item called MAP NETWORK DRIVE on the TOOLS menu. You can choose a letter, like "Y:" and map it to \\MyDiskServer\. Then go back to Analysis and READ the Y: drive to find your MDB. Now you can treat "Y:" like a normal drive. There are some kinks in this process, mainly if you move your laptop to another network, but they can be fixed by remapping to a currently connected drive.

UniqueKey and Fkey

There are at two kinds of automatic record keys in Epi Info—those that uniquely identify records (UniqueKey) and those that point to the UniqueKey of a parent record to establish a parent-child or ownership relation. The latter are called Fkey for "Foreign key" because they point to an external relationship. Each record in a data table has a UniqueKey, but only related data tables have Fkeys pointing to parent records.

In a system of Patient records having one or more Visit records each, the Patient record with UniqueKey 1 may have several Visit records with UniqueKeys in the Visit table such as 1,2,3,and 6, but all having FKEYs of 1 because they belong to Patient number 1. It is more correct to say they belong to the Record with the UniqueKey of 1 in the Patient table, as the Patient may have a hospital or clinic number of, say, 3252214, which is also in the Patient record, perhaps as PATIENTID, but not UniqueKey. If you use Epi Info Views to enter data and created Related Views, the ENTER program uses the automatic keys to maintain relationships.

Other databases, including Epi Info for DOS, use more explicit keys, and allow you to create a field called PATIENTID in two files and then use it to link the two sets of records. You can do this in Epi Info for Windows, as the primary or a backup method of maintaining relationships, but it takes a bit more programming to manage the explicit keys. An example is given in the previous chapter.

Cleaning Data: Finding Outliers

Producing statistics is relatively easy with most modern computer programs for this purpose. Once having learned the details with nice, clean sample files, however, the need arises to work with "dirty" data from the field or clinic, and especially with data that is continually being updated, perhaps from more than one center. We find—or would find, if we knew how—duplicate records, dates from the distant future or remote centuries of history, misspelled names, missing data, similar data under different variable names (Sex, Gender), dissimilar data under variables with the same name (Age-of child, Age-of parent, Age-of sterile pack, cheese, document, etc.) logical inconsistencies, negative ages, and other problems rarely included in classroom or sample data sets for statistical programs.

Many of these problems can be prevented at the data-entry stage with Check Code, as will be illustrated in examples in chapters to follow, but detecting problems and cleaning data should also be done in Analysis. The FREQuency command is the best general-purpose error detector. You can run it on a single field or all fields and find extreme values that make no sense, often representing keyboard eR%6ors. You can then use SELECT and LIST UPDATE to correct the records.

Finding Duplicate Records

Records can be duplicated in many ways. It is important to define the type of duplication intended —for example having the same patient record number, having the same values for day and month of birth, sex, and last name, or more simply, just first and last name. The first step with multiple field duplication is to combine values into a single field, using string concatenation after defining a new combined variable, as in DEFINE FIRSTLAST=FIRSTNAME + LASTNAME.

The short way to detect duplicates is to use SUMMARIZE, grouping by the one to several variables of interest and producing a count of another important variable in a table called Dupcount or something suitable. If there is more than one record with matching grouping variables, the count will be 2 or more. An example of this program can be run and then examined in the CLINIC.MNU system in the EXAMPLES folder

Incorrect Dates

The easiest problems to detect with dates are those in which the date is too early to be reasonable or perhaps in the future. A command like SELECT DIAGDATE > SYSTEMDATE OR DIAGDATE < 01/01/1900 can identify the aberrant dates so that you can use LIST UPDATE to make corrections.

Misspelled Names

There is no real magic for misspelled names, but the combination of detecting records with other fields duplicated and human inspection of the duplicates can help. If the database is not too large, a simple frequency of a name field may reveal patterns on the screen that allow you to detect misspellings.

Another aid to matching misspelled names is the SOUNDEX field type. This property has to be set when the Text field for a name is first created in MakeView (It is a checkbox on the left side of the dialog where a field is created). If a field called Name is created as SOUNDEX type, the entries are recorded in the Name field, but also in a field called sdxName as Soundex codes.

Name	sdxName
Smyth	S530
Smythe	S530
Smith	S530
Lee	L000
Li	L000
Lea	L000
Leanne	L500

You can find much more extensive descriptions of the SOUNDEX system by googling for SOUNDEX CODE, but the examples above show that it does for names what rounding does for numbers--names with similar sounds are given the same code. In the example, there would be three sdxNames of S530 and 3 of L000. This could be considered candidates for spelling variants of the same names, to be evaluated by other criteria. The system is used to facilitate searches during data entry (with the Soundex check box in the FIND panel of the Enter program), and is used by genealogists to find families whose names have varied over time and distance. Soundex is probably of use in detecting errors in aural perception rather than keyboard mistakes.

Missing Data

The SET command in Analysis has two features that can be used to evaluate the amount of missing data in your database. You can set the representation for missing data to an indicator like "Missing" or "...", and then uncheck the IGNORE MISSING box so that missing data will appear in frequencies and tables. You can then use the FREQuencies command with all fields (FREQ *) to show the frequency of missing data in all the fields. If the database is large, you will want to avoid doing frequencies on fields like Patient ID, which may have thousands of unique entries. SELECT PatientID=(.) followed by FREQ PatientID or LIST * will give a more tidy result, counting only the missing values or listing the records with missing values.

Variable Name Problems

Sometimes a variable name is too generic to be helpful. You may have several variables called Age or Duration, for example, and they are difficult to distinguish from one another. A partial solution to improve the appearance of Analysis output is to turn on SHOW COMPLETE PROMPT in the SET command dialog. If suitable prompts have been set up in the View, then Analysis output may display something like "Child's Age", or "Age of Cheese" rather than just AGE.

Changing or Adding a Variable Name

Suppose that you find it difficult to work with, or explain to others, variable names like CHL and CAT, and would prefer Cholesterol and Catecholamine. You can solve half the problem by adding prompts in a View as suggested above, but you really want to change the underlying variable name. You probably could do this in the Visualize Data program by editing both the View and the data table very carefully, but we do not suggest this risky procedure. The best way to change a variable name is to DEFINE a new variable with the desired name and set it equal to the original variable, for example,

```
READ Sample.mdb:EvansCounty
DEFINE Cholesterol=CHL
DEFINE Catecholamine=CAT
```

There are at least two choices for saving a newly defined variable:

- The neatest and most economical way of saving the variable is simply to save the definition and assignment and be sure that they appear at the beginning of any program where you intend to work with the variable. This avoids making a copy of the data, and is therefore quite safe. The data type of the new variable is set automatically to be the same as its source variable.

- Sometimes you need to copy or assign actual data to a new variable, perhaps because you will be sending it to someone else, and you need to include the name of your clinic or state, items that were not necessary for local use. Or, perhaps you calculated an age, duration, or statistic from other fields, and would like to include this in a permanent data table. Writing a permanent data table is the job of the WRITE command, described next.

WRITE Data

The WRITE command can be used to write new Data Tables, containing the results of calculations and variable definitions and assignments. Unfortunately it is prevented from writing to Data Tables that have Views, including the one that is currently active, so saving the results of calculations is a multi-step process:

1. Use ASSIGN to give new values to existing variables and/or DEFINE new variables and ASSIGN values. LIST and FREQuencies now display the new values, but they are temporary.

2. Use the WRITE command to create a Data Table of the new variables and any existing variables with new values. Include in the WRITE, a variable with unique values for each record, e.g., a Patient ID.

3. Use the MERGE command with the UPDATE and APPEND options to add the new data and variables to the currently READ data table or View.

The WRITE (Export) command allows users to save the data into a different Epi Info .MDB data file or into another file format offered by this command. With the WRITE command you can also specify which variables to write to the file and their order in the new file.

It is possible to READ a data table, and append its data to another table with the WRITE command. The receiving table may be empty, but it cannot be the one you just READ. Simply READ a table, and, in the WRITE command, leave all the variables selected, give a name to the output MDB and the table, check the REPLACE option (the first time) and choose OK. Appending a second dataset is the same, except that you now choose APPEND rather than REPLACE. This method has the advantage that it needs no "key" for appending, and the disadvantage that, in its total ignorance of content, it can append the same data as many times as you run it, and thus create duplicate records. It is a handy way to create a million-record table for testing purposes.

Using WRITE to Convert File Formats

With the READ command, you can read data files in a variety of formats from other programs. The WRITE command can export data in those same formats, so that the Analysis program can serve as a data conversion program when necessary. To see an example, READ the viewEvansCounty file in Sample.mdb (see the previous READ section) into an Excel file. Click on WRITE (Export) in the Analysis Commands dialog box to see the the WRITE command dialog, as shown:

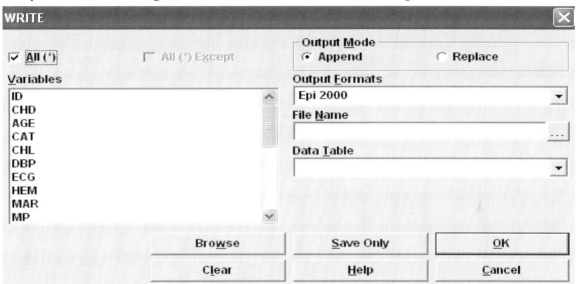

In the WRITE dialog box, the ALL (*) symbol is initially selected by default to write *all* variables from the current dataset into a new dataset. If you want to exclude some variables in the new Data table, you can use the ALL (*) EXCEPT option after first delecting ALL (*). You can also highlight and select variables by clicking. Here for the sake of simplicity, we will choose ALL variables for the new dataset .

Output Mode determines whether the data being written will Append to or Replace the existing dataset. For this example, use Replace., in case there is already a dataset with the same name. With the Append option, data will be appended to the previous data, even if already there.

In Output Formats compartment and select Excel 4.0 or another format after clicking the down-arrow button. The formats include:

Epi2000	**Access 97, 2000**	**dBase III, IV, 5.0**	**Paradox 3.x, 4.x, 5.x**
Excel 3.0, 4.0	**Epi Info 6**	**Text (Delimited)**.	

To write or read Excel files, you must have the Microsoft Excel (Microsoft Office) program on the same computer. If you do not, select another format from the list.

Pressing the button with " . . ."to the right of the FILE NAME displays a dialog box where you can select a *folder or an MDB* to save the new file. This item really should be named MDB NAME when you choose Epi2000 or Access97 or 2000, and WINDOWS FOLDER NAME when you are writing another file type.

Assuming that the FILE TYPE chosen is Excel, choose 'C:\Epi Info' for FILE NAME, (although it is not) and type "EvansCounty" (no quotes) for the TABLE NAME (which also is incorrect). The extension .xls will be added. Click OK, and EvansCounty.xls is now written (exported) to the folder 'C:\Epi Info'. To check for the presence of EvansCounty.xls, use the READ/Import command with Excel 4.0 or use Excel to open the file.

When OUTPUT FORMAT is Epi2000 or Access, FILE NAME is the name of the MDB—if it does not exist, it will be created. DATA TABLE is the name of the desired table for the data. You cannot write to the table that is currently active from the last READ command.

WRITE cannot be used to write data to a Table that has a View, hence none of the data tables with Views appear in the DATA TABLE dropdown. If you enter the name of a Table that has a View, you will get a message saying that you must use the MERGE command to write to Tables that have Views.

The MERGE Command

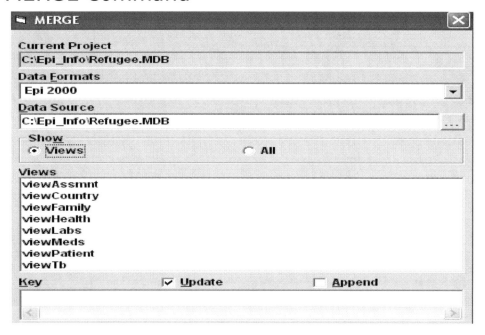

Whether in society, family, corporations, or databases, MERGing is a non-trivial operation unless the merging elements are of similar or identical structure. We will begin with an example of an "easy" MERGE, where tables of the same structure contain non-overlapping sets of records. They might be disease reports from different weeks in a surveillance system, or data from different centers that use the same View for data entry.

For data management purposes, and especially if Views are involved, you should use the MERGE rather than the WRITE command. The APPEND option in MERGE uses a key (unique identifier) that you supply, and appends only records that do not match those already in the table. If you specify that first and last names are the key (yes, multi-field keys are allowed), then a record belonging to "José Brea" will only be appended if he does not appear in the main table, and, after it is appended, running the merge a second time will not append another "José Brea". If you accidentally run the MERGE several times, no damage is done.

Imagine two people entering data from a study on separate computers. You would like to combine the two data tables into one, APPENDing one to the other.

The Use of MERGE with the APPEND Option

Master Table			Merge Table			Master Table after the MERGE	
ID	Name	MERGE APPEND with ID as the Key	ID	Name	Results in >>>	ID	Name
1	Amy		6	Fran		1	Amy
2	Betty		7	George		2	Betty
			8	Harry		6	Fran
			1	Emile		7	George
						8	Harry

Note that Amy's name was not changed to Emile, although they both have an ID of 1, but the records with non-matching IDs were appended.

The Use of MERGE with the UPDATE Option

Master Table			Merge Table			Master Table after the MERGE	
ID	Name	MERGE UPDATE with ID as the Key	ID	Name	Results in >>>	ID	Name
1	Amy		6	Fran		1	Emile
2	Betty		7	George		2	Betty
			8	Harry			
			1	Emile			

Note that Amy's name was changed to Emile, because they both have an ID of 1, but that the other records were not appended because only UPDATE was requested.

Now, suppose that we want to maintain a single master table at the national level and periodically have regional health facilities send new data for merging with the master. Some of the incoming records are new, but others are previous records that have been updated —perhaps with a corrected name or age or a new outcome. The new values (except blanks) are to overwrite previous information in the matching record.

The Use of MERGE with the APPEND and UPDATE Options

Master Table			Merge Table			Master Table after the MERGE	
ID	Name	MERGE	ID	Name		ID	Name
1	Amy	APPEND	6	Fran		1	Emile
2	Betty	UPDATE	7	George	Results in >>>	2	Betty
		with ID as the	8	Harry		6	Fran
		Key	1	Emile		7	George
						8	Harry

Amy's name was changed to Emile because their ID of 1 matched, and records 6,7, and 8 were appended because their IDs were not found in the Master Table.

Both UPDATE and APPEND options of MERGE require that at least some of the data in the master table and the merged table must have the same field names and data types. The keys can have different names, but must be of the same data type.

There must be keys in both tables, but you cannot use the built-in UniqueKey variable for this purpose. You can, however, define several fields as the keys for identifying records—first name, last name, sex, and date of birth, for example. Good database management requires that you build in a unique identifier for each record from the beginning—something like Patient ID. The multiple-field key approach can work for an emergency or one-time merge, but there is always a risk that the defined combination of keys will not be unique--on a national level, for example. Make backup copies before the MERGE and test the results.

MERGE with the RELATE Option

In addition to the APPEND and UPDATE options, MERGE has a third option called RELATE. You would never guess this from looking at the MERGE command dialog, as it does not appear there, but, if you have read the 1000 sections of the Epi Info help file, or, of course, this book, you will find this intuitive. RELATE is invoked by filling in the MERGE command dialog and Unchecking both APPEND and UPDATE. If you then click OK or SAVE ONLY, the MERGE command is placed in the program panel with the word RELATE included.

What does MERGE RELATE do? It should have been called UPDATE FKEY instead, because that is its effect. You specify one or more keys in the MERGE command for relating two Views (other than UniqueKey and Fkey), and MERGE RELATE constructs FKEYs in the specified Data Table that point to the UniqueKeys of the table that has been READ. As a message will point out, it constructs an Epi Info relationship between the two Views to agree with the relationship indicated by your explicit keys. Why would you want to do this? There are at least a couple of reasons:

- To maintain the main View / related View relationship for the Enter program so that the RELATE buttons work correctly and records in the related View are linked (via the FKEY) to their parent records in the main View.

- To preserve the Epi Info automatic relationship so that when you READ one of the Views in Analysis and RELATE the other, you do not have to specify keys. The UniqueKey and FKEY are used automatically.

So let's expand the idea of the public health surveillance system described above under MERGE APPEND/UPDATE . For single tables in the central and local agencies, APPEND and UPDATE are enough, but if your database structure includes related Views that are to be sent from the local agency to the central agency, you need MERGE RELATE. Here is the sequence for the periodic update of Central's files:

Local has two Views, called Patient and Laboratory. These have an Epi Info relation with Patient being the parent View and Laboratory the related View. Both also contain PatientID. New records arriving at Central are used to update the central Patient View with MERGE UPDATE/APPEND. The central Laboratory View is updated the same way, but then the additional step of running MERGE RELATE is necessary to restore the FKEYs in the Laboratory View based on the PatientID relationship in Central's Views. Now the records can be viewed correctly in ENTER and easily RELATEd in Analysis.

Demo: Merging Files in Three Agencies and a Laboratory

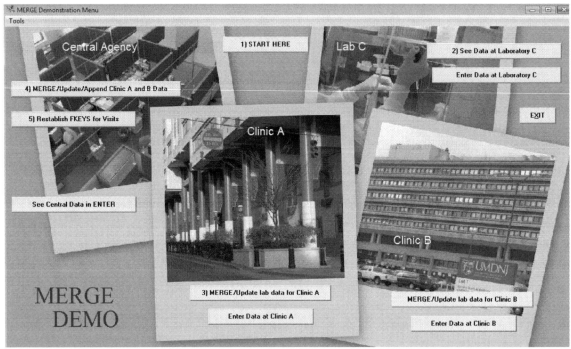

The MERGE Demo Menu

An Epi Info application is found in ..\Examples\exMERGEDEMO\ that represents a laboratory, two clinics, and a central agency sharing data by means of Epi Info data files (MDBs) and the MERGE command. The clinic databases are "relational" in the sense of having one record for each CLIENT linked to many VISIT records. To run MERGEDemo, find the file called _RUN MERGEDemo with My Computer and double click on its icon. If this does not show the menu, try _MERGE.EXE (a copy of EPIINFO.EXE in the Epi_Info Info folder, renamed to MERGE.EXE so that it runs MERGE.MNU). You should see the screen illustrated below.

Start at the top of the menu with the START HERE button and click your way around the various features and explanatory text in the order indicated by the numbers. You can use the TOOLS menu and EDIT THIS MENU to see the menu text, identify files and study how the demo works.

DELETE File/Table

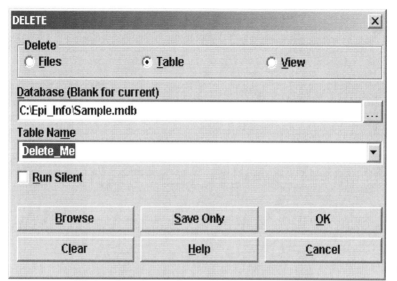

Dialog box for Delete File/Table, Epi Info

The DELETE File/Table command in Analysis can be used to delete a file, a table from within an Epi2000/Access MDB file, or a View from within an Epi2000/Access file. It is important to know that an MDB is a FILE, and that Data Tables and Views are TABLES, as deletions are permanent.

To see an example, READ viewEvansCounty in SAMPLE.MDB in the Epi_Info folder, then use the WRITE (Export) command to save the data as a new table called Delete_Me in Sample.MDB. Next, use Delete File/Table, in the dialog box click on Table, for the Database select Sample.MDB, for the Table Name, and select Delete_Me and OK

DELETE Records / Undelete Records

Using Delete Records you can either mark records for deletion or permanently remove records from the file. Records that are marked for deletion remain in the data file but are usually ignored during analyses. (Note: using the Set command the usual setting for Process Records is Normal, i.e., perform analyses only on undeleted records; two other options are to analyze both records marked for deletion [Both] or only records marked for deletion [Deleted].) The other option is to permanently remove records from the file.

You can choose criteria for determining which records to delete, such as "*" to delete all records or any other criteria, such as Age>50 or Sex="M", similar to the types of functions and mathematical comparisons described for Select (see Appendix 2). The Run Silent option, when not checked, makes a sound and pops up a small dialog box; when checked, neither the sound nor pop-up window will occur.

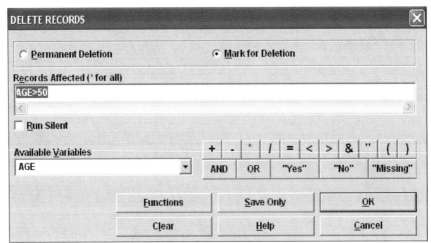

The DELETE RECORDS Dialog

Records <u>marked</u> for deletion in the Enter program or the dialog above can be undeleted using UNDELETE. Specific criteria can be given as to which records to undelete.

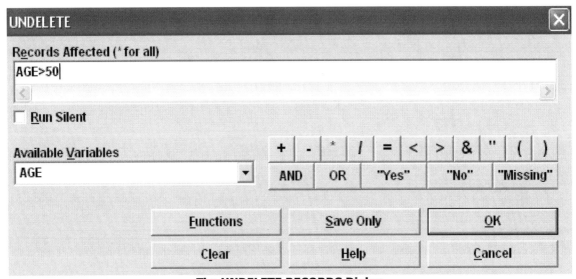

The UNDELETE RECORDS Dialog

The DELETE RECORDS command with the MARK FOR DELETION option checked affects the RecStatus field in Epi Info Data Tables. Normally, RecStatus is set to 1. If the record has been marked for deletion either in the Enter program or in Analysis with DELETE RECORDS, RecStatus becomes 0 (zero). UNDELETE changes RecStatus back to 1.

There are times when you want to PERMANENTLY DELETE records. Checking this option in DELETE RECORDS will actually delete the selected records from the MDB, and UNDELETE will not retrieve them.

The COMPACT Utility

In order to maximize the disk space saved after deleting many records, it is a good idea to run the COMPACT program from UTILITIES on the main Epi Info menu after deleting or editing a large number of records. The Compact program can also be run from the Visualize Data program or from the FILE menu in Enter. Although it asks for a password, none is needed unless you have somehow supplied one in Microsoft Access.

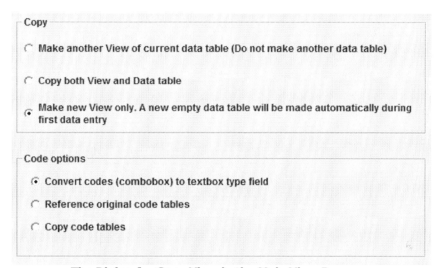

The Dialog for Copy View in the MakeView Program

Copying Views and Data Tables

As discussed in this chapter, the WRITE command can be used to make copies of Data Tables that do not have Views. There is a more flexible feature in MakeView called COPY VIEW that will not only copy a View but create a new MDB and copy all the Code Tables and the Data Table for the View. Here are the options, which should be clear after some study.

Resources

The MergeDemo example in this chapter is found in **exMergeDemo** in the **Examples** folder.

CHAPTER 18: GEOGRAPHIC INFORMATION SYSTEMS (GIS)

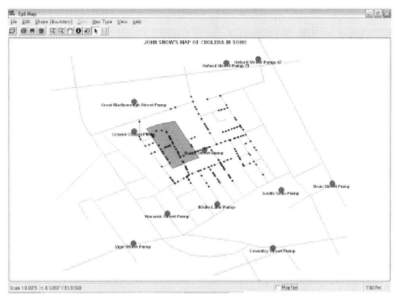

John Snow's Cholera Map in Digital Form

Introduction

Geographic Information Systems sometimes are regarded as special magic, to be managed by experts with expensive software and a vocabulary that differs from that of epidemiologic and statistical software. For public health purposes, however, geography means "place" in the classical triad of "time," "place," and "person" that is the basis of epidemiologic investigation. An epidemiologist needs not only GIS, but also a "Temporal Information System (TIS)," for time, and a "Personal Factor Information System(PFIS)" for other risk factors. These are both supplied by Epi Info (without the imaginary names) in the form of Graphs for Time and Tables and associated statistics for Personal Factors.

The Epi Map Program

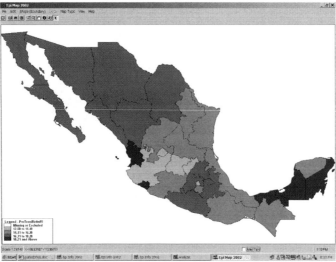

A Choropleth or Color/Pattern Map, Based on Polygon (State) Names

Adding a Shapefile to create a map

Concept
Shapefiles are an industry standard for Geographic Information Systems (GIS) used in the popular ArcView and ArcInfo programs. Shapefiles of every country in the world can be downloaded from the Epi Info website under "Maps", and the Internet provides thousands of such files. Shapefiles can be drawn or edited in either ArcView or Epi Info for emergency or custom purposes.

First, let's make a map of Mexico representing one numeric result for each State by coloring the polygons that represent the States. Run *Epi Map* from the main menu. In the FILE menu of *Epi Map* choose MAP MANAGER, and from the LAYERS card, click on ADD MAP LAYER. You should see a choice of SHAPE (.SHP) files, containing the boundaries of geographic regions. Open the one called MxState.shp and choose NAME as the field containing the names of Mexico's states.

Adding data to be represented by color density

A database containing public health data from Mexico is provided. Open the SAMPLE.MDB database and choose the table called MexMap95. The appropriate Geographic Field is STATE and the data field is PerTeenBirth95, the percentage of births in which the mother was an adolescent in

1995. You should see a map of Mexico with the adolescent pregnancy percentage for each state represented as a shade of gray.

You can experiment with features such as FIND on the EDIT menu (also represented by the binocular button). Try finding "Vera," for example. The magnifying glasses with + and - signs are for zooming to larger or smaller sizes. Click on the one with the + sign and then click and drag a rectangle over an interesting part of the map. It will zoom to fill the frame. Try panning—moving the map with the white mitten. You can restore things to normal either with the negative magnifying glass or with the world button that represents the global or home View. The "I" symbol means "information." Click it and then click on a state to see the data values for that state—both those contained in the Shapefile and those in the linked database.

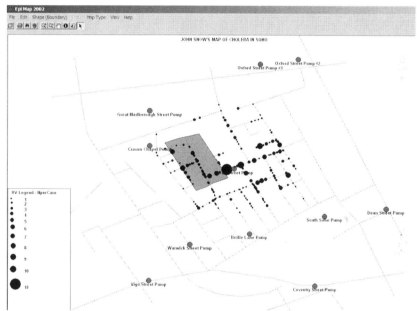

An Improved Cholera Map with Numbers of Cases at the Same Address Represented By Larger Circles

Epi Map can represent data as discrete points on the screen, as well as quantitative values within polygons. The following set of instructions will produce a map resembling John Snow's famous map of cholera cases in the Soho district of London in relation to the various public pumps used for drinking water. A popular theory of the time related cases to the presence of an old cemetery where plague victims from a previous century had been buried; hence the cemetery will be included as a separate layer in the map.

First run Epi Map from the main menu. From the FILE menu, choose MAP MANAGER. Choose ADD MAP LAYER, and then open the SOHOST.SHP file. SHP stands for SHAPE, the most common type of file used in mapping with Epi Map. Now you should see a map of the streets of Soho. From the map manager and add the cemetery by using ADD MAP LAYER and choosing SOHOBURI.SHP. To add the locations of the water pumps, use ADD POINTS and select SAMPLE.MDB and then SOHOPUMP. Another dialog asks for the x and y coordinate fields. This is an easy choice in this exercise; X Coord is the X coordinate and Y Coord is the Y coordinate. Click on NAME in the choice in the lower left so that the names of the pumps will be displayed. To make the pumps larger, choose 15 for their size, and change the color by clicking in the black rectangle and choosing a brighter color. Click OK after choosing the color, and then again for the dialog. You should see the pumps and their names arrayed on the map.

To display the cases, repeat the ADD POINTS process, this time choosing SOHODEAD from SAMPLE.MDB and 5 for the size of the symbols. Use a contrasting color and do not choose a field for displaying text. Place a checkmark in the box beside SAVE POINTS AS NEW LAYER and another checkmark beside VARY SYMBOL SIZE FOR COINCIDENT POINTS. This is a new feature in Epi Map 2002, that allows the representation of more than one case per household. Click OK and be prepared for a short wait, as the 500 + cases need to be updated many times.

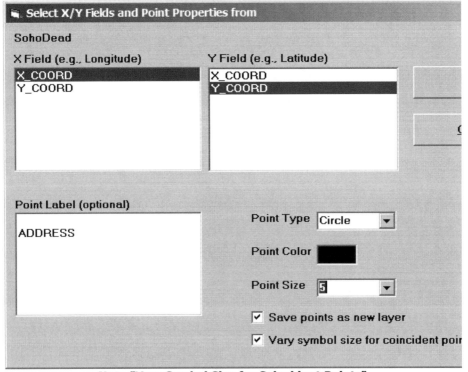

Note "Vary Symbol Size for Coincident Points"

You should see points representing the addresses where cases occurred. One household had 18 cases and is represented by the largest dot.

To see the same map without the varying symbol size, put away the Map Manager and choose from the FILE menu, OPEN MAP FILE. Find JOHNSNOW.Map and open it. This View uses the same data, but since the point do not vary in size, the multiple-case households cannot be distinguished from single-case households. The visible points actually represent households having "at least one case" rather than cases individually. One of the dots actually represents 18 cases.

Although the map suggests that the Broad Street pump was central to the location of cases, and other evidence did incriminate this pump, one must remember that the distribution of dots is a function not only of the mortality rate but also of population distribution, and that rates rather than numbers of cases would be necessary to draw a scientific conclusion. Assuming, however, that the population was fairly evenly distributed through Soho, the impression that the map gives is useful. Dr. Snow's similar map helped him convince the neighborhood council to remove the handle of the Broad Street pump, and the epidemic subsided.

Note that the elements of a map and its linkage to a data table can be saved in a .MAP file and later recalled with a single click. We have demonstrated the linking process from within Epi Map, but it is also possible in Analysis to READ a dataset containing geographic names and link it to a shapefile containing polygons of the same names to produce a map. If you have time, READ the dataset MEXMAP95 in Sample.MDB and then enter the following values into the MAP dialog in Analysis:

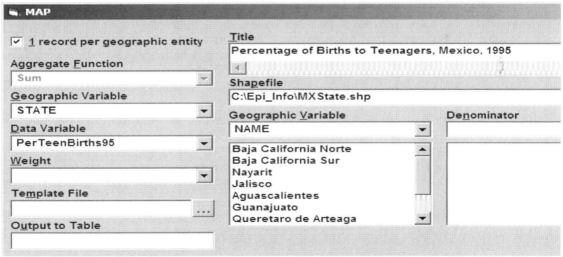

Dialog to Create a Choropleth Map with MexMap.MDB Data

The output is shown as the second figure in this chapter.

If we wish to combine place-related epidemiologic data with maps or other diagrams, it is necessary that the data be described so that they can be matched to place locations on a map. There are two main ways of doing this:

Type of Data	Linked by	Type of Map	Example
Counts or Rates	Polygon Name	Named Polygons	Case counts per county or state
Points or Cases	Latitude/Longitude or other coordinates	Any graphic that has a matching coordinate system	Individual cases on street maps

In practice, summary data is usually linked to polygons, such as states, counties or zip codes. Individual cases with exact locations can be plotted as symbols on maps of streets, or other backgrounds that do not necessarily have named polygons. Both types of GIS exercises can display counts or rates on suitable *shapefiles*, the standard for maps of polygons, lines, or points established by the ESRI, the largest GIS software provider (www.esri.com).

In this chapter, we will further explore plotting points to display cases or other individual events. Since plotting the exact residence address of an ill person may compromise confidentiality, these maps must be kept within the health department or the data can be summarized to display as counts or rates that do not reveal exact locations. For data on zoonoses or other non-human events, however, and for mortality data, point maps can be used whenever coordinates are available.

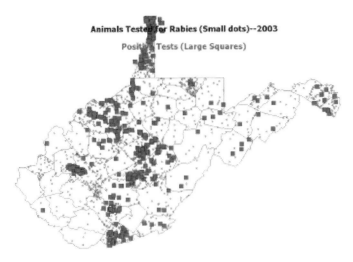

Mapping Points in Epi Map

Concept	Points are placed in a layer on a shape file using coordinates that match those of the shape file. The usual coordinates are longitude and latitude in decimal degrees. In this exercise, we will first use a dot density map to show animals tested for rabies in West Virginia. On top of this display, we will create another layer of points representing animals having positive tests plotted by their lat/long coordinates.

Displaying Animals Tested by County

As background for the display of animals with rabies, we will use a dot-density map of animals tested. To make this map, choose ANALYZE DATA from the main Epi Info menu. READ the GISDATA.MDB file in ..\Examples\exGIS\ and choose the table called RabiesTests2003. To see it, you may have to click ALL rather than VIEWS in the READ dialog.

Click on the MAP command, and fill in values as follows:

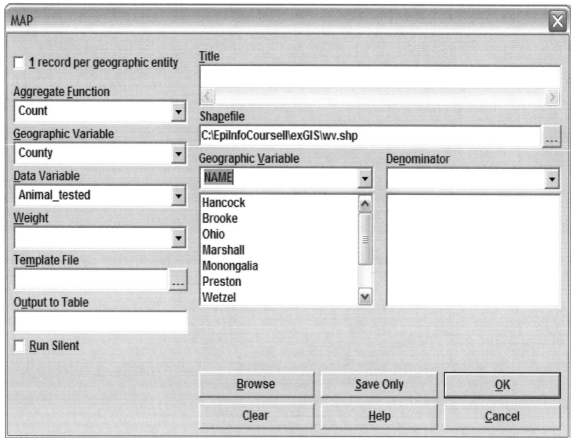

Rabies Tests Performed

Choose OK, and then, in the warning dialog, CONTINUE, and you will see a choropleth map of rabies tests performed by county in 2003. In Epi Map, choose MAP TYPE from the menu and then DOT DENSITY. In the properties pages that appear, be sure you are on the one labeled DOT DENSITY, and then click OK. You should see yellow dots representing animals tested in each county, as follows:

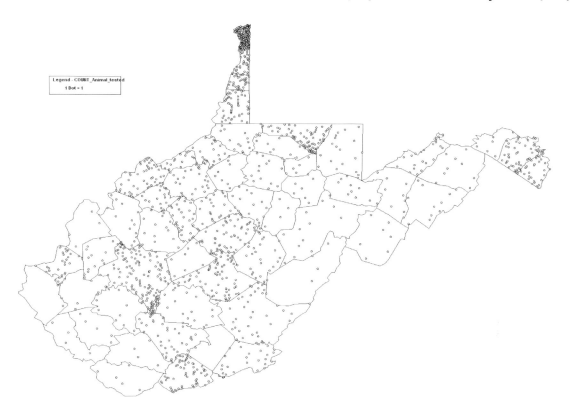

Place the mouse cursor on the legend, hold down the left mouse button, and move the legend up to a more aesthetic position. Note that, as you do so, the dots are redrawn many times, and that the number of dots in a county remains the same, but that their position is determined randomly. The tests performed, therefore, are accurately enumerated by county, but their position within the county is not displayed. This makes sense, since you instructed Epi Map to use COUNTY as the Geographic variable in the data table.

To see the name of the county with the large number of dots, click the toolbar button with the "I" (for "information") and then click on the county. County is given as NAME, but note the large number of other data items associated with the shape file (stored in its .DBF section).

Displaying Positive Rabies Tests by Point Coordinates

On this background, we will display the positive tests using latitude/longitude coordinates contained in the data table. The positive results are in a separate table called RabiesPositives2003.

Within Epi Map, with the tests still displayed, choose MAP MANAGER from the FILE menu, and click on the button ADD POINTS. Find the data file GISData.MDB and choose the table RabiesPositive2003. Another dialog pops up asking you to SELECT XY FIELDS AND POINT PROPERTIES... For the X FIELD, select DECIMAL_ LONG, and leave the Y FIELD as DECIMAL_LAT. POINT LABEL allows you to display, for example, the species of

ANIMAL_TESTED beside each point, but we found by experiment that this dataset produces too many labels to be good looking, so leave this item blank.

For POINT TYPE choose SQUARE, click on the black rectangle and change the POINT COLOR to bright red, then click OK, select 10 for POINT SIZE, and click OK again.

When you click OK, you should see the map represented at the beginning of this exercise. Note that it shows both numerator (Positives) and denominator (Animals Tested) data on the geographic background, with the positives having more precise locations than the animals tested. We have ignored the missing values, which should be considered in producing your final report, but the display is a good summary of the year's results. If you would like to display the animal species tested, repeat the ADD POINTS step, but request labels for ANIMAL_TESTED.

Try adding titles to your map by clicking on the graphics button in the toolbar—the one with the small yellow rectangle, circle, and triangle. Then click the button with the large "A" to insert a title ("Animals Tested for Rabies (Small Dots)—2003"). We found that a point size of 20 is about right. A subtitle can be inserted in red to indicate "Positive Tests (Large Squares)".

Move the legend around and note that the positive test points remain in the same locations, since they were specified by latitude and longitude, but that the randomly distributed dots representing all tests change location with each move. They are only linked to the counties by county name.

To save the image for your newsletter or annual report, choose SAVE AS BITMAP FILE from the FILE menu, and give the file a suitable name and location.

Mapping Categorical Data in Epi Map

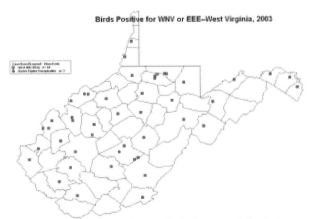

Virus Isolations from Birds in West Virginia

Concept	Epi Map can create dot density maps with more than one category, based on numeric codes. In this exercise, we insert codes in a data table for West Nile Virus (1) or Eastern Equine Encephalitis (2), and show the two categories by West Virginia county.

Preparing Data by Inserting Numeric Category Codes

Using ANALYZE DATA from the Epi Info main menu, choose READ and then EXCEL 8 for DATA TYPE. Find the file POSITIVEBIRDS2003.XLS in the exGIS folder and select the range or worksheet provided. There should be 43 records.

LIST the records to see the variables and data values. Note that latitude and longitude are given in decimal degrees and that VIRUS has two values, WNV (for West Nile Virus) and EEE (for Eastern Equine Encephalitis). It would be easy to display the values as points as we did in the previous exercise with VIRUS as the POINT LABEL, so that the two EEE values would stand out. However, sometimes there are too many values to use the categorical label display, and we would like to show the different categories as different shapes, colors, and sizes of symbols. Let's use POSITIVEBIRDS2003 to illustrate how to do this.

The categorical symbol display in Epi Map requires numeric codes for the categories. We must therefore convert "EEE" and "WNV" to 1 and 2 for example. Now that we have read the Excel file in Analysis, we can do this before writing a table in the MDB to be used for mapping.

First DEFINE a new variable with the DEFINE command, and call it VirusCode.

Choose the IF command and insert the condition VIRUS="WNV" (with quotes). In the box labeled THEN, type the command ASSIGN VirusCode=1 (no quotes). Click OK. What will this command do if the value of VIRUS is "EEE" or missing? Use LIST to find out.

Now do another IF command for VIRUS="EEE", assigning VirusCode=2. What does this one do if VIRUS is "WNV" or missing?

Note that nothing visible happens until your do a LIST or FREQuency, but that the values will remain until you do another READ or leave the Analysis program. Use the WRITE command to write all variables to a table in GISData.mdb called POSITIVEBIRDS2003. READ this table and LIST it to confirm that the new variable called VirusCode is correctly set to 1 or 2 by virus type.

Now exit from Analysis, and go directly to Epi Map by clicking the the main menu button, CREATE MAPS. Choose the Map Manager and ADD LAYER to add the WV.SHP file and bring up the map of West Virginia. Now choose the CASE-BASED button and locate GISData.mdb and the table POSITIVEBIRDS2003. A somewhat complicated dialog appears, in which you should choose NAME and COUNTY in the first two boxes, and VirusCode in the third. Now a choice of symbols and legend labels appears. Change the colors to something contrasting, the size to 10 or 20, and the shapes to two different choices. Type legend entries "West Nile Virus" and "Eastern Equine Encephalitis". When you choose OK, the two types of virus are displayed as different symbols.

As a thought exercise, give some examples of data sets for which the technique of plotting more than one kind of symbol would be useful.

Editing or Creating Shape Files

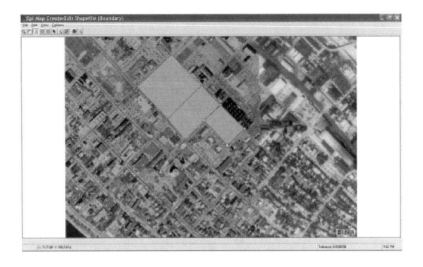

	The Partial Load feature in Epi Map can be used to customize shape files by including only selected polygons. Editing features are provided to create or divide polygons and insert lines or points. When shape files are not available, a scanned image or aerial photo can be loaded and used to guide creation of a new shape file. Use this feature for refugee camps, building floor plans, or geography that has undergone recent change.
Concept	

Creating a New Shape File by Combining Polygons from Others

From the Epi Info main menu, choose CREATE MAPS to run EpiMap. In the FILE menu, choose MAP MANAGER… and then ADD LAYER. Find the shape file called WV.shp and open it to display a county map of West Virginia. Now do ADD LAYER again and add the shape file PA.shp, and again to add OH.shp. Now you have the adjacent states of West Virginia, Pennsylvania, and Ohio. If the map is not correctly framed in the window, put away the Map Manager and click on the world View icon in the toolbar.

Our goal is to add to the West Virginia shape file just the adjacent counties from the other two states. This requires the names of the counties to be added. In order to see the names, bring up the Map Manager again and select the PA layer. Click Properties and then choose the Std Labels tab. In TEXT Field, choose NAME, and click OK. You will see the names of the counties. Do the same for OH.shp and you can write down the names of the counties you want to add to the West Virginia map, or just print the labeled map to use in the selection process.

Now remove PA and OH by selecting each and clicking REMOVE LAYER. Choose ADD LAYER PARTIAL and PA.SHP. In the list of counties in PA.SHP, hold down the Ctrl key and click on the name of each of the border counties--Allegheny, Beaver, Fayette, Greene, Lawrence, and Washington. When asked for a shape file name, use PACounties. Do the same for OH.shp, select Athens, Belmont, Columbiana, Gallia, Jefferson, Lawrence, Meigs, Monroe, and Washington, and give the shape file the name OHCounties.

So far, so good, but the combined map is a jumble of counties, and it's hard to see where West Virginia ends and the other states begin. In the map manager, select the WV layer and click PROPERTIES. In the SINGLE tab, set the Fill color to light blue or gray. Leave the other properties as they are. Click OK, and you will have West Virginia in gray or blue and the other states with clear or white backgrounds. To save the map as it is, close the Map Manager and choose SAVE MAP FILE from the FILE menu. Give the .MAP file the name WVPlus.

Click CLEAR MAP(S) in the FILE menu. Choose OPEN MAP FILE and open WVPlus.MAP to confirm that its properties were saved.

Making an Entirely New Shape File Based on an Image

At times, no shape file is available, but there are images from which one could be constructed. This may be the case with building plans, refugee camps, and areas of recent change when an aerial photograph is available.

To illustrate how to make a shape file "from scratch", open Epi Map from the Epi Info menu and in the SHAPE(BOUNDARY) menu choose CREATE/EDIT. You should see a blank screen with a toolbar at the top. In the FILE menu, choose LOAD BACKGROUND IMAGE. In the resulting file dialog, change BMP files to ALL FILES, and then navigate to find CHARLESTON1996.JPG, an aerial image of part of Charleston, West Virginia, taken from an Internet site. It is in the exGIS folder. A dialog invites you to set up a coordinate system, but we do not know the exact latitude and longitude of the image, so click OK to the arbitrary coordinates provided. To illustrate how to draw polygons on top of the image, we will trace a few blocks to construct areas called Block 1, Block 2, and Block 3.

Click on the third toolbar button, the one with the irregular polygon, to draw a polygon on one of the blocks. Then place the mouse cursor at the corner of one of the blocks and click once. Not much happens. Then move the cursor to an adjacent corner. This time, you may be able to see a thin line from the site of the first click to the cursor. Click once again, and move the cursor to the third corner of the block. This time you should see a triangle forming. Click on the corner, and move to the fourth corner. This time click twice on the same spot, and a dialog should pop up asking for the name of the polygon. Enter Block 1.

It takes a little practice to carry out this process. If you run into problems while drawing a polygon, you can start it again by pressing ESCape. Previous polygons can be selected with the arrow button, and vertices can be moved by holding down the cursor until the vertex turns red and then dragging it to a new location. There is an ADD VERTEX button that inserts additional vertices if there are not enough to modify the shapes correctly. It is possible to divide a polygon, and therefore to draw the grand outline of the map and work by successively dividing it into the inner polygon areas. This helps to assure that boundaries between areas are single rather than double lines. There is also a snap function that merges two lines that are sufficiently close together, and it is possible to set the snap distance with another button.

When you have made shapes to your satisfaction, the shape file can be named and saved with the SAVE function on the FILE menu. This creates all the files that make up a shape file, with the polygon names in the .DBF, the shapes in the .SHP, etc. Data can be linked to the new shape file by polygon name or by coordinates that match those of the drawing space. As you saw when initiating the drawing process there is an opportunity to use latitude and longitude or other coordinates for the drawing.

Resources
Sample and exercise files for this chapter are found in **exGIS** in the **Examples** folder.

CHAPTER 19: ARVCALC-CHECK CODE FOR MEDICATION DOSAGE AND NUTRITIONAL STATISTICS

Although you can do valuable work with MakeView and Enter by simply using default conditions, the data entry process can be enhanced through Check Code. You can insert conditional skip patterns, calculate durations between two dates, and perform other operations to catch errors or assist in data entry.

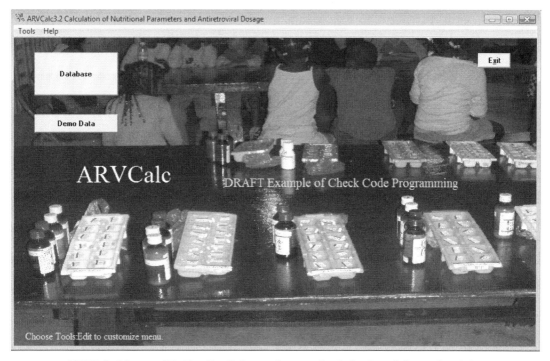

ARVCalc Menu with the English version on the left, Spanish on the right.
Each has an empty database and another with demo records.

In this chapter we will examine the more advanced features of Check Code for data entry, using calculation of medication doses and nutritional parameters as an example. The program is called ARVCalc, developed in the Dominican Republic to determine proper doses of antiretroviral (ARV) medication for patients with HIV/AIDS. Both English and Spanish versions were offered on the same menu, but the one in exARVCalc has been simplified to include only the English version.

Buttons on the menu lead to a View containing Demo Data and another View of an empty database, ready to receive new data.

Purpose and Design

Acquired immunodeficiency syndrome or AIDS is caused by the human immunodeficiency virus (HIV). Without treatment, AIDS has a very high mortality rate, but properly administered multidrug antiretroviral (ARV) therapy allows 95% 5-year survival. Internationally, ARVs are supplied by donor and/or government agencies that require documentation of use. The diagnosis of AIDS is based on clinical criteria and on the count of CD4 lymphocytes in the blood; a low count (e.g., less than 200 in adults) being considered diagnostic of AIDS. ARVs must be given in combinations of (usually) three drugs, with the choice of regimens being based on previous drug therapy, age, and the presence or absence of anemia, liver disease, and other conditions. For children, doses are calculated by body weight and/or body surface area, the latter being a challenge to calculate manually. Each ARV has its own set of conditions and instructions for administration, and list of interactions with other medications. Weight loss is one of the principal effects of AIDS (in Africa, known as"slim disease"), and weight gain and increase in CD4 count are indicators of therapeutic success. Nutritional parameters such as Body Mass Index (weight/height squared) expressed as a percentile by age are important in following children, whose height normally changes over time.

AIDS impairs immunity, and often leads to serious infections with microorganisms that are rarely problems for normal people, and/or may already be in the patient's body—the so-called "opportunistic infections." These include Pneumocystis carinii (jiroveci), toxoplasmosis, tuberculosis and other mycobacteria. AIDS patients are frequently given additional medications to prevent opportunistic infection. Prescribing depends on CD4 level, body surface area, weight, the ARV regimen, available medications, and other parameters.

ARVCalc is a calculator to determine ARV regimens and doses and the appropriate medications to prevent opportunistic infections. It has been used both in clinics and to assist in expert review of medical records. Since it creates a database of the entries, it stores the information for each patient visit, but unlike a complete clinical database, each visit is treated separately. The clinician or an assistant enters the patient's identifying data, data of birth, height, weight, and sex, CD4 count, and hemoglobin, and then chooses an ARV regimen from a series of buttons.

Recommendations and dosages for prophylaxis of Pneumocystis carinii pneumonia (PCP), tuberculosis(TB), and Mycobacterium avium complex (MAC) infection are given on page 2 of the View. They use the same kind of logic and calculations as the dosages on page 1. Both screens are shown on the next two pages.

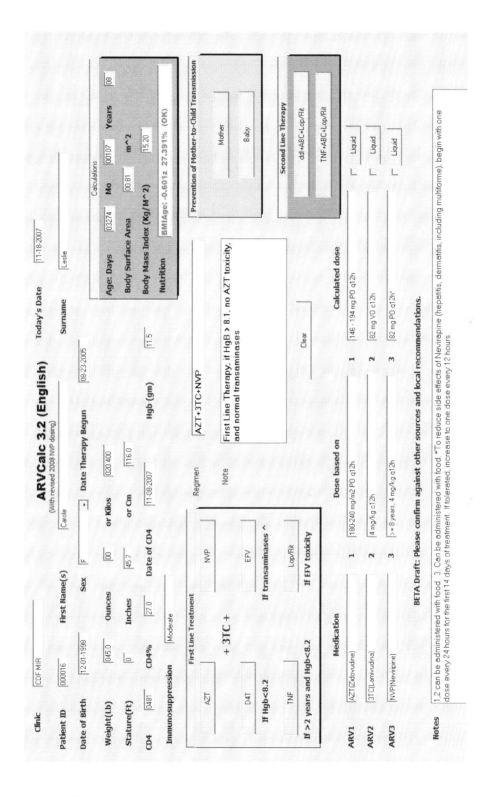

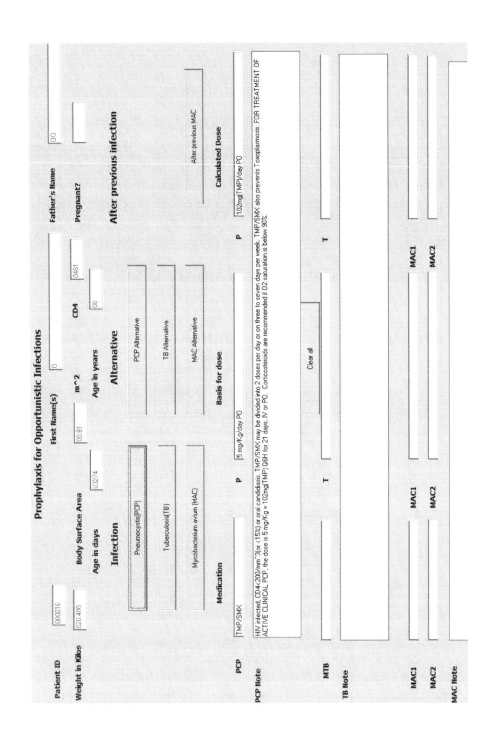

Installing ARVCalc

1. ARVCalc requires Epi Info. Please install Epi Info from www.cdc.gov/epiinfo if it is not on the computer

2. The files for ARVCalc are in exARVCalc\ in the EXAMPLES for this book.

3. To install the program for the first time, find the file called INSTALLArv.BAT and double-click to run it. If you get a message that you must have "administrative privileges," try again, but this time, RIGHT click on INSTALLArv.BAT, and choose Run As Administrator. If this succeeds, you are ready to run ARVCalc.

If you are not able to install the nutritional module, a message will pop up each time you run ARVCalc3, saying that you do not have the DLL called US2KAny. You can ignore the message and later ask someone with "administrative privileges" on the computer to Run INSTALLArv.BAT as Adminstrator (after RIGHT clicking its icon) as described above. This step only has to be done once.

Click the RUN ARVCalc shortcut to run the program. If this fails for some reason, double-click on ARVCalc.EXE instead to run the menu. The DEMO, contains a number of sample records. Click DEMO and page 1 of the a data entry View should appear. You can page through the records using the arrows in the lower left corner of the screen. Note the different regimens, doses, and preparations used and the nutritional calculations that are done from the age, weight, height, and sex. To see page 2, click its entry in the upper left corner of the screen. The DATABASE button brings up the same form with an empty database table for your own use.

Treatment of HIV infection is a very dynamic field. Indications and doses for ARVs and opportunistic infection prophylaxis change frequently, and new medications become available. Official guidelines differ between countries. If you plan to adapt the ARVCalc program for use in your own environment, please be sure to check your own guidelines and sources on the Internet, such as www.aidsinfo.nih.gov, for current information. The software we are providing with this book is presented as an example of Check Code programming, not a validated clinical tool.

Developing the View/Questionnaire

This was reasonably straight-forward, but a couple of tricks were needed. If you plan to have more than one version in different languages, the prompts on the screen are easily changed, but the underlying field (variable) names must be in one language or the other, unless you plan to have two completely separate versions. MakeView requires that field names be unique, but prompts (like "1", "2", and "3") can be the same in more than one field . You cannot have a missing or blank prompt, but we have used the underline character ("_") as a prompt, and hidden it behind another field to create what looks like a table with columns.

The database is called ARVCalc.MDB and there are two views called ARVMedication and Database.

Now let's examine the Check Code, illustrating some of the main tasks that it performs. As mentioned in an earlier chapter, seeing the Check Code requires that you run MakeView, and open the ARVCalc.MDB database and the ArvMEDICATIONS View. Click the button called PROGRAM on the left side of the screen and you will be in the Check Code page.

The first task is deciding where to put the Check Code. Here are the options:

Possible Locations for Check Code in Views			
Type of Block or Field	Happens when the cursor *enters* the field, page, or record	Separator Word	Happens when the cursor *leaves* the field, page, or record
RECORD	Yes, but only with new records	**ENDBEFORE**	Yes, but only with new records
RECORD with code in ALWAYS...END block	Yes, even when paging through previous records	**ENDBEFORE**	Yes, even when paging through previous records
PAGE	Yes	**ENDBEFORE**	Yes
Any Fields except the following:	Yes	**ENDBEFORE**	Yes
Checkbox field	No		Yes
Radio button field	No		Yes
Command Button	No		Yes
Image or Label/Title	No Check Code		
Relate Button	No		No, but see Chapter XX
DEFINED VARIABLES	Special block to hold new variable definitions for Check Code. The DEFINE command puts them here.		

Functions of Check Code in ARVCalc

Let's look a the Check Code more closely, taking one activity at a time on the first page of this View. To see the Check Code, click on the PROGRAM button in MakeView. In the dropdown list for "Choose Field Where Action Will Occur", the fields having Check Code are indicated with an asterisk (*). Click on one of these and you will see its Check Code. The code for RECORD and the DEFINEDVARIABLES section are hidden at the very end of the list, after all the pages of variables.

Set the Default Date to Today

In the Check Code block called Page 1, if today's date is missing, set it equal to the computer's SystemDate, a predefined variable.

```
*Page 1
*If today's date is missing, set it equal to the computer's SystemDate,
* a predefined variable.
If TodaysDate=(.) THEN
  TodaysDate=SystemDate
End
ENDBEFORE
```

All the code prior to the ENDBEFORE will be run BEFORE the cursor enters a new page 1.

The second line could have been:

```
ASSIGN TodaysDate=SystemDate
```

but the world ASSIGN is optional, since the program "knows" that it has two variables separated by an equals sign. Note that "=" is used in two ways in this same block of code, as a test for equality in the condition of the IF statement, and then again to assign a value to FechaDeHoy (today's date). Some languages (JavaScript) use different symbols for these purposes, but, thankfully, Check Code does not.

Showing an External Help File from a View Page

Offering a help file is generally a good idea, and, in this case, there is an help file called ARVCalc.htm. To display it, we have place a Command Button on the page and use the EXECUTE command:

```
EXECUTE 'ARVCalc.htm'
```

Since the file is an HTM/HTML file, it needs a browser for display, but the Windows file association system will bring up the default browser and pass it the name of the file. You can also run EXE or BAT files with EXECUTE, giving a tremendous range of possibilities, although passing variables back and forth from an external program would require some ingenuity.

Ensure That Important Fields Are Entered

Any field can be made REQUIRED in the field creation dialog, but this has the disadvantage that the user cannot leave the current page until a value for the field is supplied. If the information is not immediately available, the user may enter meaningless data just to be able to move on, which tends to defeat the purpose of a REQUIRED field. In ARVCalc, we have chosen a middle road, which is to remind the user if fields have missing data, but not place the page under house arrest. We chose the NAME field, as a good place to check, as a record without a name is unlikely to have serious intent. Here's the code for NOMBRES:

```
IF ID=(.) Then
  Dialog "Please enter Patient ID."
End
```

```
If Clinica =(.) Then
  Dialog "Please enter Clinic name. It will repeat automatically."
End
ENDBEFORE
```

If either the patient ID or the Clinic name is blank, a dialog pops up with a reminder, and, in the case of the Clinic name, a REPEAT LAST field, one can enter it once and then it will repeat each record until a different value is entered. The ENDBEFORE makes all this happen before the cursor drops into the First Name(s) field, but nothing actually forces the user to take our splendid advice. Medical professionals rarely enjoy being treated as two-year-olds, and we try to let them do as they wish, after being properly informed.

Calculating Age in Years or Days

When would be a good time to calculate AGE? The calculation requires two dates, Today's Date and Date of Birth. So, right after entry of Date of Birth would be a good time for the calculation.

In the block for Date of Birth, we use the following code to calculate the age in years and the age in days, and place the values in the corresponding fields on the screen.

```
*DateOfBirth
Clear BMICategory
AgeInYears=Years(DateOfBirth, TodaysDate)
AgeInDays=Days(DateOfBirth, TodaysDate)
AgeInMonths=Months(DateOfBirth,TodaysDate)
IF AgeInYears < 0 then
  Dialog "Not born yet?"
End
IF AgeInYears > 100 then
  Dialog "More than 100 years old?"
End
```

Note that these are both ASSIGN statements, and that clicking on the FUNCTION button in the ASSIGN dialog will display help for functions, from which you can choose DATE functions and discover those for YEARS and DAYS between two dates, with the earliest date placed first in the parentheses. The first parenthesis must not be preceded by a space or the function will not work. We chose to name the variable EnAños with its proper Spanish letter, since EnAnos means "in anuses" rather than the intended "in years". Usually the use of special characters in variable names, although allowed, may lead to programming errors by those not familiar with the language. Special characters are fine in data entered by the user, however. Even Asian characters can be used if the computer accepts them.

Hiding Irrelevant Fields

Now that we have ages in days and the sex of the patient, we can use the information to hide unneeded fields. The Gestational age field (Gestacion) is not useful for dosage calculation after a child is more than 6 weeks (42 days) old, and the Pregnancy is only a valid question for female patients more than 10 years old, so we hide the corresponding fields when not needed.

```
If AgeInDays < 43 THEN
  UNHIDE Gestation
  HIDE CD4 CD4Percent DateOfCD4 Immunosuppression
 ELSE
  HIDE Gestation
  UNHIDE CD4 CD4Percent DateOfCD4 Immunosuppression
 END
If Sex="M" OR AgeInYears < 10 THEN
 HIDE Pregnant
END
IF Sex="F" AND AgeInYears >9 THEN
 UNHIDE Pregnant
END
```

In case the data entry person changes either the age or the sex of the patient, we have to UNHIDE the two fields if the conditions are not met.

Wait! We're not done yet. Hidden fields will acquire missing values during data entry, but the "hidden" state is not stored in the data table. Hence, if we enter data for a 5 year old boy, Embarazada and Gestacion will be hidden, but, if we page back through the records in the file, or find the record by searching, these two fields will again be displayed (with missing values). The fix for this is to place the same code in the RECORD block within an ALWAYS...END section, as follows:

```
*RECORD
ALWAYS
 IF AgeInYears > 10 AND Sex="F" THEN
  UNHIDE Pregnant
 ELSE
  HIDE Pregnant
 END
 If AgeInDays < 43 THEN
  UNHIDE Gestation
  HIDE CD4 CD4Percent DateOfCD4 Immunosuppression
 ELSE
  HIDE Gestation
  UNHIDE CD4 CD4Percent DateOfCD4 Immunosuppression
 END
 If TodaysDate=(.) THEN
 TodaysDate=SystemDate
 End
 If Liq1>0 Then
  Unhide Liq1Dose
```

```
   else
    Hide Liq1Dose
   end
   If Liq2>0 Then
    Unhide Liq2Dose
   else
    Hide Liq2Dose
   end
   If Liq3>0 Then
    Unhide Liq3Dose
   else
    Hide Liq3Dose
   end
   Note4=""
   Note3=""
   Note2=""
   Note1=""
  END
  ENDBEFORE
```

This is exactly the same code, enclosed in the ALWAYS...END command, and designated to run BEFORE each record is presented, whether it is a new record, or one with existing data. Note, that new records will not yet have either age (Edad) or sex, and that this code will not do anything. An existing record will have Gestation and Pregnant hidden or not hidden depending on the age and sex already in the record.

Convert English and Metric Units

To make ARVCalc useful to a wide audience, we allowed Weight to be entered in either Pounds and Ounces or Kilos, and Stature in either Centimeters or Feet and Inches.

The Lb (Pounds) Field

If the user enters a value in the Lb field, and has not yet entered ounces, we jump to (GOTO) the Ounces field before converting the values to Kilograms. However, if there is already a value for Ounces (perhaps zero, but not missing), we do the calculation immediately.

```
 *LB
 IF oz=(.) THEN
  Goto oz
 ELSE
  Kilos = (Lb+(Oz/16))/2.2046
 END
 IF CM > 0 AND Kilos > 0 THEN
  GOTO BMI
 END
```

If both CM and Kilos have been calculated, we go to BMI, or Body Mass Index, where they are used to calculate several values.

Note that this all happens when the cursor leaves the Pounds field, since there is no ENDBEFORE.

The Oz (Ounces) Field

```
IF Oz=(.) THEN
  Oz=0
END
```

Now the cursor has been in the Oz field, and we assume that Kilos can be calculated. Since a missing value will yield a missing value in the calculation, we set Oz to zero if it is still missing when the user is through entering.

```
*OZ
IF Oz=(.) THEN
  Oz=0
END
if lb=(.) then
  lb=0
end
*If oz exceeds or equals a pound, distribute them as pounds and oz
If oz>15 THEN
  lb=trunc(lb + (oz/16))
  oz=oz mod 16
END
*Calculate kilos, and then go to BMI if ready or go on to get the stature measurements.
Kilos = (Lb+(Oz/16))/2.2046
IF Kilos > 0 AND CM > 0 THEN
  GOTO BMI
END
IF Kilos > 0 Then
  goto Feet
END
```

The Kilos Field

If the cursor is in this field, the user probably chose to enter the weight in Kilos, and we proceed to convert to Pounds and Ounces.

```
Lb=Trunc(Kilos * 2.2)
```

Calculate in pounds, and round down (TRUNCate)

Calculate again to find the remainder and convert this to 16ths of a pound, known in our crazy English system as Ounces.

```
Oz=((kilos*2.2)- Lb)*16
```

Note that we forgot to capitalize "kilos", but that it makes no difference, as Check Code is not case sensitive. Placing the value in the View field Oz, will automatically truncate it to the number of places in the Field Pattern, giving, for example, 6 ounces rather than an untidy 6.090909090909090.

As with the other fields, if Kilos and CM are ready, we jump to the BMI field for calculations.

```
IF CM > 0 AND Kilos > 0 THEN
  GOTO BMI
END
```

The Feet Field
```
*Feet
Clear Inches Cm
ENDBEFORE
IF Feet>0 and Inches >=0 THEN
  Inches=(Feet*12)+Inches
  cm=Inches * 2.54
  Feet=0
END
IF CM > 0 AND Kilos > 0 THEN
  GOTO BMI
END
```

Note that we disregard the contents of Inches, since the user has just entered Feet. It is always reasonable to convert feet into inches, unlike the situation where body weight in ounces may be awkward.

The Inches Field
```
*Inches
If Inches=(.) THEN
  Inches=0
END
IF Feet=(.) and Inches>0 then
  Feet=0
End
IF Feet>0 or Inches > 0 THEN
  Inches=(Feet*12)+ Inches
  cm=Inches * 2.54
  Feet=0
END
IF CM > 0 AND Kilos > 0 THEN
  GOTO BMI
END
```

The Cm (Centimeters) Field
```
*CM
Inches=cm/2.54
```

```
Feet=0
IF CM > 0 OR Kilos > 0 THEN
  GOTO BMI
END
```

Calling a Common Block of Code

In the Analysis program and in many other languages, code that will be called more than once can be placed in a block called a subroutine or procedure or function. This is not true in Check Code because there is no way to create a code block that does not correspond to a View variable. With apologies to Shakespeare, however, "A Rose by any other name is a workaround." We can cease to wring our hands, and just put the code in the BEFORE position of any other field, using GOTO to put the cursor in that field and thus call the code.

Here's how it works. We put the calculations for Body Surface Area and Body Mass Index into the BMI field's Check Code prior to an ENDBEFORE. Then, in each of the height and weight fields, we check to see if Kilos and Cms have been calculated or entered. If so, we do a GOTO BMI, calling the calculation code and placing the cursor in the BSA field.

Here's the code in the Kilos field, after calculating Oz and Lbs, for example:

```
IF CM > 0 AND Kilos > 0 THEN
    GOTO BMI
END
```

The same IF statement appears in the Check Code for each of the weight and stature variables, so that whenever the Kilos and Cm values are ready, the calculations are performed.

Calculating Body Surface Area

Body surface area is used in the ARV guidelines to calculate dosages of some medications for children. Doing the calculation by hand is a nuisance because of the square root (^0.5) The formula to calculate BSA is:

```
BSA=((CM * Kilos)/3600)^0.5
```

Calculate Body Mass Index

Body mass index is defined as weight over height squared—easy to remember, until you also recall that the height must be in meters, not centimeters. This accounts for the 10000 in the numerator.

```
BMI=Kilos* 10000 / (CM * CM)
```

If a Value Has Changed, Take Action

If entries for weight and stature change the BSA, we want the dosage calculations that follow to be derived from the new data. On the other hand, if BSA has not changed, there is no point in clearing out all the medication information that may already be present. Hence, we DEFINE a variable called "prevBSA".

The DEFINE does not appear in the code for the field in which it occurred, because Check Code automatically places the definition into the DEFINEDVARIABLES block at the bottom of the variable list. The only reason to visit this block is to see what variables have been defined, or perhaps to correct their spelling or delete one.

Now we can use prevBSA as follows to save the existing value of BSA. Then we do a new calculation, based on CM and Kilos, and compare to see if the new calculation is "close" to the old value (here defined as within 0.005). If not, then the medication dosage fields are CLEARed (set to missing), because the calculated doses may have changed.

```
*BMI
Clear BMI
*Calculate BSA and BMI. Medication fields if changed
IF CM > 0 AND Kilos > 0 THEN
  prevBSA=BSA
  BSA=((CM * Kilos)/3600)^0.5
  IF ABS(prevBSA-BSA) > 0.01 THEN
    Clear F1 F2 F3 DF1 DF2 DF3 NF1 NF2 NF3 Notes Note  Regimen
  END
  If AgeInMonths >= 24 then
    BMI=txttonum(myNutCalc!BMI(Kilos,CM ))
  END
END
```

The following will be explained in the next chapter. It returns the Percentile for age from a separate nutritional module

```
IF (Sex > "") Then
 If (Kilos > 0) OR (CM>0)then
  BMICategory=myNutCalc!NUTANYAGE(Sex,AgeInMonths,Kilos,CM)
 end
 ELSE
  Dialog "Please enter a value for Sex, either M or F"
 End
 goto CD4
ENDBEFORE
```

Summary of Weight and Stature Check Code

Managing 4 fields for English units and 2 for Metric units, and maintaining equivalence among them requires quite a bit of complexity in the program, although it should look simple from the user's point of View. The end result is that we have Kilos and Body Surface Area, both of which may be used in determining drug dosage, depending on the medication, and the source of the guidelines. The original measurements remain in the computer record, and can also be printed and inserted in the patient's paper chart if desired. Advice on printing is given in a later section.

Also in a later chapter, we will insert code to calculate Percentiles and assist in evaluating the BMI, as the expected median values change with age during childhood and adolescence.

Evaluating the CD4 Count and CD4 Percent

CD4 cells (Cluster of Differentiation) or T lymphocyte helper cells are damaged by the AIDS virus, and reduction in their count is the immunologic criterion for diagnosis of AIDS, the other criterion being the presence of defined types of clinical findings. Generally in adults, a CD4 count below 200 is taken as sufficient evidence of AIDS to start antiretroviral treatment, but the normal CD4 level differs with age in children.   Here is the code from the CD4 field that evaluates the age of the subject and places a category in the Immunosuppression field.

```
*CD4
Clear Immunosuppression
If AgeInYears = 0 Then
  SIDA_AIDS=750
  Normal=1500
else
 IF  AgeInYears >0 and AgeInYears < 6 Then
  SIDA_AIDS=500
  Normal=1000
 else
  IF  AgeInYears >=6 Then
    SIDA_AIDS=200
    Normal=500
 end
 end
end
IF (CD4 < SIDA_AIDS) OR (CD4Percent<15) then
    Immunosuppression="Severe/AIDS"
Else
 If ((CD4 >= SIDA_AIDS) AND (CD4 < Normal)) OR (CD4Percent < 25) then
    Immunosuppression="Moderate"
 end
END
IF CD4>= Normal Then
    Immunosuppression="No"
END
```

Using the age in years, we set the AIDS-defining lower value and the normal value of the CD4 count. Then labels are assigned as "Severe/AIDS" if the patient's count is below the lower value, "Moderate" if between there and normal, and "No" if Normal or above.   Criteria based on the CD4Percent, if entered, are allowed to override the absolute count, as they may be more accurate when the total lymphocyte count is abnormal.

Choosing a Medication Regimen

The user makes a choice of regimen for a new patient by clicking either the AZT button or the one for D4T. All of the recommended initial regimens contain 3TC, and it is included automatically. Simply clicking AZT does the calculations for zidovudine, lamivudine, and nevirapine (AZT+3TC+NVP), the recommended first-line regimen in the Dominican Republic, and many other countries, IF there are no contraindications. Let's look at the Check Code that screens for problems when the AZT button is clicked.

```
*AZT
IF AgeInYears = (.) OR BSA = (.) THEN
  Dialog "Please enter age or date of birth, weight, and height."
  GoTo lb
END
IF AgeInDays < 540 THEN
  Dialog "Normally, treatment for AIDS prior to 18 months requires confirmation with PCR
viral load or strong Clinicl evidence of immunosuppression.  Are you sure?" ynresponse
YN
  IF NOT (ynresponse=(+)) THEN
    CLEAR F1 F2 F3 DF1 DF2 DF3 NF1 NF2 NF3 Regimen Note Notes liq1 liq2 liq3 liq1dose
liq2dose liq3dose
    GOTO AZT
  END
END
IF Hgb < 8.2 THEN
  Dialog "With anemia (Hgb<8.2), please consider if D4T or TNF is more appropriate than
AZT."
END
```

First we look for missing values of age or body surface area, and terminate the calculation if they are not available, putting the cursor back in the first field for weight (lb). This one is like the bouncer at a club—no ID card, and you can't come in.

The next filter is a little less draconian. If the patient is less than 18 months of age (540 days), we gently ask if the diagnosis of HIV/AIDS is really confirmed, since the usual inexpensive serologic test for HIV can be falsely positive up to that age. The bouncer simply presents an informational flyer with the club rules and lets you in.

Finally, the bouncer looks at the hemoglobin that you have provided, and raises an eyebrow and a comment if the patient is anemic. Again, however, he leaves it up to you to decide on the therapy.

The logic here ignores the CD4 count, which is also important in deciding on therapy. This is a somewhat complex topic, since the AIDS-defining CD4 count differs by age in childhood, and criteria for treatment may change or differ between clinics.

We have chosen to make the program a tool for dosage, rather than a complete diagnostic guide. The latter would require more pop-up messages and data on symptoms, and run the risk of seeming more like a straitjacket than a friendly tool to the physician.

Calculating Doses for One Drug

Having survived the initial screening, or perhaps having decided to click on D4T because the patient is anemic, we are ready to do the dosage calculation. Here's what happens for AZT:

```
*Now do the calculation for the first ARV
*Put the name of the medication in the left column of the table.
 F1="AZT(Zidovudine)"
*Set up the footnote that will appear at the bottom of the screen, but keep it in a separate
variable until all three drugs are chosen.
 Note1="1,2 can be administered with food. "
*Place a description of the primary AZT+3TC+NVP regimen in the center of the page.
 TNote1="First Line Therapy, if HgB > 8.1, no AZT toxicity,"
*Place the dosage guideline in the second column.
  NF1="180-240 mg/m2 PO q12h"
*Calculate the minimum dose as 180 mgm x Body Surface Area
  Dose=(180 * BSA)
*Calculate the higher dose
  Dose1=(240 * BSA)
*Apply the maximum adult dose and do not exceed it even if the patient is unusually
heavy
  IF Dose >300 Then
   Dose=300
  END
*Do the same for the upper dose level
   IF Dose1>300 Then
   Dose1=300
  END
*Place the results in a nicely formatted text string in the third column. The FORMAT
function can use patterns like ### or ##.# to  control the number of digits and the decimal
place.

  ASSIGN Df1=Format(Dose,"###") & " - " & Format(Dose1,"###") & " mg PO q12h"
  *Calculate the Liquid dose
  Liq1Dose="10=" & Format(Dose/10,"#0.#") & " ml."
*The calculations for Lamivudine and Nevirapine then follow...
```

Calculating Doses for Three Drugs and Finding Space for All the Check Code

Calculating for the other drugs is similar in principle, but somewhat hampered by the fact that there are no "subroutines" or "functions" in Check Code, as there would be in many languages. We would like to be able to call the calculations for AZT from more than one other field, and then combine the results with those for 3TC and NVP, for example, but alas, there are no callable blocks in Check Code that can return control to more than one calling field. Although we could have used the technique described earlier, in which a dummy field is used to hold extra Check Code, we decided that it was easier to copy some of the code to other blocks, leading to some redundancy and risk of errors. But any program that calculates doses requires a lot of care and testing to avoid potential disaster, and we elected to cope with some untidiness by being especially careful when duplicating code.

Displaying Comments and Advice

Comments and advice are programmed into the code for each ARV button. For that particular button, they may result in pop-up messages. For the combinations of three ARVs however, the advice and comments are constructed from the contents of "Note" variables that are combined into a single text string at the end of the calculations. At the end of the AZT block, after placing the doses for AZT, 3TC and (if the third line is empty) NVP, in the table, the Check Code extracts whatever names are in the left column and constructs a name for the Regimen. Then it assembles text for the NOTE field from the three individual notes and for NOTES, the advice at the bottom of the page, from the individual notes.

```
D1=Substring(F1,1,3)
D2=Substring(F2,1,3)
D3=Substring(F3,1,3)
IF D3="Lop" THEN
  D3="Lop/Rit"
End
Regimen=D1 & "+" & D2 & "+" & D3
Note=TNote1 & TNote2 & TNote3
Notes=Note1 & Note2 & Note3 & Note4
*End of the AZT code; put the cursor back on the AZT button.
GOTO AZT
```

Allow Changing One Drug In the Combination

The program would have been simpler if clinicians were allowed to choose ANY three drugs from a list. This would be a disservice to patients however, as the protocols are quite specific for which drug combinations should be given early, and then in case of failure or complications. Quite a bit of this structure is imposed by the position of the buttons, the comments offered, and IF statements within the code. Thus, when you choose AZT or D4T, and lines 2 and 3 are empty, the likely choices are filled in automatically, thus excluding mono or duo therapy (except for prophylaxis) without having to mention malpractice.

When complications occur, as for example, jaundice with Nevirapine, the next drug down (Efavirens) can be chosen. Only the drug on line 3 is replaced (provided the patient weighs more than 10 kilos). The notes for the three drugs, two of which are already present, are combined with those for Efavirens, and the note fields are refreshed with the new combinations. To confirm that all legal combinations are allowed in any order, try experimenting with the various buttons.

Second line therapy is intended to use different medications from the first line (although lop/rit is often used for both because it is "such a good drug". Hence the second line therapy buttons are quite separate from the first group. Medication for HIV positive pregnant women and their babies to prevent perinatal transmission is undergoing rapid changes in the Dominican Republic , and we have not yet updated these buttons. If the mother has AIDS, however, triple therapy is appropriate, after consulting the guidelines about Efavirens, which is contraindicated in early pregnancy.

Prophylactic Medication for Opportunistic Infection

Page two contains the calculations for OI prophylaxis, an important part of HIV therapy. There are a number of choices, but the techniques for programming are the same as those on Page one.

Printing the Record

After completing the form, one can choose PRINT from the FILE menu or press Ctrl-P and obtain a reasonable image on whatever printer is the default. With ARVCalc and many other forms, the screen is horizontal and the paper is vertical, so results are better with what is called "landscape" rather than "portrait" mode. You should be able to adjust the printer settings from the print dialog. If the computer is used mainly for printing from the screen, you can adjust the default printer settings to give this and other effects permanently as described in the chapter on Output.

Conclusion

This chapter has presented antiviral medication for AIDS and HIV, as an example of the larger problem of drug dosage, particularly in children, where the necessary calculations are based on body measurements and are not easily done in one's head.

You now have the tools to begin eradicating the dangerous and unnecessary practice of relying on human memory for doses and drug interactions that is so common in the medical profession.

This chapter also describes Check Code techniques for dealing with weights and measures in English and Metric systems, of categorizing laboratory values that vary with age, and for simulating a subroutine or procedure call in Check Code.

Resources

Sample and exercise files for this chapter are found in **exARVCalc** in the **Examples** folder.

CHAPTER 20: CALLING WINDOWS DLLS FROM CHECK CODE OR ANALYSIS

Calling a Windows DLL from Check Code: EpiWeek

(From the Epi Info Help file, version 3.4.1, with editing and additions)

Epi Info allows the use of Windows Dynamic Link Librarys (DLLs) from Check Code, or, to a limited extent, from Analysis PGM code. This is a useful way of extending the built-in functions of Epi Info to include customized statistical calculations, table lookups, date manipulation, or possibly interfaces with external equipment such as a camera or laboratory instrument. DLL's are written in languages like C++ or Visual Basic and compiled for use in Microsoft Windows.

DLLs can contain both properties and methods. *Properties* are data values used by the DLL to store starting values or preferences. Examples might include what day to consider the first day of the week, language choices, or confidence levels. Property values stay the same until explicitly changed, and may have default values that are used if none are specified. *Methods* perform calculations or other functions when executed. They may or may not return values to the calling program. In some languages methods are called functions, subroutines, or procedures.

Epiweek DLL is an illustrative DLL that calculates the epidemiologic week. The user enters a date, and the DLL returns the epidemiologic week and year or just the week number to place in a field in the current record. The setps in calling a DLL from Check Code in an Epi Info View are:

1. DEFINE a variable as a DLL object and assign it the name of the DLL
2. Set properties, if needed
3. Call methods

There is an Analysis limitation in that DLLs cannot be used with field or standard variables, meaning that they are not useful for record-by-record processing

Declare a DLL Object

The Epiweek DLL must be declared in the DEFINED VARIABLES section of Check Code before it can be used.

To define a new DLL use the following syntax:

DEFINE <VarName> DLLOBJECT "<Name>.<class>"

- <VarName> any valid EpiInfo variable name you wish.

- <Name> is the internal ActiveX project name. In this case the internal name is "EIEpiwk" (but there is no way you would know this without documentation).

- <Class> refers to a class inside the DLL to be created. The Epiweek DLL contains only one class, called "Epiweek".

The code to DEFINE the DLL variable in enter is:

DEFINE Mytest DLLOBJECT "EIEpiwk.Epiweek"

Unfortunately the ENTER program will pop up an error message every time you access the View if the DLLOBJECT is missing, misspelled, or not properly registered in Windows. Since Epiweek.dll is installed and registered when Epi Info is installed, you should not have this problem.

Set Properties, If Needed

Not every DLL contains properties, but Epiweek.DLL offers several options that can be set. There are default values if you choose not to do so.

The EpiFirstDay Property

Epidemiologic weeks are usually complete weeks. The ministry of health of the country defines the day of the week to be considered the first epidemiologic day. As a result, some countries may consider the first day of the week Sunday while others may consider the first day of the week Saturday or Monday. The EpiFirstDaySetting property allows you to decide which day of the week is considered to be the first day of the epidemiologic week.

The following Check Code will set the first day settings:

<VarName>! <PROPERTY> = <Expression>

- <VarName> is the name of a DLLOBJECT variable previously defined, in this case, MyTest.

- <Property>is the name of a property defined in the DLL. In this case the property name is "EpiFirstDay".

- <Expression> is the value to which the property is to be set. It must be the type expected by the DLL. In this case, it expects a day number where Sunday=1.

The default value for this property is 1. It means that if you do not set this property, the DLL will consider that the epidemiologic week starts on Sunday by using the default value of 1.

Since we wish to start our epidemiologic weeks on Sunday, we can skip this setting, or set the property as follows:

Mytest! EpiFirstDay = 1

The Property EpiFirstWeek

Some countries may define the first week of the epidemiologic year as the week which includes January first. Other countries may consider the first epidemiologic week of the year the first full seven-day week. It is possible to change the definition for the first week of the year by setting a property called EpiFirstWeek.

> <name>! EpiFirstWeek = <number>

<Name> Is the name that you assigned to the DLL in the defined variables area

<Number> depends on what type of week you wish to use. In this case, 1 will set the first epidemiologic week as the week that includes Jan 1st, 2 defines the first epidemiologic week as the first week with four or more days, and 3 will define week number 1 as the first seven-day week of the year. If no value is set, EpiFirstweek will assume that the first week of the year is the first week with four or more days (default value of 2).

Calling a Method

Methods usually perform a calculation or other action, and may or may not return a value. Usually methods need some parameters to perform the computations. The parameter(s) to be passed to the method should be included in parenthesis. If no parameters are needed, you must include the parenthesis anyway.

Methods which do not return results are executed using the following syntax:

<name>!<method>(parameter1[, parameter2, ,...])

The Version Method

The method called Version takes no parameters and returns no results; it only displays a message box with the date of the DLL. We can call the method through the following code:

> **mytest!version()**

although the following would also work:

> **ASSIGN TEXT1 = mytest!version()**

Note: You do not need to include an ASSIGN statement because the method does not return a value.

The EpiYearWeek Method

The general syntax for executing DLL methods which return results is as follows:

<VarName> = <DllVarName>!<Method>(<Expression>, ...)

- <VarName> is the name of a variable to receive the result of the method. It is not used if no result is returned. It can be either a database avariable or one DEFINEd in Check Code.

- <DLLVarName> is the name of the DLLOBJECT variable previously defined (MyTest).

- <Method>is the name of a method defined in the DLL. In this case the method name is "EpiYearWeek".

- <Expression>is a parameter of the type expected by the DLL. If there is none, use empty parentheses. If there is more than one, separate them by commas, and be sure theymatch the required number and type of parameters. In this case, a date is expected.

Unlike the previous method, Epiyearweek takes one parameter and returns a string representing the epidemiologic week as YYYY:WW. Since the value is a text string, you cannot assign the result to a numeric variable. In the example below, TEXT1 will receive the value corresponding to the year and epidemiologic week of the onset date.

Assign Text1=Mytest!EpiYearWeek(OnsetDate)

The Epiweek Method

If the year of occurrence is not relevant, you can use the Epiweek method instead. The advantage of using Epiweek is that the value is returned as a number and it can be stored in a numeric field. Epiweek takes one required parameter that must be a date. The week is calculated relative to the year of the date provided. We calculated the epidemiologic week using the following code:

ASSIGN week = Mytest!EpiWeek(OnsetDate)

An optional numeric parameter allows the week to be computed relative to a specified year. Passing two parameters is useful to create histograms because the week numbers are sequential across multiple years. An alternative syntax to calculate the epidemiologic week for an outbreak starting in September 1, 2001 could be:

ASSIGN OutbreakWk = Mytest!Epiweek(OnsetDate, 2001) -Mytest!Epiweek(9/1/2001) + 1

The source code for EpiWk DLL is available, and is included with the source for this chapter. There are three modules, EIEpiWk.DLL, EIEpWk.VBP, and EpiWeek.CLS.
To work with them you need a Microsoft Visual Basic environment, as the bare source looks much less complicated in the Visual Basic editor. The modules can be compiled to a true Windows DLL, and then must be registered so that it can be accessed from a program like ENTER.EXE.

Making Your Own "DLL" in a Text Editor

Windows offers another method for producing customized modules with properties and methods. It is produced in an environment called the Windows Scripting Host, designed mostly for geeks to control networks or upgrade user's software. It allows you to produce a DLL-like module simply by writing either JavaScript or Visual Basic Script as plain text in a word processor like Notepad or Wordpad. This method has the advantage (or disadvntage) that the code is open for all to read or alter, and does not need to be compiled. The "Black Box" effect is gone.

Let's examine an example of a Windows Scripting Component. If you have installed and run the ARVCalc example in the previous chapter, you have already seen US2KAny.WSC in action. The viewARVMedications in ARVCalc.MDB calls US2KAny.WSC, a windows scripting component that does calculations for nutritional anthropometry. The View first calculates the Body Mass Index in a View as weight/(height*height), using kilos and centimeters. It then calls US2KAny.WSC and the Method BMIAge, with the person's sex, age in months and BMI (with an optional language preference --EN or ES) The WSC returns a text string containing a percentile based on the z-score, and a text value such as "normal", "overweight", or "underweight".

The first and last parts of US2KAny.wsc are shown later in the chapter.

Registering the US2KAny.WSC file In Windows XP 32-bit edition is relatively easy, but Windows Vista and Windows XP 64-bit edition require that you copy the file to a folder called SYSWOW64 inside the WINDOWS system folder (e.g., C:\Windows\SYSWOW64).

If registering the WSC is successful, you are ready to click the DEMO button and enter some sample data or use the left arrow at the lower left to page back through existing records and see the results of the calculations.

Enter a Date of Birth, sex, height and weight. After you enter the last one of these, you should see the BMI calculated, and then the BMI category. The latter is calculated by the WSC. If the patient is over 20 years old, you get only text output, but children get the calculated Percentile from the NCHS tables and formulas from the NHanes survey.

Have a look at US2KAny.WSC with Notepad or the printed version at the end of this chapter to see the code that is actually run in interpreted, not compiled form. It is JavaScript inside an XML wrapper that claims it is a DLL, and is treated as such by Windows. The XML part is made by a wizard, so you don't need to worry about it, but you can edit the file and change the JavaScript (or Visual Basic Script, if that's what you chose in the wizard).

Now use MakeView to look at the Check Code within the DemoDLLview in the DemoDLL.MDB. The interesting part is in the BMI field and in the variable definitions, where the WSC is treated exactly as if it were a DLL. You may also be interested in the code in various fields that prepares the measurements for calling the DLL, interconverting feet and inches with centimeters and pounds and ounces with kilograms. Finally when everything is ready, the cursor jumps to the BMI field, where the BEFORE Check Code contains the following:

```
IF CM > 0 AND Kilos > 0 THEN
  BSA=((CM * Kilos)/3600)^0.5
  BMI=Kilos* 10000 / (CM * CM )
  AgeMonths=MONTHS(FechaDeNac,FechaDeHoy)
 *Here is the call to the WSC via the DEFINEd variable called myBMICalc.
 *The method *called is BMIAge, and the parameters passed are
```
• **Sex, AgeMonths, and the calculated *BMI.**
```
  BMICategory=myBMICalc!BMIAge(Sexo,AgeMonths,BMI)
END
ENDBEFORE
```

We have added an extra parameter for the DLL call, that can be set to "ES" to return the Spanish equivalents for underweight, overweight, etc. The default is English, but you can also give "EN" for this parameter. Other languages can be added later in the WSC.

Making Your Own WSC

First download the Windows Scripting Component Wizard that Microsoft supplies gratis at

http://www.microsoft.com/downloads/details.aspx?familyid=408024ed-faad-4835-8e68-773ccc951a6b&displaylang=en

If this link doesn't work, look for Windows Scripting Component Wizard with Google.

When you run the Wizard and answer its questions, it will make a skeletal WSC in which you can insert your own JavaScript or Visual Basic Script. We chose JavaScript because we are considering using the same code in an internet version.

To generate the unique number required for each distince WSC, you will also need a program called GUIDGEN which can be found from:

http://webhome.idirect.com/~jhonz/Utilities.HTM

If you make changes in the code, it is a good idea to reregister the WSC, but it is not necessary to change the GUID number.

Microsoft has a lot of documentation on Windows Script Components, but here is a reasonable article for the How To's:

www.topxml.com/conference/wrox/2000_vegas/text/brianm_wsc.pdf

The Code for US2KAny.WSC

```
<?xml version="1.0"?>
<component>

<?component error="true" debug="true"?>

<registration
        description="US2000"
        progid="US2KAny.WSC"
        version="1.00"
        classid="{0c470e66-a6f7-4b60-a2f2-b0bce44d5a7a}"
>
</registration>

<public>
        <method name="BMIAge">
                <PARAMETER name="mf"/>
                <PARAMETER name="months"/>
                <PARAMETER name="numvalue"/>
         <PARAMETER name="language"/>
        </method>
</public>
```

```
<script language="JScript">
<![CDATA[

var description = new US2000;

function US2000()
{
        this.BMIAge = BMIAge;
}

...FOUR PAGES of code here to return results. You can see it all by
   examining US2KAny.WSC in a text editor.....

]]>
</script>
</component>
```

A WSC to Generate Global Unique Identifiers (GUIDs)

Idea and Program by Roger A. Mir, MSSE, BSCS, MCSD

Epi Info provides an identifier called UniqueKey for every record. UniqueKey, however, is only guaranteed to be unique within the same dataset. You have the option to start the generation of UniqueKey at a particular number when you first generate a data table in MakeView or Enter. Hence, you can start records generated by ten data entry clerks with numbers starting with an different multiple of a thousand. This allows easy merging of the uniquely labelled records, but works only until each of the clerks enters more than a thousand records, after which a merge will overwrite some valuable records.

A GUID is a pseudo-randomly generated number so large (3.4×10^{38}) that a duplicate number is "unlikely" ever to be generated in our lifetime, our world, etc. If there are 5×10^{22} stars in the observable universe, every star could have 6.8×10^{15} unique GUIDs[1] (if some sort of Johnny Appleseed character gave them out one-by-one sequentially, it appears).

Using Windows Script Components to Generate a GUID.

Using Windows' My Computer, find the file called GetUniqueGlobalID.WSC in the Examples\Ch20\ folder. RIGHT-click on the WSC file and select Register. You should receive a notice that registration succeeded. You only have to register the WSC once for the life of the computer, but it must be done before the component can be called from the Epi Info View.

---

1 http://en.wikipedia.org/wiki/Globally_Unique_Identifier

After registering the WSC you can see the demo in action, by using ENTER to access the View called GUIDDemo in GUIDDemo.MDB in the examples for Ch20. With each new record you should see the UniqueKey value generated by Epi Info, and the GUID value generated by the WSC.

To see the Check Code, Open the View in MakeView and click the PROGRAM button on the left side of the screen. The variables in GUIDDemo are: UniqueKeyAssigned, GlobalUniqueID, and Name.

In the block called DEFINED VARIABLES, you will find:

```
DEFINE myGUID  DLLOBJECT "GetGlobalUniqueID.wsc"
```

The syntax:is:

DEFINE <variable name> DLLOBJECT <"Windows Script Component file name">

In the block called RECORD

```
ALWAYS
    UniqueKeyAssigned=UniqueKey
    If GlobalUniqueID=(.) OR GlobalUniqueID="" THEN
      ASSIGN GlobalUniqueID=myGUID!GetGlobalUniqueID()
    END
END
ENDBEFORE
```

The syntax is:

```
ASSIGN <field name>=<defined variable name>!<VBScript function name>
```
Here is the code inside the separate file called GetGlobalUniqueID.WSC, constructed with the help of the Microsoft Windows Scripting Host. Note that it assigns a GUID to the module as an identifier, and that this script takes advantage of the same capability to generate GUIDs when called.

```
<?xml version="1.0"?>
<component>

        <?component error="true" debug="true"?>
        <registration
                description="GlobalUniqueID"
                progid="GetGlobalUniqueID.WSC"
                version="1.00"
                classid="{EF72B1F9-4415-42FB-A157-CD0713A84CDA}">
        </registration>



        <public>
                <method name="GetGlobalUniqueID">
```

```
                </method>
            </public>

            <script language="VBScript">
            <![CDATA[

                Function GetGlobalUniqueID()
                        Set objID = CreateObject("Scriptlet.TypeLib")
                        GetGlobalUniqueID=mid(objID.GUID,2,36)
                End Function


            ]]>
            </script>
        </component>
```

Reference:

N H A N E S - United States Growth Charts - Data Files. National Center for Health Statistics, Centers for Disease Control and Prevention (CDC)

http://0-www.cdc.gov.library.ccf.org/nchs/about/major/nhanes/growthcharts/datafiles.htm 2000: Accessed Sept 3, 2007.

Resources

Sample and exercise files for this chapter are found in exDLLs in the Examples folder. EpiWeek is included in the installed Epi_Info folder

CHAPTER 21: PHYSICAL SECURITY: THEFT, DISK FAILURE, HUMAN ERROR, AND ELECTRICITY

Problems

One of us (AD) used Epi Info views to enter, store, and analyze data in a clinic in the Dominican Republic during the four years prior to October 2008. During that time the clinic experienced :

- Separate thefts of two laptops and a monitor

- At least 6 hard disk failures

- Thousands of data entry errors, and occasional larger problems where a file was overwritten during a merging operation

- Numerous computer viruses (more than 30 in one unprotected 10-minute period on the Internet) and instances of spyware, adware, and other predators. (But never in the presence of adequate and updated Internet security software)

- Almost daily power outages and much voltage variation, at least once serious enough to melt and set fire to surge protectors

I wish we could tell you all the magic answers that we (or those responsible) should have had in place, but there are lots of documents that give recommendations, so we will outline some of the rough and ready horse-out-of-barn measures that we took, and then focus on doing backups and encryption with the help of the Epi Info menu so that data is less likely to be lost or read by others when these events occur.

Theft

The first break-in and theft occurred while we were discussing the need for bars on the doors that did not yet have them. The thief, perhaps with inside information, used a crowbar of modest dimensions on a wooden door, and gained access to the entire clinic, entering the record room through a sliding glass window that had a defective lock, and stole a laptop computer. After this, we consulted our ironmonger, who finished protecting all the doors and windows with iron bars, closed with padlocks as needed.

Now the question arose, how would a person inside the building get out in case of fire? We screwed plastic boxes to the wall near two exits with emergency keys to the exits, and labeled them with signs.

A few weeks later, the watchman next door made his rounds and noted that the clinic door was open. Investigating, he encountered a thief, who was in the process of preparing another computer for transport. Apparently he had hidden inside the clinic at closing time and used the emergency key from the wall to get out. Unbelievable as it seems, he escaped over a wall during further conversation with the watchman and a nun!

So we contracted to have an alarm installed—the kind that detects movement inside the building and sets off an external siren if it has been armed. After a while, senior staff learned how to arm and disarm the alarm and lock the iron barred door. We also installed iron bars on the internal windows of the record room, as they did not interfere with passing records or information, but secured the records better against theft. Did we solve the problem? Well, no one has hidden in the clinic after closing, and we took down the emergency keys, since the alarm can detect late workers when we exit. But the alarm battery tends to lose its charge after a weekend of no power, and some periods are without its coverage.

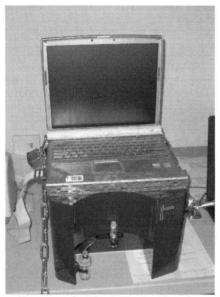

**Homemade Theft Protection for
Laptop and CD4 Counter**

To protect the remaining three laptops, we devised a harness similar to those in computer stores, but made from locally purchased battery cables or chains, u-bolts, and padlocks. The cables would probably not withstand large, compound bolt-cutters, but they prevented constrained laptops from walking away.

The next laptop—a personal one--was stolen immediately after a staff meeting when it was used for a presentation, and then ignored briefly while equipment was put away. We became more careful (this phrase gets a lot of use here) to attach laptops with a portable theft cable even during staff meetings. An employee about whom we had some misgivings moved on to other pastures, and we think this also may have been helpful.

What do we recommend for your situation? Follow the advice of those boring books on security, "assess the threats" and do something about them. Unfortunately, if this is not entirely successful, learn from the incidents, and patch the holes they make evident.

Electricity and Fire

Power outages were common, sometimes several times per day, meaning that battery backup was necessary. We purchased "Uninterruptable Power Supplies" (UPSs) for each computer that also provided protection against voltage surges. The batteries generally went bad after a year or two, and we found that laptop computers not only used less power than desktops, but had the extra advantage of having their own internal batteries that allowed them to function for hours rather than minutes when the power was off.

Periodically, we had surges of high voltage that could destroy any electronic equipment that happened to be connected and turned on at the time. Most of these were transient and were managed by the surge suppressors that we maintained for each piece of equipment. One episode, however, lasted for about 15 minutes, causing 30 or 40 fluorescent lights to glow like the sun and then burn out, setting two fires, and burning out and even melting most of the surge protectors that had equipment connected. The equipment was protected however, and surge protectors are valuable and necessary in many localities. Note that those designed for 120 volts emit smoke and die in 220 volt circuits, something we demonstrated in Mexico.

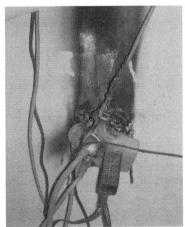

**Fried Surge Protector.
Attached equipment was not
harmed.**

CHAPTER 22: THE EPI INFO MENU

OK, enough of physical security, and back to Epi Info. The Epi Info menu can be programmed (some would say "scripted") to carry out a number of useful tasks, including those related to software security. We will use a clinic system to illustrate. First, let's review how the menu works and how to make it perform at your command (or someone else's).

The program called EpiInfo.exe, if left to itself, loads a text file called EpiInfo.mnu that is the main Epi Info menu. However if you develop a different MNU file--MyClinic.MNU, for example-- almost everything about the menu can be changed to suit your application. One way to do this is simply to make a copy of EpiInfo.MNU and rename it to MyClinic.MNU. In the Examples\exMakeMenu, we have provided a customized menu called MakeMenu.MNU that will manufacture a new menu skeleton that you can refine for your own application.

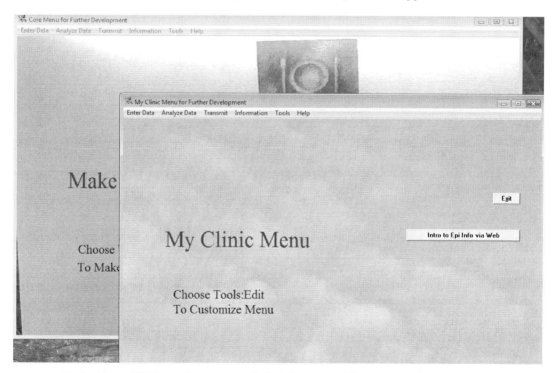

MakeMenu.MNU creates a new skeletal menu with a name of your choice.

Using MakeMenu to Make a Menu

New menus can be made using the method just described and My Computer to copy and rename files. We have provided a menu that makes menus, however, in a folder called MakeMenu in the

Examples for this chapter. To make a new menu, simply copy the MakeMenu folder to a folder where you would like to have the new menu, and then double-click on the shortcut called "Click Here to Run MakeMenu." Follow the instructions to make a menu and a desktop icon with a name that you choose, ignoring the security warnings if necessary. Then use EDIT THIS MENU in the new menu to examine the MNU file and its documentation and add your own commands. Documentation presented as comments (starting with an asterisk) in the text of the MNU file. Note that an image called SKY.JPG replaces the EPIINFO.JPG used in the Epi Info menu and the London restaurant menu in MakeMenu.MNU. Of course, you will want to provide your own theme picture and choose it from CHANGE PICTURE on the TOOLS menu.

How to Run a Menu File

If you used MakeMenu to construct your menu, and an icon was placed on the desktop, running the new menu is simply a matter of clicking on the icon. Since you may be constructing menus for others to use, and they may not have MakeMenu, here are some details about running MNU files.

The MNU file requires EpiInfo.EXE in order to run, there are several ways to put the two together, none of them as graceful as one might wish.

1. Set up a file association between the MNU extension and EpiInfo.EXE by RIGHT clicking on the MNU file's entry in My Computer and choosing Open With from the menu that pops up. You can then navigate to the Epi_Info folder and choose EPIINFO.EXE, choosing Always Use the Selected Program in the dialog. In the future, you will be able to run MNU files merely by clicking their entries, and EpiInfo.EXE will run automatically.

2. Set up a desktop icon for the MNU by RIGHT clicking the MNU and choosing Send To Desktop (Make Shortcut). Then RIGHT click on the Shortcut that appears and choose Properties. Insert the words EPIINFO.EXE before the address of the MNU with a space between the two entries, and click OK. Now clicking on the desktop should run the new MNU.

3. If you make a copy of EPIINFO.EXE, place it in the same folder with the new MyClinic.MNU and rename it so that to MyClinic.EXE, the menu will run if you click on MyClinic.EXE. This is a bit wasteful of disk space (385 K), but reliable and easy to understand if you are distributing an application to others.

4. From inside a menu, the MENU command will run another menu, e.g.,

   MENU MyClinic.MNU

5. From the Windows Command Prompt, you can use CD (Change Directory) to navigate to the folder where the MNU is located and then type EPIINFO.EXE MyClinic.MNU

Menu Commands

There are three main parts to the menu

1. The background picture, specified in the Edit menu, or with the PICTURE command. For details on the commands, consult the Epi Info help file.

2. The structure and wording of the menu, specified in the MNU as POPUPS, MENUITEMS, BUTTONS, and SCREENTEXT.

3. Command Blocks, each one beginning with a name and containing commands within a Begin .....End structure. This are called by clicking MenuItems or Buttons that refer to them by name. Unlike Check Code blocks, extra command blocks can be created and called from another block to perform a particular service that may be needed repeatedly.. The two special blocks STARTUP and SHUTDOWN are called automatically when the menu is first run and as execution stops, repectively.

From the EDIT menu, choose EDIT THIS MENU or use Notepad or any text editor to see the MNU text file. After making changes be sure to save the file as a text file and not an RTF or Word document. The MNU file will reload automatically when changes are saved, based on monitoring of the file date and time at frequent intervals.

What Kind of Commands Can You Put in a Menu?

1. Menu commands, which include a very capable IF..THEN..ELSE..ENDIF that can be nested to quite a depth, the versatile REPLACE command to replace unique words in any text file, including Analysis PGMs. EXECUTE will run any executable file, such as all the rest of the Epi Info programs, or a file that has a Windows association with an executable. You can also run other menus with the MENU command.

2. DOS commands, like COPY, XCOPY, ECHO, DIR, ETC. These can be included in a menu command block or placed in a separate batch (.BAT) file and run as such. The menu instructions caution against mixing Windows commands and DOS command in the same block, but sometimes, with careful testing, this can be done.

3. Windows script files in either jscript or Visual Basic Script, if you use them with cscript.exe or wscript.exe.

Variables in the Menu

Variables can be defined in the menu merely by using them in an ASSIGN command (with or without the word ASSIGN). If the variable is first used in the STARTUP block, the variable is defined as permanent. Its value is stored in the EPIINFO.INI file, located in the @@IniDir, and can be accessed from other Epi Info programs or from the menu, even after the computer or Epi Info has been shut down and restarted. Variables assigned inside menu command blocks are temporary variables, visible only inside the menu during the current session.

The value of a variable can be obtained using "@@" with the variable name. There are a number of useful predefined variables, including:

MenuDir, InstallDir, WorkDir, IniDir, ThisMenu, and SystemDate. @@MenuDir is the complete path of the directory where the MNU file is located. @@InstallDir is the directory where Epi Info is installed. @@SystemDate comes from Windows, and includes both the current date and time. Examples of the values in these variables can be seen from the HELP menu within MakeMenu.MNU by choosing PREDEFINED VARIABLES.

Menu variables can be embedded in menu commands preceded by @@, and their value is used as part of the command. Hence the command:

Copy @@InstallDir\Sample.mdb @@MenuDir\

will copy the Sample.mdb file to the directory where the MNU containing this command resides. When using @@, the interpreter must be able to identify the end of the variable name, either with a space or a backslash. Hence the command above will work just as well as:

Copy @@InstallDir \Sample.mdb @@MenuDir \

but

Assign Filename="MyText.txt"

Dialog "@@Filename is where our notes are kept."

will show "MyText.txtis where our notes are kept."

TWO spaces are required after @@Filename, as one is automatically eliminated.

Dialog "@@Filename is where our notes are kept." (two spaces after "@@Filename")

will show "MyText.txt is where our notes are kept." as intended.

Running Programs from the Menu

The EXECUTE command runs Windows (or DOS batch) programs, using, if necessary, file associations that come with Windows, the commonest of these being that EXECUTE "Somefile.HTM" will run the default browser and show Somefile.HTM.

The following runs WordPad, a Windows editor. It is not necessary to give the *location (path) for WordPad, or for Epi Info programs, because Windows "knows" *their location.

    Execute WordPad.exe

Now let's tell WordPad what file to open

    Execute WordPad.exe "@@MenuDir\MyFile.TXT"
    Execute WordPad.exe "@@ThisMenu"

Note that quotation marks in case the path or file name contains spaces. @@ThisMenu is a special menu variable that gives the path and name of the current menu.

With Epi Info databases, you may have to specify not only the MDB, but the View or Data table within the MDB. An example is given in menus created by MakeMenu in the EnterCases block:.

Execute Enter.exe Sample.MDB:Surveillance

A more precise way to specify this command would be to use the predefined variable INSTALLDIR, which provides the name of the directory in which Epi Info is installed. The command in this format would be:

EXECUTE @@INSTALLDIR \ENTER.EXE @@INSTALLDIR \SAMPLE.MDB:Surveillance

Note the lack of quotation marks and that the table viewSurveillance is called Surveillance without the "view" prefix. The @@ symbol indicates "Insert the value of the following variable here"

Unfortunately, the Analysis program requires a slightly different syntax, best illustrated by another example from menus created in MakeMenu.

Here's how to run an Analysis program that is contained inside an MDB. The sample program called STATISTICS, supplied with Epi Info, will do for illustration. The program exercises most of the statistical routines in Analysis.

Execute Analysis.exe pgmname='@@InstallDir\Sample.MDB':"Statistics" viewname='@@InstallDir\Sample.MDB':viewOswego

Note that "Statistics" is the name of the program within the MDB. This name MUST be in double quotes if the name of the program is a reserved word in Analysis (There is a "STATISTICS" setting in Analysis) or if the program name contains any spaces. Hence it is a good idea ALWAYS to put it in double quotes. The Execute command must be all on one line.

The ViewName= parameter sets the name of the MDB and View that will be considered the HOME database when Analysis runs the program. In this case the program begins with READ 'Sample.mdb':viewOswego and the ViewName parameter is needed to make sure that the default for Sample.MDB is that of @@InstallDir, the installation directory.
Note that the View name, viewOswego should NEVER be enclosed in double quotes, or the statement will not work.
To access programs in a directory other than the current one or InstallDir, it may be necessary to resort to some tricks. Analysis cannot work with a relative path like "..\", so we set the menu's Working Directory to the relative path as follows:

WorkDir="@@menudir\..\..\exSurveillance\"
Execute Analysis.exe pgmname='@@WorkDir\surveillance.mdb':"MapHepatitisARates" viewname='@@WorkDir\surveillance.mdb':viewCaseReports

The first means, "Set the special variable called WorkDir to the exSurveillance folder which is two levels up from the directory where the menu resides (menudir) and then down one level" --a little like a child of MenuDir's grandparent who is not MenuDir's parent--in other words an uncle or aunt of MenuDir. Now we can access the database that is in WorkDir:

> It is also possible to run a program that has been saved as a text file. The
> following line will run a STATISTICS.PGM program
> in the installed directory. It works with or without the "pgmname=" syntax.

EXECUTE Analysis.exe pgmname='@@InstallDir \STATISTICS.PGM'

> The following line should run whatever series of commands were active on the last exit
> from Analysis. (Analysis saves your last program as LastPgm.PGM in case you forget to do so.)

EXECUTE Analysis.exe '@@InstallDir\LastPgm.pgm'

Further documentation is in the HELP Contents, under EXECUTE for the menu and the programs Enter and Analysis.

Timing and Sequencing in Menu Commands

The DOS operating system that preceded Microsoft Window is based on text commands, executed one after the other in sequence, so that one command is completed before another is executed. Microsoft Windows, however, and Visual Basic, the language with which Epi Info is built, process commands asynchronously, meaning that they do not necessarily wait for the results of one command before starting to process the next. This leads to problems if one of the commands creates or copies a file, and the next command makes use of the new file for some purpose. Because Windows does not wait for the first command to complete before processing the second command, the second may lead to an error such as "File not found," that, with a second or two of delay, would have been corrected.

There are several commands in the Menu that attempt to fix this problem. The broad-axe approach is to insert a DIALOG box, such as

DIALOG "Proceed?"

A dialog is so-called "modal," that is, it stops the flow of commands and the next command will not be executed until someone clicks "OK" in the dialog. This is a good way to test whether a problem is due to timing and asynchronous processing. If you suspect that it is, insert a dialog temporarily. If the extra wait imposed by the dialog fixes the problem, then consider using one of the commands: WAITFOR, WAITFOREXIT (from a specified program, like Enter or Analysis), WAITFORFILEEXISTS (with an option that it be less than xx seconds old), which are documented in the Epi Info Help file. WAITFOREXIT seems to work pretty reliably; the others require some experimentation to find and verify the right choice and syntax.

If the operation being performed is only occasional, I sometimes choose to insert dialog commands that inform the user about the steps of the operation and avoid any difficulty with sequencing and timing. An example is contained in MakeMenu.MNU, in which creating a new menu requires a series of confirmations from the user, without my having to worry about whether the various WAITFORs work properly with the sequence of programmatically writing a Visual Basic Script and running it to put an icon on the desktop.

Testing MNU Programs

Because there are so many versions of Windows available, and even more kinds of "Security" software and regulations, some of your most successful tricks and workarounds in menu programs may not always work. Hence, if you intend to distribute your system, it is important to test the programs in as many different computers as possible, and under conditions shared by many users. In a single clinic, of course, you have information about the target computers, and can confine your testing to these.

In a later chapter, we give advice on debugging, but, for menus, liberal use of the DIALOG command to interrupt processing and display the value of variables is useful. The menu is unique among the Epi Info suite of programs in being able to display the value of variables in a dialog, and this is a powerful ally for debugging.

Managing Files: Creating, Copying, Joining

There are many ways to create text files. A simple way is to use a word processor like WordPad or Notepad and save the file in text (TXT) format. Another way is to use a DOS ECHO command with the redirection symbol (>) as follows:

ECHO Error in line 39 > Error.Log
ECHO Error in line 42 >> Error.Log

The first line creates a new file or overwrites the previous one; the second line appends the text to the file if it already exists.

Copying files from one place to another requires the path and name of the existing file, and the destination. There are various parameters that can be given with a "/" after the command to specify what happens if the destination file already exists, etc. Instructions for DOS commands like COPY (and XCOPY) are easy to find on the Internet by googling, for example, for [DOS COPY tutorial] (without brackets or quotes). Here's a simple example:

COPY @@MenuDir\DATA\MASTER.MDB   D:\TodaysBackup\

You can also practice using DOS commands in the Windows Command Prompt, the dark little window available under Accessories in the Windows Program Menu. After finding a command that works, you can insert it in a block in the MNU. To get information about a DOS command, type   /? after the command and you should see a list of options.

The COPY command can join several files, with the following syntax:

COPY File1+File2+File3 DoIt.pgm

This could be used to put together a customized program from selected pieces.

DIALOG with "The User"

The DIALOG command in the menu has several forms that are documented in the Epi Info help files. Since it is different from the DIALOG command in Check Code and Analysis programs, it is important to consult the help file and use the correct syntax for the menu version of DIALOG. As mentioned above, one important use for the DIALOG command is to interrupt the flow of commands so that Windows does not go skating on past a task before it is complete.

To find the documentation, pull down the HELP menu in Epi Info and then CONTENT. Searching for DIALOG will bring up three apparently identical entries for DIALOG COMMAND, of with the third one is applies to the MENU dialog. As they say in computerese, the content is "rich", meaning bewildering, but there are a number of useful features, and the rest are available for study and experimentation.

Let's interrupt the flow of commands with a simple DIALOG:

DIALOG "Continue?"

This might be used to slow things down while files are being copied from one place to another so that they are available for the next command. The dialog has an OK button and execution of commands resumes as soon as the user clicks OK.

The form of DIALOG that specifies BUTTONS is especially useful because specifying a variable and one or more BUTTONS will automatically place a CANCEL button in the dialog, as in:

DIALOG "Continue?", goahead, BUTTONS="OK";

This time a CANCEL button is displayed automatically, and clicking CANCEL will cause the menu to skip all the remaining commands in the same command block. It is a simple way to bail out of a series of commands, perhaps after warning the user about a time-consuming process or a missing file. You will find several examples of this use of DIALOG in the ARVCalc and exClinic systems in following chapters.

Note that the variable "goahead", does not need to be pre-defined, but it may be best to give it a unique name to avoid confusion with permanent variables defined elsewhere in the menu or in other programs.

REPLACE to Customize Programs and Other Files

The REPLACE command is only available in the menu, and offers a way to insert phrases or files into programs, HTML output, or other files so that they can be customized for a particular computer or set of responses from the user. Both Analysis programs and Check Code work best with exact Windows path and filenames embedded in commands. Here is a one-line program called TEST.PGM that might be located in the same folder with the menu from which you intend to run it:

READ Sample.mdb:Oswego

TEST.PGM may work when run from the menu, if Analysis happens to be "pointed" at the Epi_Info folder as its default, but, if you have directed Analysis elsewhere during another exercise, it may not be able to find Sample.mdb. The solution is to keep a source copy of TEST.PGM called, for example, TEST.SRC, and use REPLACE in the menu to insert the correct path on the current computer, as follows:

REPLACE Sample.mdb,@@installDir\Sample.mdb FROM @@MenuDir\TEST.SRC TO @@MenuDir\TEST.PGM

Recall that "@@" means, "the value of" the variable name that follows, and this should make sense.

TEST.SRC will remain intact, but TEST.PGM might become:

READ C:\Epi_Info\Sample.mdb:Oswego

and could be run from the same menu block with the following command:

EXECUTE Analysis.exe pgm=@@MenuDir\TEST.PGM

Since REPLACE can also substitute an entire file for a word or phrase, it can be used to insert either textual or programmatic "boilerplate" into a file such as an Analysis output HTM file.

REPLACE allows you to write custom programs dynamically from within the menu, and is a key component of the SAFE system described in a later chapter.

CALL a Block as a "Function" or Subroutine

As illustrated in the exClinic system, it is possible to use the CALL command to jump to another block of commands. After that block is executed, control returns to the line after the CALL command, so that the called block behaves like a function or subroutine in other languages. In order to pass values of variables to the called block, however, they must be defined and have values. In the Clinic system, for example, the name of an Analysis program is passed as the variable PGM so that a block of commands called "DoAnalysis" can run the named program from the menu.

(Very) Artificial Intelligence: The IF Command

The IF command in menu programs will be your friend UNLESS you forget the ENDIF at its conclusion and use END instead. Then strange things happen because the command block terminates within the IF statement and the menu becomes confused. It is otherwise quite flexible, and allows one IF statement to be nested within another to several levels. (A nested IF in the ELSE clause must be the first line after ELSE.).

IF is useful for checking whether a file exists (IF EXISTS("MyFile") ....) and issuing a DIALOG message in the ELSE clause if not. You can also give the user a choice with DIALOG, and then use the IF command to execute the choices, depending on the result contained in a variable set by the DIALOG.

Both the ARVCalc and exClinic examples in later chapters contain many examples of IF commands. While you are programming, it may be useful to insert temporary DIALOG commands (e.g., DIALOG "One") in the IF and ELSE blocks to test how the logic is working.

Resources

Sample and exercise files for this chapter are found in **exMakeMenu** in the **Examples** folder.

CHAPTER 23: CLINICAL COMPUTING—A COMPLETE SYSTEM

Background

The example in this chapter was developed in La Romana in the Dominican Republic for an HIV/AIDS clinic. It was put into service in January 2006. Three years later, it contained data for 1500 patients and about 20,000 visits, individual patients having as many as 99 visits. The original system was built in Spanish, and the example presented here as exClinic has been translated and/or rewritten in English.

Because exClinic is entirely built with Epi Info for Windows (version 3.5.1), it illustrates many of the features that can be used to build a complete system. The difficulties that were encountered along the way illustrate the problems that must be solved in developing clinical computer systems.

Plan for This Chapter

Because exClinic is a complicated application, the details will be presented at two levels. For those who merely want to try it out and see what it does, the Menu, Data Entry, and Analysis sections will be described from a user's point of view. Most sections are followed by notes about the location of the Epi Info code and the functions that it illustrates.

Since all the code is provided in the example, along with obfuscated records from 340 patients and 2800 visits, you are invited to explore the nooks and crannies, and experiment with alternative solutions to the problems.

Installing the exClinic Demo System

To see the sample clinic system in action and examine the files, copy the exClinic folder from \Examples for this book. If you have installed Epi Info for Windows, Version 3.5.1, it should not matter where you install exClinic, although it should be on the local disk drive of a computer with Windows XP, Vista, or Windows 7. Other systems may work, but have not been tested.

Copying the exClinic folder will create contained folders that are part of the system. The main menu,CLINIC.MNU, and related files are in the exClinic folder. A folder called DATA contains Master.mdb, a database with 340 sample patient records and 2800 visits. PROGRAMS contains Analysis programs for each of the Reports offered by the menu. When a report is requested, necessary programs are copied to the ANALYSIS folder and run against a copy of the database called ANALYSIS.MDB. Encrypted copies of the ANALYSIS folder are kept in the COPIES folder. Backup copies of the entire system can be made with with a single menu choice. A computer name can be set from the CHOOSE COMPUTER NAME in the CONFIGURATION menu to identify the backup files.

If you have not previously established a Windows association of .MNU files with EpiInfo.exe, RIGHT click on the name or icon for CLINIC.MNU. Choose OPEN WITH and then navigate to the Epi_Info folder and select EpiInfo.exe. After performing this step, subsequent clicks on CLINIC.MNU should run the program automatically and show the following screen.

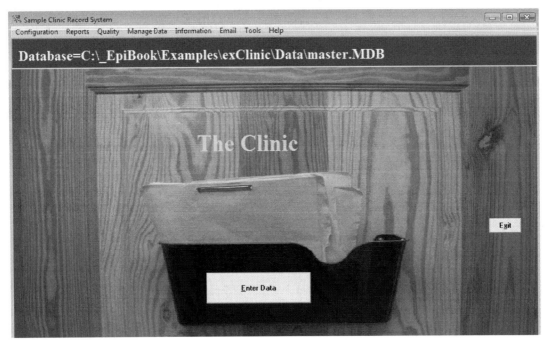

Do not be disappointed if the Database is not indicated above the picture of the clinic door and the words "The Clinic" are missing or replaced by a dot. You can use the CONFIGURATION menu to set these up as described below.

Configuration

The first part of the menu to explore is the CONFIGURATION menu. Click to make it drop down and then choose ENTER CLINIC NAME, giving whatever name you would like to your facility. Similarly, in COMPUTER NAME you can choose a name for the workstation, such as "RegDesk1" or "ER", if there will be more than one computer on a network.

CHOOSE DATABASE selects the database that will be brought up when you click the ENTER DATA button in the middle of the screen. After choosing the database, its name and location will appear at the top of the screen in a panel. Initially the database is set up to be the one in the exClinic example, but eventually you may choose to make a copy of the MASTER.MDB file, delete the data and establish your own database. We have supplied an empty database called NewDB.MDB in the DATA folder, along with Master.MDB, which contains sample data.

Details of how the CHOOSE DATABASE function works are contained in the menu block by that name in CLINIC.MNU and in the technical notes at the end of this chapter.

What the Menu Does

The usual activities of the system are carried out with the ENTER DATA button, and the three menus for REPORTS, QUALITY evaluation, and MANAGING DATA. You can access search engines in INFORMATION and configure EMAIL for your own preferences by editing the CLINIC.MNU with the EDIT THIS MENU option in TOOLS. Editing the MNU file also allows you to program your own functions in the menu and incorporate other Analysis programs and/or databases that you may create.

Exploring Data Entry

The Patient Record View

Click the ENTER DATA button to see the first page of a Patient record. As always in Epi Info, the Enter program opens the next new and empty record in the database. Look at the lower left corner to see how many records exist—about 340 in the demo. Use the left arrow (<) to page back a record or two until you find record number 339.

Note the demographic and initial intake information, and then click the VISIT button to see the visit records. Since you are on the fifth visit record, click the left arrow (<) to move back to previous visits. Note that these have different Date-Of-Visit values, but that the Clinic ID and the Treatment ID and basic demographic information have been carried over from the Patient record. The Body Surface Area(BSA) and Body Mass Index (BMI) have been calculated for the height and weight recorded at each visit, an important activity in administering ARV's to children. The doses for the patient's three ARVs in liquid preparations are calculated and recorded, and advice and warnings for these three medications appear on the right side of the screen.

Return to the Patient record screen by clicking the BACK button in the left panel. Now click NEW to begin entering a new record. Enter the name as "Domi" with Family Name of "Indom" and press the Enter key. (You may have to enter 0000 in the Treatment ID to get to this point). A search is automatically conducted for Domi's name and an existing record (#333) is found. To retrieve the record, double click on the left side of the line where it is listed.

The Patient Record offers only a few special features. It coordinates Treatment ID numbers with the Group value, since only Group 1 patients are on Highly Active Antiretroviral Therapy (HAART) and have Treatment ID numbers other than zero. Try to change the Group choice to see how this works. There are two sets of calculations in this page. One produces Age from Date of Birth and the Date of entry into the system. The other calculates Body Mass Index from the patient's initial weight and height. When you click the Visit button, additional Check Code gathers the values of selected variables and assigns them to global variables so that they are available in the related Visit view automatically. This will be explained in a later section.

The Visit View

Since one patient may have many visits, the Visit view is related to the main Patient Record view. In the Patient Record for "Domi INDOM," click the VISIT button to bring up a new Visit Record. Note that this is Domi's second visit. Use the (<) button to see the first visit, which, we learn, was on May 6, 2008. At that time, Domi weighed 198 pounds (90 kilos) with a normal Body Mass Index of 25.4. Although his CD4 count of 261 was low, it did not qualify him for HAART at that time and place (guidelines vary by country and over time), and he was not started on HAART.

Click the NEW button to enter a new Visit record. Let's assume that the Date of Visit is today; you can enter the Date of Visit or simply press the Enter key for today's date. Note that a number of calculations occur, including Age and Months in Center. Clearly Domi is long overdue for a visit, and a warning pops up about the need for another CD4 count. Domi's appearance has changed radically, and you find that today he weighs 124 pounds. Under Body Measurements, enter today's date and for Pounds, enter 124. We see that the Body Mass Index has dropped to a somewhat alarming 15.9. Now change the date for the CD4 count to be today's date, and enter the low value of 49 that just came back from the laboratory. For the Hemoglobin, enter today's date and 7.9. Domi not only has AIDS (defined in many places as CD4<200), but is also severely anemic.

Your physical exam shows white exudate in the tongue and pharynx (thrush), muscular wasting, and cervical, axillary, and inguinal lymph nodes, findings that you should record in the box under the ENTER NOTES button. Clearly Domi should be started on HAART; click the HAART Regimen field to see the choices. They are listed in rough order of priority for new patients, and you can see descriptions in the box to the right in the HAART group of fields. Let's pretend that you are a little tired and do not notice the hemoglobin of 7.9. Click the 01 AZT+3TC+NVP choice to choose the normal starting regimen. Now enter 14 days in the FOR ____ DAYS field and click the PRESCRIBE NOW button. A warning appears that this may not be a good choice (AZT itself causes anemia, and choosing it might be considered malpractice). Since you are the doctor, you can still make this choice (perhaps you are on a mountain top and have only these three drugs), but normal wisdom suggests that you go to choice #02. This time, there are no complaints, and doses are displayed in the boxes for the usual triple therapy. Because Domi is an adult, the dosages are given for capsules and tablets, although you can choose liquid preparations if he is so ill that these are needed. Note that the dosage of Nevirapine is to be adjusted to once per 24 hours for the first 14 days, as shown in the notes on the right side of the screen.

Prophylaxis against opportunistic infections is essential for a patient with such a low CD4 count (49). Click the PCP button for Pneumocytis Carinii Pneumonia prophylaxis. One tablet of Trimethoprim/Sulfamethoxazole per day is recommended, but other choices can be seen if you click PCP several times.

Click VITS several times until you arrive at Adult Vits/Fe, the routine prescription for adult AIDS patients.

You ask Domi if he has ever had tuberculosis treatment and his chest film does not show active TB (or PCP). Since more than half of the surrounding population is tuberculin positive, you click TB to prescribe prophylactic INH.

Mycobacterium Avium Complex or MAC bacteria are a serious hazard for AIDs patients with CD4 counts under 50, and you click the MAC button and choose weekly Azithromycin as the most convenient prophylaxis.

The date of next appointment is calculated automatically from the number of days prescribed, with allowances if it falls on a weekend, but you can change it by changing the Next Appt In field at the bottom of the screen.

In order to have a paper copy of the Visit page, you pull down the FILE menu at the top of the page and choose PRINT. The first time you do this, you may want to set printer preferences to Landscape (horizontal) mode and black-and-white printing. If you do this from the Windows Printing Control rather than from inside Epi Info, and then set your printer to be the default printer, the changes will persist between sessions, and clicking on PRINT or pressing Ctrl-P will be enough to print the current screen in a format suitable for the paper record. We have already used the MakeView program to set the background of the form to white, thus saving a good deal of ink or toner for the printer.

To return to the Patient Record, choose the BACK or the HOME button on the left side of the screen (Both do the same thing when there is only one level of related forms.) In the Patient Record, fill in the Case Report Sent with a "Yes" and supply the Notification Number. Change the Current HAART Regimen to D4T+3TC+NVP, and give today's date for Date ARV's Initiated.

If you wish to enter a new patient record from the beginning, click the NEW button at this point. In any case, by finding the record belonging to Domi Indom, and entering a complete Visit record, you have seen essentially all of the features of data entry in this system. Nearly all can be modified by changing the field specifications or the Check Code behind the scenes, with the help of the details contained in the later parts of this chapter.

> **Technical details and references to the files containing the Epi Info programming code will be given in indented, bold type in the following sections.**

Obtaining Reports with Analysis Programs

The REPORTS section of the menu provides an easy way to run customized Analysis programs that perform common tasks. Each item in this menu will be described with its own heading.

> **Examine the code in CLINIC.MNU, at the block called DoAnalysis to see how to run Analysis programs from the menu. DoAnalysis is called from other blocks in the menu after setting variables containing the name of the Analysis program (PGM), the name of the main database (MainDB), and the name of the output file produced by the PGM (Outfile). DoAnalysis copies the program file named as PGM to the Analysis folder and**

executes Analysis.exe with the PGM After the program runs, an opportunity to view Outfile in a browser is presented.

Copy Data for Analysis

In order to protect the main database, and to be sure that you are analyzing the latest data,   COPY DATA FOR ANALYSIS is the first item. It provides an easy way to copy the Main (Master) database or other files from one place to another. To begin doing Reports, choose this item. It will copy the Main database to the folder called Analysis within the exClinic folder, giving it the new name of "Analysis.MDB". The rest of the Reports act on this standard file name and location; hence, it is important to perform the Copy Data step first.

Examine the code in CLINIC.MNU in the block CopyDataForAnalysis to see how to test for the existence of a file, make a backup copy, copy a file from one place to another, and verify the existence of the copy.

Patient List

This choice produces an alphabetized list of patients' names and record numbers for use by the front desk clerks who must have a record number to pull a physical record from the filing cabinets. The list is printed out periodically and provided to the clerk at the desk. This is an example of using the program called EpiReport, the report generator, with an Epi Info Analysis program.

After clicking on Patient List, an Analysis program runs to extract the names and save a list that is then formatted by EpiReport and presented as a Print Preview. When you see the preview, choose the Print option to obtain the printed list.

Examine the code in the PatientList.PGM program in the Programs folder to see how to produce a sorted list of patient names and Clinic numbers using EpiReport, the Epi Info report generator. Note the use of the REPLACE command to insert the path for the database into the file called PatientList.epx, which, together with PatientList.ept, does the report in EpiReport.exe. The report files require the exact and literal path, so that it must be inserted each time the report is run on a different computer.

Patient Summary

Choose this item to produce a summary of patients who have records in the Clinic. The Analysis program called PatientSummary.pgm produces frequencies, tables, and graphs for a number of parameters in the database. When you run the program, dialog boxes offer a choice of starting and ending dates in case you want to focus on only a specific period like the past year or past month. Then you have a choice of ADULT or PEDIATRIC patients or ALL AGES. Let the program run until it halts by itself and gives instructions. Examine the output, by scrolling up in Analysis. You are invited to continue your own analysis, using the Analysis commands on the left side of the screen.

Look at the last two graphs in the output, one for patients on HAART and the other for patients not on HAART. It is easy to see that the ages vary from very young (depending on whether you chose Adults, or Children or Both) to the late 80's. Unless you remember placing two octogenarians on HAART, you may want to explore these records more carefully by using FIND with on Age ">80" in data entry or by using SELECT Age > 80 in Analysis, as they could represent data entry errors or misclassification. Patient Summary is a good way to detect outliers that need to be evaluated for data quality.

Examine the code in PatientSummary.PGM to see how to summarize data using Frequencies, Tables, and Graphs.

Managing Report Output
When you click the EXIT button in Analysis, the output file, PatientSummary.HTM, for example, will be shown in the default browser on your computer. It is an Internet web page in HTM format, and can be copied to another location with Windows Explorer or by using SAVE AS within the browser. You can also read the program in Microsoft Windows or OpenOffice, since both will import HTM files and allow editing, printing, and saving in various formats. When you exit from the exClinic menu, you will have a choice of zipping and encrypting the Analysis folder with a password. If you plan to do this, it is more convenient to copy the HTM file to another location that is easy to access. For the most part, PatientSummary.HTM and VisitSummary.HTM do not contain private information such as patient names, although this is your decision, particularly if the clinic serves a small community.

Visit List

Prior to computerization, our clinic had its own paper format for keeping track of patient visits, consisting of a row of monthly calendar boxes for each patient into which appointment dates were inserted. This report reproduces the same idea, recording up to a year of Visits in the format *Day of first appointment (number of appointments if more than one)* for each month

Special symbols are used for patients lost to followup (A) or deceased (X). Because the format is basically a spreadsheet, the program produces a CSV file that can be read by either Microsoft Excel or OpenOffice Scalc, and asks Windows to run your default program for CSV files. An extra file is produced in HTM format for those who prefer to view it in a browser.

Examine the code in ListVisits.PGM to see how to produce a calendar containing date of first visit each month and the number of visits in the month for each patient. The results are shown in a comma-delimited (csv) file and displayed in the default spreadsheet program on the current computer.

Visit Summary

This program produces summary data on Visits, with graphs of visit counts over the period requested, and visits for both patients on HAART and those who are not. The average number of visits per month per patient is determined, although you probably already know who is the winner, with 10 visits per month. Keep in mind that the demo data we are using is selected from a much larger dataset (using the MOD operator to eliminate selected ID numbers), and should not be taken too seriously.

Examine the code in VisitSummary.PGM to see how to obtain a starting and ending date and use frequencies and graphs to display summary values of interest.

Absent and Overdue List

Responsible and effective medical care includes followup of patients on long-term therapy, and especially of AIDS patients. The Absent and Overdue list program produces a list of patients who have not been seen for more than 90 days. The interval is set within the program, but could be easily changed or made the subject of a user dialog as the program is run. Normally the current date would be set to the current date (SystemDate), but for the sake of demonstration with this database, it is set to August 1, 2008 (08/01/2009).

Examine the code in OverDueList.PGM to see how to find the interval between the last and the penultimate Visit.

Residence

This program uses a map of the clinic's "catchment area" to indicate place of residence for each patient. You will note that most patients come from the La Romana province, where the clinic is located, but that many patients come from other provinces. This entry illustrates many features of Geographic Information Systems, including Shapefiles and map templates.

In interpreting the map, it is important to notice that many of the residence cities do not map to the categories in the index file, and are therefore listed as missing values for residence. This can be corrected with a bit more work. Note that the dot density map provides one dot for each patient, but that the dots are randomly distributed within a province, and will be in different places each time the map is constructed, or even when you click and drag the legend to a different location. This assures confidentiality, but is not the same as placing "pins" or other markers on exact geographic coordinates.

Examine the code in Residence.PGM to see how to use RELATE with a code file to convert city values to province, and then relate these to a shapefile (.SHP) to produce a map. This example also uses a template file called TEMPLATE1.MAP to store parameters for a map so that a dot density map is produced rather than the default choropleth or color/pattern map.

Weight and CD4

AIDS patients who have lost weight and those with low CD4 counts gain both weight and CD4 cells as they are successfully treated. This program and the overall mortality can be used to measure outcomes of treatment. It is not uncommon for patients weighing 75 pounds and on death's door to increase their weight to 130 pounds and their CD4 count from, say, 50, to several hundred. Running this program gives an idea of the mean levels of increase in CD4 and body weight. Since patients may not be weighed at every visit, and height may be hard to measure if the patient can't stand up, there are many missing values, and this small sample should not be considered representative.

Examine the code in WeightAndCD4.PGM to see how to identify patients with values for more than one visit and calculate the difference in values between the initial and latest visit.

Mortality

This short program removes the few patients who do not have HIV and presents frequencies of Status to find the percentage Deceased from the total number. Confidence intervals on the percentages are included. A second frequency of Status is done after selecting only those patients on antiretroviral therapy (HAART).

Examine the code in Mortality.PGM to see how to convert missing values to an explicit value and then do frequencies to determine Mortality rate with confidence limits.

Encrypt Analysis Folder

You will recall that COPY DATA FOR ANALYSIS makes a copy of the current main database as Analysis.mdb in the Analysis folder. Unless the the computer is completely protected from theft and unauthorized use, both the main database and the analysis copy should be encrypted whenever you exit from the menu. ENCRYPT ANALYSIS FOLDER offers the opportunity to protect files in the Analysis folder at any time. It first offers the opportunity to delete individual files such as graphics from repeated analyses. Then it uses the EpiLock program to ZIP all the files in the Analysis folder and then to Encrypt the files, producing an ELH file in the Copies folder. This process leaves unencrypted files in the Analysis folder, however, and these must be deleted.

The normal deletion process, using the DEL command in the CMD or DOS window leaves the contents of deleted files on the disk until they are overwritten by others, and the files can be recovered using commonly available software (search the Internet for "Recover deleted files", to find such programs, but beware of those that say they are "free," but at some crucial stage are not.).

The Internet also offers a number of programs that do secure deletion of files, basically by overwriting zeroes or ones repeatedly. The number of times the files are overwritten can be set to meet various security standards. We downloaded a program called SDELETE.EXE and placed it in the Epi_Info folder. When you run the demo version of ENCRYPT ANALYSIS FOLDER, the menu will detect whether you have SDELETE and offer choices accordingly. If you do not have SDELETE or choose to use the DEL command instead, the files will be deleted, but can be recovered with one of the recovery programs. After SDELETing, however, the chances of recovery are essentially zero, even with sophisticated resources.

Examine the code in CLINIC.MNU in the block called ENCRYPT ANALYSIS FOLDER to see how to use the EpiLock program first to "zip" and then to encrypt the contents of the Analysis folder. The zipped file is deleted securely by EpiLock, but the remaining files in Analysis must be deleted by another program or by the DEL command in DOS/WINDOWS. This illustrates how to incorporate an extra program to do a specific task in the menu system.

Data Quality Measures

The QUALITY menu contains three functions that call on Analysis programs to find problems in the database. An alternative is to use the ENTER program and the FIND function to locate, for example, records having missing values for important fields. This allows you to correct the problems directly from ENTER.

The programs in the QUALITY menu produce lists of records having potential errors. The lists can be printed and used to find the problem records in the main database with the ENTER button. Note that it will not help to correct errors in the Analysis.mdb database, as it is merely a temporary copy for analysis. The real database is the one indicated at the top of the menu and reached via the ENTER DATA button.

Duplicates

The DUPLICATES program checks for two kinds of duplicate records—those with the same Clinic ID number (ID2), and those having the same first and last name. Running the program against the sample database (after using COPY DATA FOR ANALYSIS) produces one duplicate record by ID2, but there are many records with the same first and last names. Note that many have different birthdates, ages, and other details, and are not really duplicates. The artifact is the result of the way sanitized names were constructed in preparing the sample database. If a patient's first name was "Pablo", his last name was constructed as Lopab. Hence there is more than one Pablo Lopab in the database, but they have different record numbers and other items. On the bright side, it makes a nice demonstration for the DUPLICATES program.

> Examine the code in DUPLICATES.PGM in the PROGRAMS folder to see how to detect duplicates in almost any field, and produce a list of duplicated records.

Errors in Relational Linkage Keys

You have probably noticed that we have been using two sets of "keys", to link Visit records to their Patient records. One set uses the Clinic ID Number in both Patient and Visit records, with one such ID per patient. The other set, behind the scenes, is constructed automatically by Epi Info for related Views, and consists of the FKEY in Visit records that contains the UNIQUEKEY of the Patient record. When you READ the Patient view in Analysis and RELATE the Visit view without specifying a key, the UNIQUEKEY/FKEY link is used. If all is in order, the Clinic ID in each Visit record should match the Clinic ID in its linked Patient record; if not, this program lists the details so that you can find and correct the problems.

> Examine the code in KEYERRORS.PGM in the PROGRAMS folder to see how to compare explicit key linkages with automatically generated Epi Info key linkages.

Errors in Dates

There are several kinds of errors that can occur in dates. The easiest to detect are those outside the range of possibility, either in the past or in the future. They can arise from entering 209 instead of 2009 for the year, for example. Reversing the month and day is common, and may be difficult to detect when both are 12 or less, unless there are other values with which it can be compared. For many dates, a value in the future (>systemdate), is not valid.

> The DateError program screens for:
> InitialDate < 01/01/2000 OR InitialDate > systemdate
> DateARVInit < 01/01/1990 OR DateARVInit > systemdate
> DOB < 01/01/1900 OR DOB > systemdate
> StatusDate < 01/01/2000 OR StatusDate > systemdate
> DateHIVTest < 01/01/1985 OR DateHIVTest > systemdate

FirstCD4Date < 01/01/2000 OR FirstCD4Date > systemdate
DateOfVisit < 01/01/2004 OR DateOfVisit > systemdate
DateOfVisit = (.)
If such values are found, the values and record numbers are printed out so that corrections can be made in the main database.

Data Management Functions in the Menu

Copy Database

This menu item asks for a source file and a destination, copying the source to the designated destination.

CopyDatabase is implemented in the CopyDatabase block of CLINIC.MNU.

Merge Databases

This item is designed to merge additional data into the Master database, perhaps from several clinics that submit data to a central database, or perhaps from a copy of the current database in which corrections have been made. Suppose that the main database is AAA.mdb and the additional source database is B.mdb. Records in AAA.mdb:Patients are updated from B.mdb:Patients by ID2 and any records that do not match are appended. The same is done with the Visit tables as a second process. The third merge reads the now updated AAA.mdb:viewVisits and does MERGE RELATE with AAA.mdb:viewPatients to update the FKEY field in viewVisits. The process is complicated and hard to understand, but you can see the code in the

MergeDatabases block of CLINIC.MNU and the program MERGEDATA.PGM.

Encrypt Data

This entry provides a way to choose a file for encryption and then to use EpiLock to encrypt it with a password of your choice.

EpiLockE is the block in CLINIC.MNU where this is implemented.

Decrypt Data

A file can be unencrypted, if you know the password, with the assistance of the EpiLockD block of CLINIC.MNU and the EpiLock program.

Make Backup

Choosing this menu item copies all the files in exClinic to a backup location that is named in the variable BackupLocation, defined in the Startup block of the CLINIC.MNU menu as:

```
Assign BackupLocation ="%SystemDrive%\@@ComputerName Backup\"
```

Within the BackupLocation, files are assigned names from the ComputerName and a sequential number from 1 to 9. After the ninth backup the numbers are recycled so that no more than 9 backups are maintained.

If no Computer Name is entered from CHOOSE COMPUTER NAME in the CONFIGURATION menu, the backup directory will default to something like C:\Backup\, otherwise it will include the name of the computer that is chosen, C:\Workstation1Backup\, for example.

The code is in the MakeBackup block of CLINIC.MNU, where it is easy to change the number that Nextnum must exceed before being reset to 1, for example.

Passing Variable Values from One View to Another

You have noticed by now that the Patient View passes values of ID, ID2, DOB, Name, FamilyName, Sex, and InitialHeight and other values to the VisitView and they automatically populate the corresponding fields in Visit. To do this, you must DEFINE variables in the Check Code of the Patient view as being of type GLOBAL. Open the PATIENT view in MakeView and click the Program button in the left panel to go to the Check Code page. In Field Where Action Will Occur, scroll all the way to the bottom and examine DEFINEDVARIABLES. You will see a number of variables with names like GlobalID, GlobalSex, GlobalFamilyName, etc. After each, there is the word GLOBAL. It is this word that makes the variable global, not the "global" that appears in its name. GlobalID could just as well have been called "LunarID", but it must be defined as GLOBAL. One of the lines, for example, will be:

DEFINE GlobalID GLOBAL

The values of the global variables must be set to the corresponding field values in the Patient view, using code like the following:

```
GlobalID=ID
GlobalName=Name
GlobalFamilyName=FamilyName
GlobalSex=Sex
GlobalDOB=DOB
GlobalID2=ID2
GlobalHeight=InitialHeight
GlobalDateARV=DateARVInit
GlobalInitialDate=InitialDate
GlobalHAARTRegimen=HAARTRegimen
GlobalCenter=Center
```

The problem is that the only good time for this action to occur is when you click the VISIT button to go to the related Visit view. Simple--just put the code in the Visit button. Unfortunately the MakeView program in Epi Info provides no easy way to put Check Code into the button that leads to a Related View. You can, however, put the code in a Command Button field and instruct the user to click this button just before clicking the VISIT button. This is easier if both buttons are on a page by themselves. You can also put a command button ON TOP of a Relate button and use HIDE and UNHIDE to make it appear like a single button that requires two clicks. The first click runs your Check Code and hides the command button; the second click goes to the related view.

Roger Mir, a very persistent and resourceful programmer, discovered by experiment, that one CAN put Check Code into a relate button, using copy and paste in the Visualize Data program (Visdata). Here's how:

Develop the Check Code in another field or in the Notepad or Wordpad editor, select it (Ctrl-A for All), and copy it to the clipboard with Copy (Ctrl-C). Minimize the editor.

From the Epi Info main menu, choose Visualize Data from the Utilities menu, and then Open the MDB containing the related views, in this case MASTER.MDB as an Epi Info project. (We suggest that you make a copy or use ANALYSIS.MDB if this is a practice session.) Double click on TABLES, and you should see a list of the tables in the database, including viewPatient. Double click the small icon that looks like a table and you should have a spreadsheet-like view of the View table. If you were ever curious about the structure of Views, here is a chance to explore. We are here only to paste a few lines of Check Code, however. Find the line where NAME is VISIT and the TYPE is RELATE, and scroll over to the Checkcode column. This is where the code belongs, and where you would normally Paste (Ctrl-V) the code from your clipboard. If you are actually doing this, be sure you remove any existing code from this cell first (Ctrl-A to select, Del key to delete). After closing VisData, your new Check Code should function, but more is needed in viewVISIT before you can see results.

To add Check Code to viewVISIT that makes use of the global variables set in viewPATIENT, you must use MakeView and first open the Patient view. Then hold down the Ctrl button and click the VISIT button. The VISIT view will appear, ready for programming or editing. Here we want to set the fields in VISIT from the global variables, and want this to happen BEFORE data entry begins in each record. Hence we choose the RECORD block in Check Code and make sure that BEFORE is chosen so that ENDBEFORE appears after our code. Now above the ENDBEFORE, you insert assign statements of the type:

```
ID=GlobalID
FamilyName=GlobalFamilyName
etc.
```

(The word ASSIGN is optional.) These are just the opposite of the statements in Patients that set the values of the global variables to the values of the local viewPATIENT variables. Now when you run the Patient view in Enter, clicking the Visit button should show the Visit view with an ID, FamilyName, etc. already populated with values from the PATIENT view.

Developing a Simple Local Area Network

Early in our clinic's history, we shared a building with another clinic where several computers and a server had been installed by an international development agency and connected by Ethernet cables and a 24-port switch. Apart from email, the system had a heavy-duty accounting package that was used intermittently and a partially completed installation of SQLServer and Ministry software for HIV/AIDS surveillance. The antivirus software on the computers was two years out of date, and numerous viruses were detected by more recent software. The server had a tape drive, but there were no tapes, and backups were not available. Since there was only one computer with a tape drive in the clinic, there would have been no way to restore backed up files to another machine if the server failed.

We installed new antivirus software and managed to remove the viruses after downloading a specialized "cure" for a particular virus. Then we added a router/firewall between the first computer and the DSL modem supplied by the telephone company.

After a short time, the server died, probably from a hard disk or motherboard problem, and was taken back to its parent agency for repair, where it remained for several months. I was rescued from having to understand and administer a server-based network. Given sufficient time and Internet access, I could have assumed the role of cable geek in the back room, but I was relieved not to be cast in this role.

About this time, construction of a separate HIV/AIDS clinic was complete, and we moved to another building. We deliberately avoided purchasing a server, feeling that the learning curve was not worth the payback, and also that we needed either two servers or none at all, in our location remote from the country capital. We contracted with a local company to install about 20 ethernet cables to the rooms, connected by a large local area network switch, and with a router to the telephone company modem for (DSL) Internet access. Initially we had 4 laptop computers, each of which was used independently for a particular purpose. Pediatric records were on one computer and the adult database on another. One or two computers were reserved for staff use in browsing email and the Internet, so that we could restrict Internet access to the data computers using the Internet security software.

When the adult database system that we describe in this chapter was ready for use, we developed a menu that could be used on each computer. The menu provided access to an Epi Info View for Patients and a related View call Visits. Data entry and analysis were initiated through menu items. Now that we had software and staff with the skills to use the computers, we finally felt the need for a common data storage area, and multiuser data entry into the same database, one of the capabilities of Epi Info.

We decided to base the system on a FILE SERVER, which is basically a network-capable hard drive, rather than a full server, which would have its own software, user accounts, antiviral software, and other complexities. Epi Info would run on each peripheral computer, but not on the server, and the data files would reside on the server, but could be copied to other computers in encrypted form or to CDROMs or another hard disk for backup. The best thing about the file server approach was the price, as the network hard drive was in the $200 range rather than the several thousand need for a true server and its software. We bought two of the same brand (Buffalo Link Stations) so that we could keep one at a remote site and bring it up to date each week as a possible replacement for the one in the clinic.

Setting up the file server was fairly easy. After a bit of trial and error, reading the instructions, and consulting Google to see what problems others had had, we connected it to our network switch, and after enough rebooting, and incantations to a Microsoft Windows Wizard named "Setting Up A Home or Small Office Network", the file server appeared in MyComputer on one of the workstations as \\LinkStation. We found we could read and write files to it just as to a local hard disk. We copied an MDB file over and were able to do data entry on two computers at the same time in the same View without trouble. Analysis, however, refused to deal with the network address \\Linkstation\ . It demanded to have a drive letter. We found that this required "mapping" a drive letter with the NET USE command in DOS (reached by opening the "Command Window" in Windows), as follows:

NET USE R: \\Linkstation

Analysis then happily referred to files on R: Since NET USE is DOS command, we inserted it in the Startup block in the Menu to run each time the menu starts up.

Setting Up a File Server for Multiple Users

It is quite possible to have several computers with systems similar to exClinic, but with data entry all referring to a single MDB on a common file server. The Enter program provides record locking so that two users that make changes in the same record do not overwrite one another's entries in unpredictable ways. All that is necessary to set this up is to have several computers on the network run local copies of Enter.EXE, but Open the same MDB on the network server.

Our strategy for analysis earlier in this chapter was to make a copy of the main database renamed to Analysis.mdb and do analysis with this temporary copy. The same thing can be done on a network. If the database is large, analysis will be faster if the database copy is on a local computer; if not, it can be kept in a separate folder on the file server.

For each computer on the network, one might set up the following Folders or Directories on the File Server:

- Analysis
- Copies
- Programs

or, alternatively, use the same organization of folders on the local computers' hard disks. Much depends on the security risks perceived for the local computers and the server, and the speed of the network that connects them.

 If the database is maintained on the network file server and perhaps accessed from several computers, it is not a good idea to have one user encrypting and deleting the Master database while another user is trying to enter data. In fact, EpiLock will refuse to encrypt an MDB file that is being accessed by another program—a good thing. But on the negative side, EpiLock may actually take its name seriously, lock up and require Ctrl-Alt-Delete to access the Windows Task Manager and stop the EpiLock task.

We therefore recommend other security measures for databases that are located on a network. A couple of choices are possible:

1. Many file servers and all network servers have provision for password protection on individual files or directories, and this can be set so that a password is required to access the shared database.

2. Microsoft Access® can be used to set a password for an MDB. This requires that you allow Access to upgrade the file to the Access 2000 format (from Access 97), but then you can set a password. Both the Enter and Analysis programs will bring up the password request, and the correct password will be required to open the file.

Encryption

As described in an earlier chapter, the EpiLock program in Epi Info performs encryption of files with a password supplied by the user. The files can be decrypted with the same password. With the aid of a customized menu, we were able to set up the following sequence of events for a data entry session with a local database.

- If there is no data file available, decrypt the file from the Data folder where it is stored

- Access the necessary View, using the Enter program.

- Enter data from the desktop

- On exit from the Enter program, run EpiLock to encrypt the MDB and delete the unencrypted copy.

Here is the code:

Backup of Data Files

There are many automatic backup programs available, some as free utilities that come with hard disks or file servers. If configured properly, they should work with a network that has minimal interruptions, but the only way to be sure is to read back the saved files and compare them with the originals.

Unfortunately, restoring files from a backup copy requires either a clone of the relevant computer, or the risky procedure of overwriting the original files. This is a little like removing the piece of floor on which one is standing to test whether a promised replacement is indeed satisfactory. This probably explains why there are so many systems in the world that are only *believed* to be carefully backed up.

A long time ago, I watched a contract truck load up the backup tapes from a large government institution for off-site storage. Some of the tapes fell out of the box onto the recently wet ground. The driver picked them up and threw them back in the box, but I wondered if the data center managers really were aware of what happens at the back loading dock.

Automatic backup is important and helpful, but we decided to use a semi-automated method implemented in the Epi Info menu to make backup copies of the data files on the file server after every data-entry session, and then to back up the server once a week by writing the files to a CDROM stored on-site and occasionally to another stored off-site. In retrospect, this seems the bare edge of minimal, and more recent systems would probably involve backup of encrypted files to the Internet to supplement the local backup copies.

How Should the exClinic Example Be Used?

We have given a working example of exClinic for a single computer and discussed some aspects of extending its use with a Local Area Network, but every situation is different, and many systems use a mixture of software and strategies to accomplish what is needed, and adapt to the skills of those who will set up the system, the resources and topography of the system, and an analysis of security threats.

In planning a system, the first task is to have a clear idea of what is wanted—a set of ideal and/or future goals. After having fun with this phase, you come back to Planet Earth and do an inventory of resources and limitations, combining the two views to produce a realistic plan. An assessment of possible security threats and a security plan should follow, with plans for backup, antiviral software, training of personnel, and other necessities. There are many outlines for "Planning a computer system" available on the Internet via Google.

The simplified example in this chapter illustrates many principles and methods for using Epi Info, but should not be taken as a complete, plop-into-place system. It can be used as part of a modified system or for comparison with other systems. At the very least, it is free, and not accompanied by a lot of exaggerated claims. If you find it useful, please send us an email and describe your experiences.

Technical Notes

Stripping the Extension from a Filename in the Menu

Because a clinic might have several different database (MDB) files (morning and afternoon clinics, surgery and medicine, etc), the Clinic system provides for choosing the Main Database in the CONFIGURATION menu. Obtaining the user's choice of files is easily done with the FILE DIALOG command in the menu, but the Epi Info menu does not provide good tools for stripping a part of a text phrase such as the extension of the filename.

After many experiments, we found the following method for obtaining the choice of files as the variable MainDB, stripping the extension(s), and obtaining a CoreDB file name that can be used to build a name either for the MDB or the encrypted version:

The method uses the REPLACE command in the menu to construct a small menu called SUB2.MNU that runs and then exits, placing the CoreDB name in a permanent variable that is visible to the main Clinic.mnu. Hence we obtain the two variables, MainDB and CoreDB that are needed for further manipulation of the files.

The code is found in the ChooseDatabase block of the menu.

After studying the code, you will be wondering what is in the menus called Subx.MNU. Here is Sub2.MNU after choosing a database called Master.MDB. Note that the menu has only one active command block, STARTUP, and that it performs an EXIT after doing its one task, which is to set the variable CoreMDB to the value inserted by the REPLACE command to replace the phrase "%Core%". Hence, a menu can act like a script that can be run by another menu, and we have solved the problem that REPLACE can only act on another file, not on a text phrase within a variable. Here is Sub2.mnu after the replacement that removes ".MDB" from the filename:

```
MENU Sub
begin
  Popup "one"
   begin
   end
end
Startup
begin
  Define CoreMDB Permanent
  Assign CoreMDB="C:\_EpiBook\Examples\exClinic\Data\Master"
   exit
end
```

Resources

Sample and exercise files for this chapter are found in **exClinic** in the **Examples** folder.

CHAPTER 24: CUSTOMIZING THE OUTPUT OF ENTER AND ANALYSIS

Printing from ENTER

Using the PRINT function on the FILE menu in Enter will bring up your printer's dialog, where you should be able to set properties. To make the properties persist from session to session, however, you should set the properties from the Windows control panel for printing, and make your chosen printer the default printer.

To do this, in Windows, click the START button and then choose "Printers and Faxes." If you don't see it, try searching in the "Control Panel" for this item. Within Printers and Faxes, find the default printer-- the one with a check mark--and RIGHT click on it, choosing Printing Preferences, or, if that doesn't look right, Properties (printer driver software varies). Experiment with the settings, but probably choose black and white or gray scale to save colored ink, and set the pages to Horizontal or Landscape. You will find that printing from ENTER will use these properties forever until someone changes them back or changes the default printer.

Customizing Analysis Output

Editing the HTML Output

The HTML or Web page output of Analysis can be loaded directly into many free and commercial programs, including OpenOffice and Microsoft Office. Within both the word processing and spreadsheet applications of these suites, it is possible to edit Analysis output files and save them either as HTML (HTM) files or in other formats. Use the ROUTEOUT command in Analysis to send output to a file with a suitable name, for example, ROUTEOUT 'Oswego.htm' with REPLACE if you want a new file or APPEND if you want to append to any existing Oswego.htm.

The SET Command

The SET command is described in Chapter 9. The value chosen for display of missing values, whether missing values are included in the output, and the setting for Statistics from "None" to "Advanced" all affect the appearance of Analysis output files. For output that will not be viewed in a browser, it may be best to turn off "Hyperlinks," since they are mainly for navigation within the output window of Analysis. You can save the settings as commands by using the SAVE ONLY button at the bottom of the dialog, a handy feature when preparing programs for others to run.

HEADER

The HEADER and TYPE (actually TYPEOUT) commands can place text on the output screen and in the current output file. HEADER has a number of choices for location of the text that you specify in the dialog for the HEADER command. Some of these repeat for each output command given, and others are one-time events. The color and size of each can be set. HEADER 0 sets the color and size of the plain text in the output, for example. We have included samples in the program, HEADERS.PGM, in the folder exOutput in the Examples for this book.

In order to run the example, first run Analysis from the ANALYZE DATA button, and then click the OPEN button in the Program Editor. In the OPEN dialog, choose CHANGE PROJECT and navigate to ..\Examples\exOutput\Oswego.mdb. Click on TEXT FILE and find the program, HEADERS.PGM.. Choose this program and click OK to bring it into the Program Editor. To see the results, click the RUN button in the Program Editor. You can experiment with the HEADERs by making changes in the program and using RUN again.

Displaying Text or Including HTML Files with TYPE (TYPEOUT)

The TYPE command displayed in the left panel of Analysis becomes TYPEOUT within a PGM. It can be used to insert text into the output of Analysis or to include a text file in a particular format. To experiement with these features, use the OPEN button in the Analysis program window and then CHANGE PROJECT in the dialog to find the folder ..\examples\exOutput\. Then click the TEXT FILE button in the OPEN dialog, find TYPEOUT.PGM, and click OK to load it into the program editor window. Run the program and then examine its commands to learn about the TYPEOUT command features.

The file called WHITE.HTM can be included in any Analysis program with TYPEOUT followed by 'WHITE.HTM' in SINGLE quotes to convert Analysis output to white and save a lot of ink when printing. We suggest that you copy WHITE.HTM to the folder where Epi Info is installed (e.g., C:\Epi_Info) so that Analysis can find it easily.

Customizing Graphs, Maps and Templates

Graphs can be extensively customized when on the screen in Analysis by right-clicking on the map and exploring the various options. EpiMap has its own set of menus and these can be used to customize a map and save it as a .MAP file that can then be used as a TEMPLATE in the MAP command of Analysis. Experimentation and the help files are the best way to become familiar with the many features available.

Using CREATE REPORTS

The CREATE REPORTS button on the main menu leads to a program that can accept many kinds of data sources and produce various kinds of output. An example is found in exClinic, where EpiReport is used to format a list of patients enrolled in a clinic.

Unforturnately, Epi Report is very sensitive to changes in location of the files, and a great deal of care is required to make examples work on more than one computer if the directory structures are not the same. It is possible to produce good-looking reports with embedded graphs and tables, but, for many, the results are not worth the time invested. If you do have good examples of Epi Report use, please let us know so that we can include them in a future edition.

Using Excel or OpenOffice as a Report Generator

An alternative to using Epi Report is to use a free or commercial spreadsheet program to generate reports. Microsoft Excel ™ is the long term standard for spreadsheets, and the Scalc program in OpenOffice is not only free, but capable of very nice reports.

Spreadsheet Programs as Report Generators

Microsoft Excel and the free OpenOffice Scalc can both acquire data from HTM files using a feature called "Link". This means that the HTML output of the Analysis program can be linked to a preconfigured spreadsheet to produce customized output. Epi Info can be used to process the data and produce a suitable table or list as an HTM file. Here are the important parts of a program written by Dr. Leonel Lerebours Nadal, who developed and has refined this technique extensively.

```
READ 'Refugee.MDB':viewPatient


   *Things happen here to select  which records will be processed


ROUTEOUT 'reportlist.htm' REPLACE
sort todaydate
LIST  TODAYDATE LASTNAME FIRSTNAME SEX AGE RACE HEAD RELATION
CLASS COLUMNSIZE=300,1,2 NOWRAP
closeout
DIALOG "The LIST has been made.  Now the spreadsheet to which it links will do
the formatting."
EXECUTE NOWAITFOREXIT "Refugee/Refugeelist.ods"
Exit
```

The program is part of exRefugee. To run it, copy the folder called exRefugee from Examples into the Epi_Info folder (often C:\Epi_Info) and click on the icon within the folder labelled.

Resources

Sample and exercise files for this chapter are found in **exOutput** and **exReports** in the **Examples** folder.

CHAPTER 25: NUTRITIONAL ANTHROPOMETRY

Nutstat is a program for recording and evaluating measurements of length, stature, weight, and head and arm circumference for children and adolescents. It can be run as a standalone program or linked to an Epi Info 2000 questionnaire view.

The program calculates percentiles, numbers of standard deviations from the mean (z-scores), and in some cases, percent of median, using data from the following sources:

- The CDC/WHO 1977/1985 reference curves for age, sex, height, and weight (1)

- WHO reference data for arm circumference (8)

- The 2000 U.S. National Center for Health Statistics reference curves for age, sex, height, weight, head circumference, and body mass index.

The main screen of NutStat is configurable to use either English or Metric units and to perform calculations with the desired reference dataset. Measurements entered on the screen are automatically stored in a Microsoft Access database and can be retrieved by patient name or identification number. Data from one person or from the entire population can be displayed graphically in several formats. NutStat databases can be read by the Analysis program to produce summary tables, lists, frequencies, and graphs, or to perform more complex data manipulations.

Existing data in Microsoft Access files can be imported to produce a standard NutStat database with appropriate statistics. An Add-Statistics feature adds the results of calculations to external Microsoft Access data files that are not necessarily in the NutStat format.

Entering or Editing Measurements in Nutstat

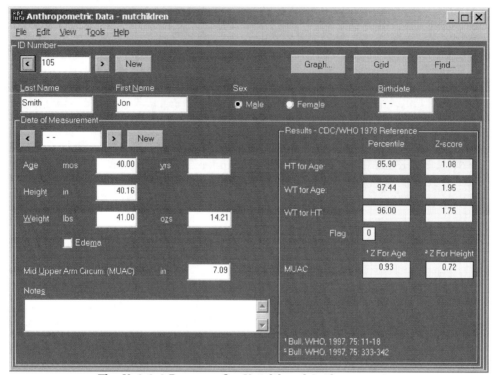

The Nutstat Program for Nutritional Anthropometry

The main screen for *Nutstat* is divided into three general sections, separated by frames. The outer frame contains the ID level data, corresponding to the records for a single person. Clicking the navigation buttons at this level will navigate through the IDs (persons) in the table.

The DATE OF MEASUREMENT frame displays the data associated with a set of measurements on a single date. A person can have many measurements on different dates. The navigation buttons in this frame will navigate to the other measurement dates for the current ID. The RESULTS frame contained in the DATE OF MEASUREMENT frame contains the calculated statistics for the current measurements. The statistics are calculated upon exit from the relevant data fields.

The GRAPH button will display a graph when clicked. The format of the graph is determined by the selections made in the GRAPH tab of the Customize screen. The graph options can also be displayed upon clicking the GRAPH button if that option has been selected in the Customize screen.

The GRID button will display all of the measurements for a single person in grid format. The values can be viewed but not edited in the grid.

The FIND button provides methods of searching for records based on ID Number, First Name, Last Name, Birth Date, Measurement Date or any combination thereof. The ID Number, First Name and Last Name fields will accept Access wild card characters. The results of a search are displayed in a grid. Double clicking on a record in the grid will close the Find screen and load the record into the Main screen.

The DELETE button will delete the current measurement date and data. If the measurement date is the only one associated with the current ID Number, the ID Number and data will be deleted as well. NOTE: The records are actually deleted from the table and not just marked for deletion, as in other Epi Info programs.

Entering data from one child's measurements

Run the *NutStat* program by clicking the NUTRITION button on the main menu. The program should obtain the name of the last database accessed from the EPIINFO.INI file and load this database automatically. If you do not see record number 106 and the data table name NUTCHILDREN at the top of the program, use the OPEN command on the FILE menu to open first the NUTRI.MDB database and then the table called NUTCHILDREN.

Click the left arrow next to the IdNumber several times until you see a record belonging to Alouetta Delia. Alouetta has four records in the table. To see the others, click on the left-pointing arrow in the DATE OF MEASUREMENT box and look at each of the earlier records. Click on the GRAPH button. Choose "Z-Scores" as the graph type and click OK to see a graph of her results compared with the International growth reference curves. Age is shown across the bottom of the graph and the left axis shows by how many standard deviations the child's measurement differs from the International average reference standard for that age and sex. The advantage of z-scores (standard deviations) is that both height and weight can be plotted on the same graph. In interpreting the graph, it is important to know that two standard deviations in either direction from 0 is approximately the 95th percentile and three is near the 99th percentile. Hence, in Alouetta's second set of measurements, her height is nearly at the 99th percentile for girls her age, but her weight is slightly below the norm; she must have been tall and slender at age 4 (48 months) when this set of measurements was taken.

To move to another child's record, choose the next IDNumber by clicking on the right arrow in the IDNumber box. By clicking repeatedly, you will discover how many children there are in this database. Click on the second button to the right of the IDNumber to create a new record and IDNumber Note that clicking the left arrow from the new record will return to the last completed record in the table.

In the new record, enter a name, sex, and birth date. Note that the age is calculated automatically after you press Enter. Now enter values for height and weight (for a 10-year old, 140 centimeters and 40 kilos will do). Note that the statistical calculations appear as soon as you press Enter in the weight field. The body mass index is calculated automatically (but we are awaiting new standards before calculating the age-specific values for body mass index).

Enter 15 centimeters or 6 inches for arm circumference and note the z-scores. Now click on New in the IDNumber box to save the record and go on to the next.

From the File menu, choose Customize to see the options available. On the Units tab, choose either the English or Metric system of measurement, click on Arm Circumference to deselect it, and then choose OK. Note that the main screen now displays only the measurement units selected and that Arm Circumference no longer appears. Return to Customize and set up the main screen in the configuration you find most useful for your own environment.

NutStat offers a choice of the CDC/WHO international growth reference curves of 1978 or, for the United States, the year 2000 CDC growth reference curves. To make this choice click OPTIONS on the TOOLS menu and then choose CDC/WHO 1978 or CDC 2000 growth curves from the tabbed dialog.

Configuring Nutstat

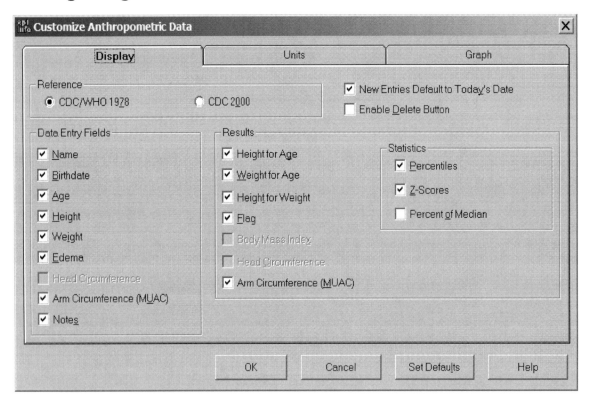

The configuration screen for *Nutstat* is accessed through the VIEW-CUSTOMIZE menu item. The configuration screen consists of three sections separated by tabs.

The tab labeled DISPLAY contains the names of nearly all of the fields on *Nutstat*'s main screen. A field can be added or removed from the main screen simply by checking or unchecking the check box next to the field name. The reference standard that is used to calculate the statistics can also be changed on this tab. If the reference standard is changed, the user will be prompted if they want to update all of the existing records with statistics calculated with the newly selected reference standard. WHO/CDC and NCHS statistics are stored in separate columns in the data table so that statistics calculated with one reference standard will not replace statistics calculated with the other reference standard. (Note: the NCHS reference set expected in the year 2000 is not yet available.)

The tab labeled UNITS allows the user to switch between Metric and English units for the data entry fields. This tab also allows the user to select the format for the date fields and whether the age should be entered in months or years and months.

The tab labeled GRAPH allows the user to select which graph will be produced when the GRAPH button is clicked on the main screen. If a graph is dependent on a data from a field that is not being displayed on the main screen, the graph will not be included in the list.

PERCENTILE LINE RESOLUTION controls the number of points that are used to create the growth curves. The higher the resolution, the smoother the curves, but the longer it takes to produce the graphs. On slower computers, you may want to select a lower percentage of points to display. If the SHOW BEFORE GRAPHING check box is checked, the graph options will be displayed every time the GRAPH button is clicked on the main screen.

Printing From Nutstat

Nutstat uses templates to determine the format of the output when printing. The FILE:PRINT menu item will use the last selected template to produce the printout. Printed output can be previewed by selecting FILE:PRINT PREVIEW. The Print Preview screen will display the data associated with the current ID Number.

The Print Setup screen is accessed by way of the CUSTOMIZE button on the Print Preview screen. The Print Setup screen consists of three sections separated by tabs.

The GENERAL tab enables the customization of the information contained in the beginning and end of the document. Text entered in the HEADER text area will be displayed in the top right corner of the first page of the document. The PATIENT INFORMATION list box will display all of the checked items directly below the Header information. An image can be added by entering the path name of a Bitmap, Icon, or

Windows Metafile image in the IMAGE FILE text box. The image will be displayed in the upper right corner of the first page of the document. The size of the image can be adjusted by changing the value in the IMAGE SIZE combo box. A Text or Rich Text file with additional information can be appended to the document by entering the path name of the file ADDITIONAL INFORMATION FILE

The GRAPHS tab allows the addition of graphs to the document. Checking the check box next to a graph will cause it to be inserted into the document. A title or description can be added to a graph by selecting it in the list and adding the title and/or description in the GRAPH TITLE and GRAPH DESCRIPTION text boxes respectively.

The TABLE tab allows the addition of a table. Fields are added to the table by moving the field name from the AVAILABLE FIELDS list to the SELECTED FIELDS list. The text entered in the TABLE TITLE field will be added as the title for the table.

The SAVE and SAVE AS buttons on the bottom of the screen are used to save the current settings on the screen in a template file. The OPEN button is used to open a previously saved template. Clicking the OK button will save the current settings on the screen to the default template, refresh the Print Preview screen with the new settings and close the Print Setup screen. Since the OK button always saves the settings to the default template, it is only necessary to use the Save and Save As buttons if multiple templates are desired. Clicking the Cancel button in the Print Setup screen will close the screen without refreshing the Print Preview screen or saving the changes to the default template.

Generating Reports With Nutstat

The *Nutstat* Report Generator is reached from the FILE:REPORT GENERATOR menu item. The first screen to display after selecting the menu item will be the REPORT GENERATOR – SOURCE screen. This screen has two textboxes that capture the template path name and the data source. The template path name can be entered directly into the text box or located by clicking the BROWSE button.

The Data Source text box is read only. The data source can be changed by clicking the CHANGE button. This will display the DATA SOURCE screen, which is similar to the FIND screen. The data source can be selected based on ID Numbers, Birth Dates, Measurement Dates or a combination thereof. The TEST button will display the records in the data source in a grid. Clicking OK will refresh the Data Source text box on the REPORT GENERATOR - SOURCE screen with the new data source and close the DATA SOURCE screen. Clicking the CLOSE button on the menu bar will close the Data Source screen without updating the data source.

Clicking the OK button on the REPORT GENERATOR –SOURCE screen will display the DATA REPORTER screen. This screen allows customizing the report. The LAYOUT WINDOW toolbar button pops-up a window that lists all of the fields in the data source. The fields can be added and grouped in the report simply by dragging and dropping them into the appropriate list. The PROPERTIES toolbar button pops up a window that allows several formatting properties to be set. The report template can be saved by way of the SAVE or SAVE AS item in the File menu.

External Data Features of Nutstat

Nutstat has two features that deal with external data--ADD STATISTICS and IMPORT. The purpose of the Add Statistics feature is to add statistical data to an existing table. The purpose of the Import feature is to import data from an existing table into a new table that has the data structure that is required for Nutstat to use it. The table can be an Epi 2000 table or a table from Microsoft Access.

ADD STATISTICS and IMPORT are accessed via the FILE:EXTERNAL DATA menu item. The first two screens to be displayed after selecting either feature will capture the database and table name for the table to be imported or added to. The third screen that is displayed will capture all of the information needed to process the incoming table.

The frame with the label SELECT THE FIELDS TO USE is common to both ADD STATISTICS and IMPORT. It is used to link the fields in the table with the type of data they contain. The list box labeled INPUT FIELD contains all the fields in the source table. The list box labeled FIELD TYPE contains all the field types that the process can use. To link a field to a field type, select the field and field type in the list boxes and click the link button. For some field types, a UNITS dialog box may pop up to capture the unit of measurement that the data in the field is in. After the unit is selected (if necessary) the field, field type and unit of measurement will be added to the Linked Fields grid.

The only field types that are required are the SEX and DATE OF MEASUREMENT fields (marked by asterisks) when importing. None of the other field types are required, but, if a statistic is dependent on a field that is not linked, it cannot be calculated.

The frame labeled SELECT THE REFERENCE STANDARD TO USE is common to both IMPORT and ADD STATISTICS. It is used to select the reference standard to use when processing the data in the table. Currently, only the WHO/CDC 1977/1985 reference is enabled.

The frame labeled SELECT THE STATISTICS TO ADD is unique to the ADD STATISTICS feature. It contains check boxes that indicate whether a statistic should be added to the table. The check boxes are only enabled if the required field types for the statistics have been linked. Hovering the mouse pointer above a check box will display a tool tip that lists the field types required for the respective statistic.

The OUTPUT DATABASE and OUTPUT TABLE text boxes are unique to the Import feature. They capture the path and name of the database and the name of the table that the data will be imported into. If the database or table does not exist, it will be created when the Import is preformed.

The PROCESS' button is common to both IMPORT and ADD STATISTICS. Clicking this button starts the processing of the data. A dialog box with a progress bar will display after clicking the process button to indicate the progress of the process.

Nutstat as Part of an Epi Info 2000 Questionnaire View

N*utStat* can be run from within an Epi Info questionnaire view as though it is a related table. *Nutstat* is represented by a button on the questionnaire that can be clicked to bring up the nutritional entry screen.

 To set up the relationship and the button, right click on the screen of a questionnaire in *MakeView*, enter a name for the button to be created ("Growth," for example), and then click on the button labeled CREATE RELATED VIEW. In the next dialog, selection criteria can be entered so that the button is active only under certain conditions, or it can be made active at all times. A reasonable condition might be that an AGE field contain a value between 0 and 18 years, since most of the calculations in *NutStat* are limited to this age group.

Overview of 1985 CDC/WHO Growth Reference Curves

The following sections were written by Kevin Sullivan, PhD, Department of Pediatrics, School of Medicine, and Department of Epidemiology, Rollins School of Public Health, Emory University, Atlanta, Georgia and Nathan Gorstein, World Health Organization, for the Epi Info 6 manual.

The anthropometric calculations described in this chapter are based on the growth reference curves developed by the National Center for Health Statistics (NCHS) and CDC using data from the Fels Research Institute and US Health Examination Surveys.1 These growth curves are recommended by the World Health Organization (WHO) for international use.2

NCHS is in the process of developing new growth reference curves for the US. When these become available, they will be incorporated into the *NutStat* program so that both sets of curves will be available.

To calculate anthropometric indices, information is needed on each individual's sex, age, weight, and height. From these data it is possible to form different indices, including those that relate to height-for-age (HA), weight-for-age (WA), and weight-for-height (WH). These indices can be expressed in terms of Z-scores, percentiles, and percent of median relative to the international growth reference population mentioned above. The following abbreviations will be used throughout this chapter:

HAP	Height-for-Age Percentile
HAZ	Height-for-Age Z-score
HAM	Height-for-Age percent of Median

WAP	Weight-for-Age Percentile
WAZ	Weight-for-Age Z-score
WAM	Weight-for-Age percent of Median

WHP	Weight-for-Height Percentile
WHZ	Weight-for-Height Z-score
WHM	Weight-for-Height percent of Median

Interpretation and Uses of Anthropometry

Anthropometry can be used to assess nutritional status at both the individual and the population level. Ideally, individuals should have several weight and height measurements over time so that growth velocity can be assessed. A decline in an individual's anthropometric index from one point in time to another could be an indication of illness and/or nutritional deficiency that may result in serious health outcomes. In some situations, a single set of measurements may be used for screening populations or individuals to identify abnormal nutritional status and priority for treatment.

At the population level, data are most commonly available from cross-sectional surveys in which the prevalence of low anthropometric indices can be assessed by determining the proportion of the population that falls below a cutoff value. In addition, the mean or median anthropometric value of a population can be compared with the reference value to assess the status of the study population relative to the reference population.

The two preferred anthropometric indices for determining nutritional status are WH and HA, as these discriminate between different physiological and biological processes.[2,3] Low WH is considered an indicator of wasting (i.e., "thinness") and is generally associated with failure to gain weight or a loss of weight. Low HA is considered an indicator of stunting (i.e., "shortness"), which is frequently associated with poor overall economic conditions and/or repeated exposure to adverse conditions. The third index, WA, is primarily a composite of WH and HA, and fails to distinguish tall, thin children from short, well-proportioned children.

The distribution of the indices can be expressed in terms of Z-scores, percentiles, and percent of median. Z-scores, also referred to as standard deviation (SD) units, are frequently used. The Z-score in the reference population has a normal distribution with a mean of zero and standard deviation of 1. For example, if a study population has a mean WHZ of 0, this would mean that it has the same median WH as the reference population. The Z-score cutoff point recommended by WHO, CDC, and others to classify low anthropometric levels is 2 SD units below the reference median for the three indices. The proportion of the population that falls below a Z-score of -2 is generally compared with the reference population in which 2.3% fall below this cutoff. The cutoff for *very* low anthropometric levels is usually more than 3 SD units below the median.

Percentiles, or "centiles," range from zero to 100, with the 50th percentile representing the median of the reference population. Cutoff points for low anthropometric results are generally < 5th percentile or < 3rd percentile. In the reference population, 5% of the population falls below the 5th percentile; this can be compared with the proportion that falls below this cutoff point in the study population.

The calculation of the percent of median does not take into account the distribution of the reference population around the median. Therefore, interpretation of the percent of median is not consistent across age and height levels nor across the different anthropometric indices.2

Traditionally, in the United States and some other countries, percentiles are used as cutoff points. In other parts of the world, either Z-scores or percent of median are used, although WHO favors the use of Z-scores.2

Z-scores and percentiles are directly related. Both rely on the fitted distributions of the indices across age and height values and are consistent in their interpretation across anthropometric indices. Z-scores are useful because they have the statistical property of being normally distributed, thus allowing a meaningful average and standard deviation for a population to be calculated. In addition, Z-scores have a greater capacity to determine the proportion of a population that falls below extreme anthropometric values than do percentiles.

Percentiles are useful because they are easy to interpret (e.g., in the reference population 3% of the population falls below the 3rd percentile). Percentiles, however, are generally not normally distributed in either the reference or the study populations.

The more common cutoff value used is < -2 SD. The prevalence of < -2SD can be compared with other countries as shown in Table 1.3 For example, in a survey of children, if the prevalence of weight-for-height <-2 SD if found to be 16.7%, this would be considered to be a *very high* prevalence of low WH. If the prevalence of low height-for-age is found to be 18.9%, this would be a low prevalence of stunting. The prevalence of low anthropometric indices should be presented by one-year intervals for children less than six years of age, or, if age is unknown, for children <85 centimeters compared with those ≥85 centimeters, which approximates comparing the children <2 years of age to those ≥2 years.

**Prevalence of low anthropometric values (<-2SD) compared
to other surveys of children five years of age or younger**

Relative Prevalence of Low Anthropometric Values

Index	Low	Medium	High	Very High
Low WH	<5.0%	5.0-9.9%	10.0-14.9%	>15%
Low HA	<20.0%	20.0-29.9%	30.0-39.9%	>40.0%
Low WA	<10.0%	10.0-19.9%	20.0-29.9%	>30.0%

Limitations of Growth Reference Curves

HA and WA indices can be calculated for individuals from birth up to 18 years of age. WH indices are calculated for males to 138 months (11.5 years) of age and less than 145 cm (57 inches) and for females to 120 months (10 years) of age and less than 137 cm (53 inches). WH cannot be calculated for children less than 49 cm (19.3 inches). For children less than 2 years of age, recumbent (i.e., lying down) length measurements are assumed; for children 2 years of age and older, height refers to standing height.

No anthropometric indices are calculated if sex is unknown or miscoded because there are separate growth reference curves for males and females. If weight is unknown, only HA will be calculated; if height is unknown, only WA will be calculated; and if age is unknown, only WH will be calculated. When age is unknown, children shorter than 85 centimeters are assumed to be less than 2 years of age; otherwise, WH is calculated with the assumption that the child is 2 years of age or older.

How to Reduce Anthropometric Errors

Below are some basic steps to follow to ensure that age, weight, and height data are collected accurately.

- Make sure the equipment is correctly calibrated on a regular basis.

- Thoroughly train those who collect the data.

- To reduce errors on the child's age, collect information on both the child's age and the dates of birth and measurement. The year of birth is frequently given incorrectly. Compare the calculated age with the age provided by the child's caretaker. If there is a large discrepancy between the two age values, the age provided by the caretaker is probably closer to the true value. Check the year of birth and see how the anthropometric indices change if you correct the year of birth to correspond with the stated age.

- After the age, sex, weight, and height information are collected, check the data against a growth chart or by calculating the anthropometric indices on a computer. Children with extreme values should be remeasured.

- For research projects, data should be entered twice and compared or otherwise confirmed as correct.

What the Anthropometric Calculation Program Does

The following values are needed:

- SEX - coded as 1/M/m for males, 2/F/f for females

- AGE - in months

- WEIGHT - in kilograms

- HEIGHT - in centimeters

The program performs the calculations and returns the following values:

	Percentiles	Z-scores	Percent of Median
Height-for-Age	HAP	HAZ	HAM
Weight-for-Height	WHP	WHZ	WHM
Weight-for Age	WAP	WAZ	WAM

A record FLAG, coded 0 to 7, described below.

The first nine fields contain the results of the anthropometric calculations. For the Z-scores, a code of 9.99 means that the index could not be calculated because of missing data or data values that were out of the appropriate range. An example of the latter would be an age of 18 years or older. A code of 9.98 for Z-scores denotes that the Z-score was greater than or equal to 9.98 and most likely indicates an error in measurement. For percentiles and percent of median, a similar coding scheme is used (99.9 and 99.8 for percentiles and 999.9 and 999.8 for percent of median, respectively).

A tenth field, the record FLAG field, is used to identify records where there are missing data points or a strong likelihood that some of the data items are incorrect (based on extreme Z-scores). The criteria for "flagging" an anthropometric index are as follows:

Index	Minimum	Maximum
HAZ	-6.00	+6.00
WHZ	-4.00	+6.00
WAZ	-6.00	+6.00

Two additional criteria for "flagging" a record are combinations of data items:

(HAZ > 3.09 and WHZ < -3.09) *or* (HAZ < -3.09 and WHZ > 3.09)

It is recommended that all "flagged" records be verified for accuracy. Common errors include incorrect data entry, incorrect age/dates, weight or height measurements entered incorrectly or in the wrong units, and missing/blank data. When anthropometric data are being analyzed in the Epi Info *Analysis* program or elsewhere, it is recommended that certain indices be set to missing (and therefore excluded from analyses) based on the coding in the FLAG field (Table 2). Note that when a Z-score is flagged, the corresponding percentiles and percent-of-median values are also flagged.

Record Flag Coding Scheme				
	Index Flagged			
Flag Code	HAZ	WHZ	WAZ	Notes
0				No indices flagged
1	Y			Only HAZ flagged
2		Y		Only WHZ flagged
3	Y	Y		Both HAZ and WHZ flagged
4			Y	Only WAZ flagged
5	Y		Y	Both HAZ and WAZ flagged
6		Y	Y	Both WHZ and WAZ flagged
7	Y	Y	Y	All three indices flagged

Y=Index flagged, blank means index not flagged.

Interpretation of the flags is as follows:

Flag 0: This means that none of the indices were flagged. However, this does not necessarily mean the information is correct. Either sex, age, weight, or height could be incorrect but not extreme enough to be flagged.

Flag 1: HA is flagged but not WH or WA. This could be an extremely short or tall individual. Assure that the height information entered onto the computer file is correct. If height is incorrect, then WHZ would generally be close to -3.09 or 3.09 (a WHZ value beyond these would produce a flag error number 5). The other alternative is that the age information is incorrect, which would make the WAZ extreme (near -6 or 6).

Flag 2: WH is flagged but HA and WA are not. First, check the age and height of the child and make sure they are within the limits described in the section *Limitations of Growth Reference Curves.* If the child is within the age and height limitations, then either height or weight may be incorrect. If height is incorrect, then HAZ would be expected to be near an extreme value (but not extreme enough to be flagged), and if weight is incorrect, then WAZ would be close to an extreme value (but not extreme enough to be flagged). Finally, this could truly be an exremely thin or obese child.

Epi Info and OpenEpi

Flag 3: HA and WH are both flagged but WA is not. This is an indicator that height may be incorrect or missing.

Flag 4: WA is flagged but not HA or WH. If the weight is incorrect, then WHZ would be near an extreme value (but not extreme enough to be flagged), and if age is incorrect, then HAZ is likely to be near an extreme value (but not extreme enough to be flagged).

Flag 5: HA and WA are flagged but not WH. This is an indication that the age information is incorrect, missing, or out of range.

Flag 6: WH and WA are flagged but not HA. This is an indication that weight is likely to be incorrect or missing.

Flag 7: All three indices are flagged. This can occur if sex is unknown or incorrectly coded; or at least two of the following are missing, incorrectly coded, or beyond the limitation of the growth curve: age, weight, or height.

Other Considerations

As mentioned above, the subroutine that calculates anthropometry assumes that age is in months, sex is coded as 1/M/m for males and 2/F/f for females, weight is in kilograms, and height is in centimeters. However, with Epi Info, you can calculate age from two dates (i.e., date of birth and date of measurements) and convert US. measurements (e.g., inches and pounds) entered on the screen to metric within a .CHK file (described in more detail later in this chapter).

When possible, it is always preferable to have age calculated from the birth date and the date of the measurement(s). The reference curves are based on "biologic" age rather than calendar age. Biologic age in months divides the year into 12 equal segments as opposed to calendar age in which months have from 28 to 31 days. Although this makes little difference in older children, it can have an effect on the anthropometric calculations for infants. To calculate biologic age, the number of days between the two dates is calculated by the program. The age in days is divided by 365.25 and then multiplied by 12. Entering age by rounding to the nearest month and/or the most recently attained month can have a substantial effect on the anthropometric calculations, especially for infants.[4]

Other Anthropometric Software and Sources of Information

For additional information on the use and interpretation of anthropometry, please refer to the articles by: WHO Working Group on the Purpose, Use, and Interpretation of Anthropometric Indicators of Nutritional Status;[2] Gorstein et al.,[3] Dibley et al.;[5] Waterlow et al.,[6] and Beaton et al.[7] Much additional information on anthropometric statistics may be available from:

Division of Nutrition

Center for Chronic Disease Prevention and Health Promotion

Centers for Disease Control and Prevention

1600 Clifton Road NE, MS A08

Atlanta, GA 30333 U.S.A.

and

Nutrition Unit

World Health Organization

1211 Geneva 27

Switzerland

The US National Center for Health Statistics

http://www.cdc.gov/GROWTHcharts/

Acknowledgments

Special thanks to Phillip Nieburg, M.D., M.P.H., Norman Staehling, M.S., Ronald Fichtner, Ph.D., and Fredrick Trowbridge, M.D., Centers for Disease Control and Prevention, for their assistance.

This chapter was taken from the Epi 2000 Manual, from the Help files of Epi Info for Windows, and from the Manual for Epi Info for DOS, all of which were published by the Centers for Disease Control and are in the Public Domain. The trademark Epi Info is the property of the Centers for Disease Control.

CHAPTER 26: THE STRUCTURED APPLICATION FRAMEWORK FOR EPI INFO (SAFE)

Many of the exercises and examples for learning Epi Info are necessarily fairly simple. Constructing a larger system, such as those used in public health surveillance, requires planning and a more formal design. EpiInfo.EXE (the menu), the Enter program, and Analysis,exe can be used together in a system, in which each of the programs complements the strengths and weaknesses of the others.

A group of authors at the Global Immunization Division, Centers for Disease Control and Prevention, Atlanta, GA, USA, has published a description of such a system, called SAFE, with design considerations and a description of how it is used in various programs in Europe, Africa and Asia. The title and abstract are as follows, and the entire article is available on the CDC website.

Ma J,Otten, M, Kamadjeu R, Mir R, Rosencrans L, McLaughlin S, Yoon S. New frontiers for health information systems using Epi Info in developing countries: Structured application framework for Epi Info (SAFE). Int J Med Inform. (2007), doi:10,1016/j.ijmedinf.2007.02.001.

BACKGROUND: For more than two decades, Epi Info software has been used to meet the data management, analysis, and mapping needs of public health professionals in more than 181 countries and 13 languages. Until now, most Epi Info systems have been relatively simple, mainly because of a lack of detailed and structured guidance for developing complex systems. OBJECTIVE AND RESULTS: We created the structured application framework for Epi Info (SAFE), which is a set of guidelines that allows developers to create both simple and complex information systems using accepted good programming practices. This has resulted in application code blocks that are re-useable and easy to maintain, modify, and enhance. The flexibility of SAFE allows various aggregate and case-based application modules to be rapidly created, combined, and updated to create health information systems or sub-systems enabling continuous, incremental enhancement as national and local capacity increases. CONCLUSIONS: SAFE and Epi Info are both cost-free and have low system requirements-characteristics that render this framework and software beneficial for developing countries.

PMID: 17369080 [PubMed - as supplied by publisher]

The full text of the paper is available (gratis) at:

ftp://ftp.cdc.gov/pub/NIPGID/SAFE/SAFE%20Documentation/Paper/

It is possible to download an example(Measles_Surveillance.zip) of SAFE from:

http://ftp.cdc.gov/pub/NIPGID/SAFE/SAFE%20Development/

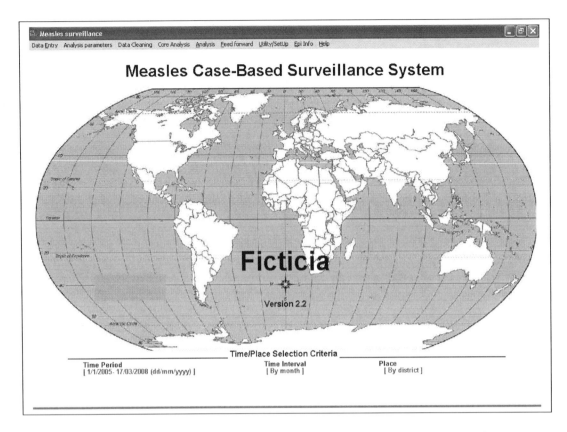

Main menu of the first example. Another example (District_ICS_Sierra_Leone.zip) is found at

http://ftp.cdc.gov/pub/NIPGID/SAFE/SAFE%20Development/

I (AD) have downloaded the examples, but never installed or worked with SAFE in the field. Hence, please consider the following explanation as only a distant view of a large set of programs.

The menu of the second example is shown on the next page:

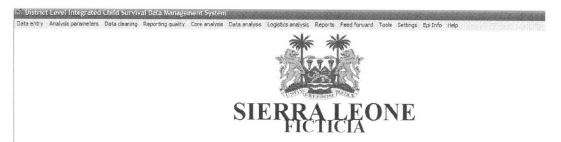

To run the second program, you first adjust the parameters shown. I had to broaden the time interval so that it incorporated the sample data provided, for example. After setting these parameters, you can then choose a type of report from the many options in the other menu headings.

SAFE Feature	Purpose	How Implemented
Modularity	Allow adding and removing components without disturbing others, e.g., adding a TB or Malaria module to immunization	Additional Views and PGMs or pieces of PGMs can be added, using the other standard features
Standardization	Allow data to be merged from many stations. Enable use of programs written elsewhere, Preserve programmer's mental health.	Standard variables Standard folders Standard chunks of analysis
Simplicity of Use	Completely menu driven programs for all standard analyses.	Analytic choices all collected from user in menu, then used to assemble a PGM from standard pieces.
Ease of Deployment	Make it possible for one programmer to	Standardization as above. Folder

	install and maintain scores or hundreds of installations.	locations and dataset names stored as variables in EpiInfo.INI file and can be edited in one place.
Flexible DataAnalysis	Enable useful analysis by person, place and time, with graphs and maps, in the agency where data originate.	Use of the Menu's REPLACE to copy and customize blocks of PGM code and DOS COPY to paste the blocks together before running Analysis. Use of permanent variables to transmit user choices to Analysis.

A program that constructs other programs dynamically is sometimes called a "factory". In a sense the SAFE software sets up a software factory for analysis of surveillance data. As the user interacts with the menu, SAFE pulls the generic parts of a program from a folder called SOURCE. In the article, C_Set_Time_Period.src, is a module that contains the Analysis SELECT command to select records between the start date and end date specified by the user in interacting with the menu. The dates can be passed with the REPLACE command or as values of permanent variables.

From a conceptual point of view, SAFE is analogous to a design for a franchise chain of sandwich shops. A truck comes each day and delivers ingredients for the sandwiches that are kept in standard locations. Let's suppose that the raw bread dough mixture represents DATA from which a certain number of RECORDS (rolls) are produced daily. "Users" come through, and each one specifies a number of choices to the clerk. According to specification, the clerk grabs a roll (white, whole wheat, or Italian), and begins applying ingredients to produce a customized "program" or completed sandwich. Some of the ingredients come from the freezer or refrigerator, and have to be customized (unwrapped, dumped into a bin, etc.) before they are applied to the sandwich. It may be necessary to substitute (REPLACE) some components (all Swiss cheese or double meat). The final steps, heating in an oven, and/or wrapping in waxed paper, unify all the components into the final sandwich, as the COPY command does with pieces of PGMs. In about 5 minutes, the customer (local epidemiologist) has a highly customized sandwich (PROGRAM) for local use.

Well, perhaps your experience with Subway® or Blimpie® is different, but I think the analogy is helpful. In the early years of computerized public health surveillance, each health department had its own forms and computer programs, and "cooked" its own analysis, if any, like individual Mom-and-Pop restaurants in different towns. In recent years, the "franchise" approach has appeared, with standard data definitions, forms, etc. Some people are happier with home cooking, but it is clear that a lot more sandwiches can be assembled by the standardized "factory"approach, particularly in developing countries, where skilled cooks of Western cuisine may be in short supply.

The ideas in the SAFE framework are excellent, but I find in talking with the authors and examining some of the samples that there are differences in style. Some SAFE programmers prefer to assemble programs from small pieces as in a sandwich shop or auto assembly line, but others find that it is easier to provide a whole program (complete sandwich) and use REPLACE and permanent variable values to inject the necessary place, time, and disease information. Both approaches make the best use of two Epi Info programs—EpiInfo.exe for flexible user interaction, processing of text, and use of Windows tools; and Analysis.exe for running programs to clean and merge data and reduce individual records to summary information. EpiReport, EpiMap, and the graphing module each play a role in producing and formatting the output.

In other chapters, we describe how additional techniques for data backup and encryption can be incorporated into a menu-driven system. After encryption, files can be sent by email or uploaded to an Internet site from a menu with appropriate calls to communication software.

Since the output of the Analysis program is in web page format (HTML), there is ample opportunity for post-analytic customization by applying internet techniques like Cascading Style Sheets (CSS), using the EpiInfo menu to edit the HTML output with REPLACE, having the effect of inserting "Apply the style sheet to put 3-D shading and a pleasant tan background in all the tables.".

Many thanks to Roger Mir and Jinghong Ma for their helpful comments and materials for this chapter.

CHAPTER 27: DEMO: AN EPI INFO™ DATABASE ON THE INTERNET CLOUD

Taha Kass-Hout, MD, MS, BioSense Program Manager, Centers for Disease Control and Prevention (CDC), Atlanta, USA

Eduardo Jezierski, VP Engineering, InSTEDD, Palo Alto, California, USA

Disclaimer: The findings and conclusions made in this manuscript are those of the authors, and do not necessarily represent the official positions of the Centers for Disease Control and Prevention (CDC).

Modern management of disease outbreaks requires collaboration across jurisdictional and organizational boundaries. While Epi Info™ (1, 2), CDC's suite of tools for field collection of disease surveillance and outbreak information, has over 1 million instances worldwide (3), there exists no easy way to exchange data, making analysis of disease surveillance and outbreaks more time consuming for epidemiologists. Furthermore, the problem is made more complex by the proliferation of diverse ad-hoc tools for data collection on multiple platforms, from online surveys to use of spreadsheets. The non-profit organization known as InSTEDD (Innovative Support to Emergencies, Diseases, and Disasters) has been facilitating the development of a set of open source tools to enable data sharing. Partnering with US Centers for Disease Control and Prevention (CDC), InSTEDD demonstrated (4) the ability to rapidly, safely, and securely exchange Epi Info™ data in a virtual — or cloud — computing environment (over Internet infrastructure [e.g., Government cloud (5), Amazon's EC2/S3, Google cloud/App Engine]). A cloud environment is one in which servers and resources are remotely maintained and their use is 'virtually' available to users, drastically reducing or eliminating the need for capital investment and additional IT support.

InSTEDD's Mesh4x (http://code.google.com/p/mesh4x) allows for data synchronization among different data sources regardless of technology platform or network connectivity. By including the Mesh4x adapters for Epi Info™, epidemiologists can make their data available to all users in their distributed project team or across different jurisdictions. In this chapter we demonstrate the utility of Mesh4x to share data over the Internet cloud where an epidemiologist determines which subset of her data are exchanged. This technology raises the potential to share data (e.g., during outbreak investigation) where multiple epidemiologists are then allowed access to see each other's data, update the information as the outbreak unfolds, and securely exchange data with one another.

Demonstration

A near-real time data exchange between multiple instances of Epi Info™ was enabled by configuring Mesh4x for Internet cloud use. A client-based tool (Figure 1) was developed to easily be used by an epidemiologist to build and configure without requiring any prior technical knowledge. Many epidemiologists are familiar with the foodborne outbreak in Oswego, New York, U.S.A. on April 18th, 1940. In this outbreak, over half of the participants at a potluck church supper developed a gastro-intestinal illness. A survey was created and interviews were conducted with 75 of the 80 people known to have been present to determine the source of the contamination. The actual church supper was held in the Oswego county; however, we demonstrated value of data synchronization by an imaginary scenario (6) where interviews and data entry were conducted in different localities. Therefore, we populated fictitious addresses spread across five counties in New York upstate region (Oswego, Jefferson, Lewis, Oneida, and Wayne) then used Mesh4x tool to synchronize data across multiple Epi Info™ instances.

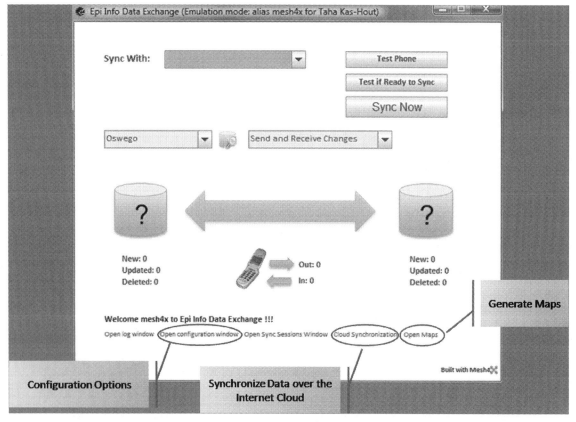

Figure 1: Mesh4x Client for Epi Info™ (Epi Info™ Data Exchange)

Download the Mesh4x client for Epi Info™

You can download the Mesh4x client and sample Oswego database here (under "Demo Version", file size is ~36.6MB): http://code.google.com/p/mesh4x/wiki/EpiInfoMesh4x. Unzip the content of the file to your C drive (C:\mesh4x). You can also participate in the active discussion group here: http://groups.google.com/group/mesh4x

Set Up a Collaborative Mesh and Share your Data

You can create a mesh (a collaborative space (supported by cloud service authentication (Basic or SSL), users can further encrypt their storage (e.g., MS Excel, MS Access, Google Docs/Spreadsheets, MS SQL Server, MYSQL)) where you can share and synchronize data with others) by visiting this site: http://sync.staging.instedd.org/mesh4x

Give your mesh a name such as Epiinfo (case sensitive) as shown in the following figure:

Create or update you own Mesh:

by: | name: Epiinfo | title: Epi Info Mesh | description: State's Epi Info Mesh | format: rss20

Add

Then, you will need to create the data feed (i.e., the data you want to share with others); enter the name of your data and add your initial at the end of the name; for example, for the Oswego database we can enter "OswegoTK" in the name field) as shown in the following figure:

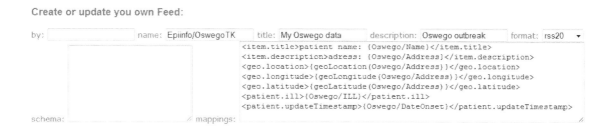

You can also define the variables you want plotted on a map by entering the mapping parameters in the "mappings" field. Here is an example of the variables that can be plotted on a map (please refer to the sample file "example_Oswego_mappings_to_Cloud_feed_creation.txt" in the "C:\mesh4x\properties" folder:

```
<item.title>patient name: {Oswego/Name}</item.title>
<item.description>adress: {Oswego/Address}</item.description>
```

```
<geo.location>{geoLocation(Oswego/Address)}</geo.location>
<geo.longitude>{geoLongitude(Oswego/Address)}</geo.longitude>
<geo.latitude>{geoLatitude(Oswego/Address)}</geo.latitude>
<patient.ill>{Oswego/ILL}</patient.ill>
<patient.updateTimestamp>{Oswego/DateOnset}</patient.updateTimestamp>
```

Currently, there is no data in your collaborative space in the cloud:
http://sync.staging.instedd.org/mesh4x/feeds/Epiinfo/OswegoTK

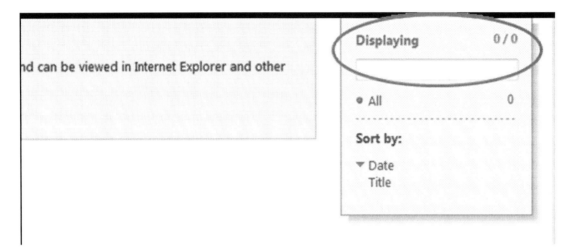

Start the mesh4x client (Figure 1) by double clicking "epiinfo.jar" file in the "C:\mesh4x\"
folder, this will launch the "Epi Info™ Data Exchange" window. Click the "Open
configuration window" option at the bottom of the "Epi Info™ Data Exchange" window to
configure the location of the sample MS Access database. Select the "Data Sources" tab in
the configuration window as shown in the following figure, assign the name "Oswego" in
the first field, browse for the sample data file "Epiinfo.mdb " in the "C:\mesh4x\data"
folder by clicking on the symbol (···) in the next field, select the Oswego table from the
drop down list, and then click "Save".

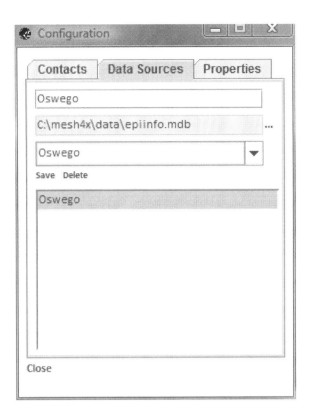

Close the "Configuration" window once the steps above are completed by clicking "Close" at the bottom left of the window.

Click the "Cloud Synchronization" option at the bottom of the "Epi Info™ Data Exchange" window (Figure 1), enter the URL for your mesh data feed you created earlier in the URL field (http://sync.staging.instedd.org/mesh4x/feeds/Epiinfo/OswegoTK) then click the button "Synch Now"

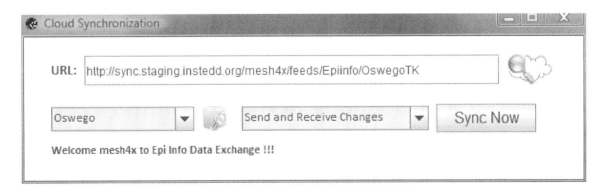

In your web browser, refresh the page for the above URL (or click the icon with the cloud and magnifying glass next to the URL field in the figure above) and you should now be able to see all of the 47 records.

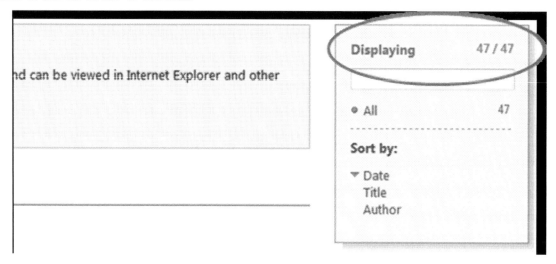

You can update the data in Epi Info™ then repeat the steps above and your data will be updated in the cloud. You can share the URL with other team members and they can share their data as described above (you only need to create the mesh group and the data feed once though). As records are being updated or new records are added, each member can simply synchronize their data with the cloud and everyone on the team will be in sync with the latest information.

Generate a Google Earth map

You can create a map and display it in Google Earth (or KML map layers) (A free copy of Google Earth can be downloaded from http://earth.google.com). Click the option "Open Maps" at the bottom of the "Epi Info™ Data Exchange" window, the "Epiinfo Map Exchange" window will appear; click on the green icon right next to the URL field to download the mapping schema you defined in an earlier step.

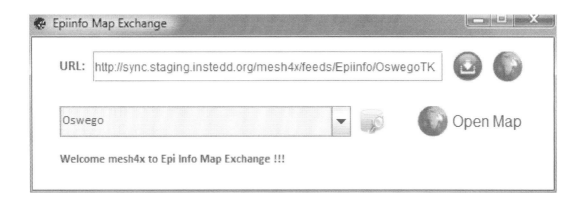

Next, click on the "Open Map" icon in order to automatically geo-code the addresses you have in your local database and generate a Google Earth map for all the cases as shown in the following figure:

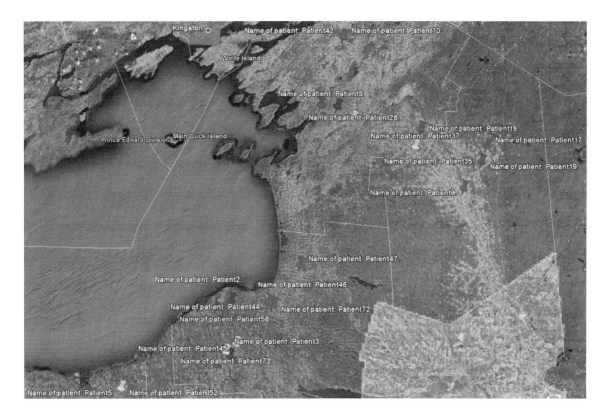

Conclusions

The impact of sharing data is that decisions can be made earlier and based on more complete analysis. Analyzing only subsets of the information about a population affected by an outbreak can lead to erroneous conclusions about the nature of the event and wasting time and response resources. We describe an application providing a lightweight solution for sharing public health data based on cloud computing and peer-to-peer architectures. The significant value of this application is demonstrated, whereby epidemiologists can rapidly stand up a collaborative environment for data exchange and system interoperability, especially when conducting an outbreak investigation or responding to a disaster under austere operating conditions.

References

1. Epi Info™: http://www.cdc.gov/epiinfo
2. CDC takes its epidemiological software open source; Government Health IT, Dec 12, 2008
3. J. Ma et al., New frontiers for health information systems using Epi Info in developing countries: Structured application framework for Epi Info (SAFE), Int. J. Med. Inform. (2007)
4. Epi Info™ and Mesh4x Prototype: http://kasshout.blogspot.com/2008/12/epi-info-and-mesh4x-prototype.html
5. Towns S. 2009. Google to Launch Government Cloud. Government Technology http://www.govtech.com/gt/724044 (accessed November 22, 2009).
6. Oswego in the Cloud: Scenario Script: http://www.slideshare.net/kasshout/oswego-in-the-cloud-scenario-script

CHAPTER 28: SOLVING PROBLEMS—SEARCH AND DON'T DESTROY

Bugs

There are several known bugs in Version 3.5.1 that lead to problems. They include:

Inability to use MAKE VIEW FROM DATA TABLE in MakeView without first choosing the Epi Info Data type as Access 95 in the SETTINGS section of the main Epi Info menu.

In the Analysis RELATE and MERGE commands, the BUILD KEY feature of the dialog will not allow more than one entry in each key box. The Enter key is not recognized. Ctrl-Enter, however, works just fine, and you can enter several field names easily with this key combination.

According to the Epi Info helpdesk, deleting a variable in a View with more than 200 fields can cause corruption of the database. There are a couple of solutions if you want to work with a very large questionnaire.

1. Review the content and see if it is all necessary. The world is full of unanalyzed data that was collected just because "it might be useful."

2. Break the content into logical entities of less than 200 variables and make each one a related view, accessible from a button on the main form. The main form can contain a page of identifiers and demographics with a second page that offers buttons leading to a number of related Views. This approach makes it easier to manage data entry and will not present the same problems in deleting fields.

Quirks and Limitations

In programming MNU files, you must use ENDIF after IF. Using END by mistake will produce errors or locking up, but no helpful error messages.

The commands WaitForExit and WaitForFileExist in the menu sometimes work as described in the help files and sometimes do not, leading to strange timing problems and hangups. It safer to insert a Dialog command so that there is a manual pause, although this may not make the user experience as smooth as it should be.

In MNU programming, mixing DOS and Windows commands may lead to problems, but sometimes it works. You can usually get away with a block in which Windows commands come first, and then DOS commands are placed at the end. Experiments and testing are recommended.

Analysis will not allow values of variables—a path name, for example—to be used as part of program commands. As a simple example, try defining a variable called MyPhrase and assigning it the value "Hi, there". Then give the command Dialog MyPhrase, or Dialog "MyPhrase". The first of these is an error, and second displays "MyPhrase". In a menu program, you can use Dialog "@@MyPhrase" , and the value, "Hi There", will be displayed. This means that the only way to get an Analysis PGM to work on different computers may be to REPLACE some of the words in the PGM file from the Menu before running the PGM.

As described in the chapter on The Complete Clinical System, the commands FindText and SubString, important for managing text phrases, are not available for menu programming, and something so simple as removing ".MDB" from the end of a file name requires a complicated workaround to put the phrase into a file, use the REPLACE command to do the work, and then feed the result back as a variable value by using a fake menu as a "script."

Check Code has an undocumented limit on the amount of code in one field You can work around this limitation by defining one or more text fields and hiding them under a button or elsewhere. Say that FieldA has too much code. The solution is to put the extra code into the hidden FieldB, followed by ENDBEFORE. Immediately before ENDBEFORE, place a GOTO and the name of the next field (possibly another hidden field).

When Things Are Acting Funny

Downloads in progress
If you have Windows updates turned on, there will be times when the computer refuses to respond because it is downloading updates. This can happen with antiviral and other software also. Try hovering the mouse over the small icons at the lower right corner of the screen to see if information pops up.

No Idea, but Reboot Cures It
Rebooting can cure a series of problems, and is worth trying whenever you don't understand what is going wrong.

Windows Task Manager
You can use Ctrl-Alt-Delete to bring up the Task Manager and see what is running and using memory and CPU resources. If you find ten copies of a program or process, all running at once, you may have made a mistake in coding, or clicked too many times on an unresponsive icon. You can stop these processes from the Task Manager or by rebooting.

Date and Time
The date and time in the lower right corner of the screen represent the SystemDate as represented in Epi Info code, but is also used by Windows in managing files. If it is wrong, strange things can happen, such as files saved right now being considered older than those made last week. If it is not current, reset it so that it is. If the computer "forgets" again and is an older computer, there may be a small battery on the motherboard that needs replacing to maintain the "BIOS settings".

Run Registry Clean Program

There are many good and many fraudulent programs on the Internet that claim to clean the Windows registry, remove excess files, and generally do miracles. Some of them are free or reasonably priced, but beware of those that offer a free scan, and then announce that, for a price, you can also have the program fix the problems. Use Internet searching to find a "review" of programs that you want to evaluate.

Disaster Recovery

Disasters include viruses, hard disk crashes, motherboard failures, unwise deletes (your own, your children's, or your cat's), effects of evil or half-baked software, power surges, fires, liquid spills, full disk, etc. Here are a few reminders to consult when disaster occurs. Many more are available on the Internet and there are books on the subject.

Prepare in Advance

Make backups, have extra hardware, ….yeah, yeah, yeah....not much help at this point.

Stop and think,

Then stop and think again. Panic and random action can make things worse, and may destroy backup copies that you have.

Gather Information

Assess what you have. Make a list of possible backups that you have made or might have made, including distribution copies or those emailed to yourself or others or uploaded to your website. Search for the missing files elsewhere on your computer in case you put elbow to keyboard and moved them inadvertently. If the files have been deleted in Windows, they should be in the Recycle Bin and can be recovered.

Make Backup Copies Of Damaged Documents

Do not turn the computer off until you have saved everything relevant to the problem, even if all you can do is print what is on the screen. Save copies of what you have to physically separate media and put these away before beginning repairs. Start a notebook page and record everything you can about the problem, including error messages, recent installations, and symptoms.

If the Computer Does Not Function

There are many reasons why a computer won't boot up. Probably the worst is total hard disk failure, but an undamaged hard disk can be copied to another computer and the data rescued. Your best ally is a skilled repair person, but you should make it clear that you want to save the data. Do not allow a computer warantee facility to simply give you a replacement computer with a new hard disk, unless it is proven that the old one is unrecoverable. In practical terms, recovering a truly crashed hard disk can cost thousands of dollars and is not usually worth this amount, but there are many problems short of a total crash that allow at least some recovery. In either case, a prior backup is/was a great idea.

A Practical Example

While writing this chapter, I tried to save the book manuscript, and an error message popped up. "Unable to Save." After the third time, I knew it was time to begin the steps mentioned above, the first being, "Don't panic or do something stupid." Then, assess the situation. Yesterday's copy was OK, so the most that could be lost is the chapter you are reading. It is still on the screen, so I try printing it. It prints and therefore is not completely lost. I try saving the main file in the RTF format, and then the Microsoft Word DOC format, both with success. Then I select the chapter, and copy it to an empty document, and it saves nicely. Whew! So now, I just open yesterday's file and copy the new chapter into place, saving it with today's date.

Take a History

Before or after the patient has been revived, we take a history, looking for any recent changes or events, new versions of software, etc. It turns out that I had run the Registry cleaning program mentioned above, just to confirm that it is helpful. It said I should close FireFox, but FireFox was not open, so I continued, leaving the manuscript open in OpenOffice. The scan completed successfully and made some fixes.

What happened is clear in retrospect. The Registry cleaner and file eraser apparently erased one or more temporary files or registry settings created by OpenOffice when a file is open, and made it impossible to save the current document. Nice illustration of the principles mentioned above— keep lots of backups, stop, think, save what you can, put things back together.

Therapeutic Trial (Shotgun Therapy)

Once you have followed the advice above about not panicking and saving every last scrap of data that can be saved, there are a number of therapeutic maneuvers to follow that have low risk, and may resolve the situation quickly. These include:

1. Rebooting Windows. Shut down the system and then restart it again. Be sure that the computer is not downloading updates when you do this, as it may cause problems with the update.

2. Scan the system for viruses. You do have a virus protection program, don't you? If not, the purchase is long overdue!!

3. Uninstall Epi Info, using the icon in the Windows Control Panel and the "Add or Remove Programs" feature. Then download the latest version of Epi Info from www.cdc.gov/epiinfo and install it.

4. Identify a registry scan and file cleanup program that is well reviewed by others on the Internet with the help of a Google or other search. Be sure that the repair features are either free or reasonably priced, as many of these programs use the bait-and-switch

technique of offering a free scan and then telling you after the nuisance value of installation and scanning, that you must pay for the repair features.

Gathering Information

After you have written down or printed all the error messages and symptoms, use an Internet search engine like www.google.com to find others who have had the same problem. Exact words or number from error messages often will turn up hints. The net is full of half-baked speculation that sounds authoritative, but you can use it as a starting place, and it can often point your next steps away from or toward particular solutions.

There are several sources of Epi Info information, starting with the CDC helpline, at epiinfo@cdc.gov and including the websites referred to under Resources in the last chapter of this book.

Inside Epi Info—Where's the debugger?

A debugger is a program that lets you execute computer code line by line and shows values of variables and output as you do so. There are a couple of tricks that can accomplish this in Epi Info programs, but they differ for the Menu, Check Code, and Analysis environments.

In a menu program, you can inset DIALOG commands that display their own location and the value of relevant variables, for example:

DIALOG "Line 6 of menu block COPYFILETONETWORK. Destination =@@Destination"

This would show a dialog box with the first sentence about location, and then the value of @@Destination as "Z:\exClinic\Analysis\Analysis.mdb"

In Check Code, the Dialog Box can mark a location, but it cannot display the value of a variable. Hence, about all you can do is insert something like:

DIALOG "AZT code, after dosage calculation"

Although this is how we discovered the limitation on the amount of Check Code in a single field, it otherwise has limited usefulness, unless you need to confirm that one block did a GOTO to another.

In Analysis, there are better tools for debugging. The dialog boxes are the same as in Check Code and can only display messages, not variable values. But if you Open the program in the program editor, or create it there, you can place the cursor on a line of code and then click RUN THIS COMMAND. The single line of code will run and the cursor will move to the next line. Repeat RUN THIS COMMAND and see the results of another line. Using this technique you can work through an entire program line by line. Although you can't display the values of variable, you can detect values as follows to confirm your guesses:

```
IF MyVar=(+)  then
   Dialog "MyVar =Yes"
END
```

Resetting Goals

Having done everything above to resolve the problem, it may be time to go for a jog, or sit by the window and think about alternative ways of doing what you intend. Explaining the goals and barriers to someone else may help. See if what you are doing is worth the effort or can be done another way.

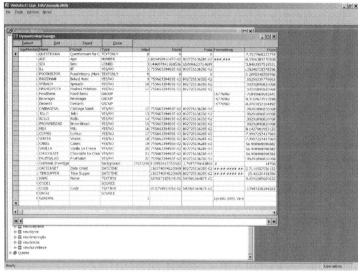

VisData

Seeing Inside Epi Info Tables

VisData is a utility program for viewing and performing useful operations on database files or tables. Choose Visualize Data from the UTILITIES menu. Choose OPEN EPIINFO PROJECT from the FILE menu and then the SAMPLE.MDB database. You should see a tree that contains Properties, Tables, and Queries. Click the plus sign next to Tables to see all the tables contained in SAMPLE.MDB. To see the contents of a table, double-click on its icon to display a grid view of the data.

Explore the contents of a code table, the Oswego data table, and viewOswego, a questionnaire View table. Note that the View has a special format that is unique to EpiInfo, but that the data table consists of simple rows and columns with variable names compatible with Microsoft Access and other database programs. Chapter 31 gives the detailed structure of Epi Info views, which you should alter only after saving backup copies of the MDB, and even then, at your own risk.

VisData is a useful utility for seeing the internal details of databases. Microsoft Access, if you have it, can be used for the same purpose, but care is needed to be sure that MDB's are saved in a format that is compatible with Epi Info, preferably Access 2000.

CHAPTER 29: EPI INFO AND CLINICAL AUDIT: AN EXERCISE

Clinical Audit is a process for assessment of clinical care quality that uses systematically gathered data to describe actual practices or results. Ideally the results are compared with an objective or standard ("X percent of emergency patients will be evaluated by a nurse or physician within 5 minutes of arrival"). Steps are taken to achieve the desired results, and the auditing process is repeated to assess the outcome. Although the term Clinical Audit is native to the United Kingdom, similar processes are conducted in many countries.

Epi Info and other database and statistical programs can be used to organize and process data in a clinical audit. The needs are for flexible data entry or abstraction from databases, usually involving hundreds or thousands, not millions, of records. Ready and preferably free availability of software usable by medical professionals is desirable. These characteristics describe Epi Info in both its DOS and Windows versions, and, in fact, a book has been published about the use of Epi Info 6 (the DOS version) for clinical audit (Stewart A and Rao JN, Clinical Audit and Epi Info, Radcliffe Medical Press Ltd, Abingdon, UK, 2003).

In this exercise, we will use Epi Info for Windows to process data from the Romagna Area of Italy.

Standards

There are many documents available on the Internet containing standards for evaluation of clinical diabetes care. With the help of a search engine like www.google.com, you can pick one that is most relevant for your own area. One that is recent and well documented is:

American Diabetes Association
Executive Summary: Standards of Medical Care in Diabetes—2010.
Diabetes Care January2010 33:S4-S10;
http://care.diabetesjournals.org/content/33/Supplement_1/S4.full

Data

Data files from actual practice are provided by Dr. Pasquale Falasca, Ravenna, Italy, with patient identifiers removed, and physicians indicated only by letters of the alphabet. This exercise on evaluation of care is based on these files, but they should be considered only a non-random sample of the actual files from which they came. The files for this exercise are in ..\Examples\exClinicalAudit\.

No dataset is perfect, except perhaps those gathered for a narrow and specific purpose (e.g., in cash registers), but we will try to illustrate in this exercise a number of general operations with Epi Info that can be applied to almost any patient registry or list of individuals and their characteristics.

These operations include:

- Importing data from a file that is not in the Epi Info/Microsoft Access format.

- Identifying and fixing data problems such as invalid dates, mixtures of coding systems (M/F, 1 / 2, 0 / "neg", etc.)

- Calculating ages or durations from dates

- Recoding continuous data (days or years of age) to categorical data (decade of age)

- Doing descriptive analysis (e.g., % of patients with diabetes, case load by physician)

- Selecting portions of the data for analysis

- Measuring Process variables

- Measuring Outcome/Result variables

- Finding or testing associations between variables (BMI and hypertension for example)

- Mutivariable analysis—adjusting for effects of more than one variable

- Repeating the work so far by running a program

- Saving and recalling programs for later use

- Making a data entry form for additional variables

- Making a data entry form from the existing data table

- Linking the new data form to the existing data form

- Adding variables to the dataset

- Using the Epi Info Menu to make the Audit process easy and repeatable

Importing Data from a Text File

1. PatientRegistry.csv is a comma-delimited TEXT File

2. Run Epi Info and choose ANALYZE DATA

3. With the READ command, choose Text(delimited) and the PatientRegistry.csv file.

4. Use the LIST command to see the records.

5. Use the WRITE command to write all variables, in "Epi2000" format, to a table called Registry in an MDB called PatientRegistry.MDB

6. READ the new table (choose ALL to see tables)

Cleaning Data with IF and ASSIGN

1. Detect invalid dates with FREQuencies and ASSIGN the missing value, =(.)

2. Do the same with impossible lab values (can fix with LIST UPDATE if you know the correct values

3. Mixtures of coding systems (M/F, 1 / 2, 0 / "neg", etc.)--use FREQ to identify and IF and ASSIGN to fix. Convert Sex to "M" and "F"

4. Remove text comments from quantitative fields.

Calculating Ages and Other Durations from Dates

1. Calculate Age in years from DOB [ ] and SystemDate [ ]

2. Use the ASSIGN command with the Function YEARS to place the values in AGE.

3. For help, click Functions in the ASSIGN window

4. DEFINE a variable called MonthsSinceA1C and use the MONTHS function to ASSIGN it the difference between Date_Hemo_A1C and SystemDate

Recoding Continuous Data (months or years) to Categorical Data (decade)

1. DEFINE Decade as a text variable

2. Use RECODE with Age and Decade

3. Click Fill Ranges and 0 for Start, 100 for End, and 10 for By

4. Do a Frequency of Decade to check results

Descriptive Analysis

1. Use LIST to see data and variable names

2. Use FREQuencies to find number of patients in registry by decade, sex, diabetes, physician, and other variables

3. Find the number of diabetic and non-diabetic patients for each physician

4. Find mean age of diabetic and non-diabetic patients

SELECTing Portions of the Data

1. Use SELECT with Diabetes=(+) to limit records to diabetic patients

2. Use WRITE to create a new table called DiabeticPatients containing all variables in the current dataset

3. READ DiabeticPatients and find the Mean Hemo_A1C by physician. Do the same for glucose.

Measuring Process Variables

1. For Diabetic Patients, describe MonthsSinceA1C by physician

2. Use the SET dialog to include or not include missing values

3. How many Patients have a date for Date_Hemo_A1C and no value for Hemo_A1C

4. How many patients do not have a glucose or BMI recorded?

Finding Sentinel Problems

1. DEFINE a new variable called HighRisk

2. Assign HighRisk=(+) for Smokers with Hypertension and Elevated Cholesterol

3. How many Diabetic and Non-diabetic patients are HighRisk

4. Imagine that you are one of the physicians with patients in the registry. Produce a LIST of patients meeting these criteria that contains the risk factors mentioned, ID number, age, and sex of the patients

Measuring Outcome/Result Variables

1. How many patients have had a Stroke_TIA?

2. What other outcome variables would you like to see added to the registry?

Defining and Calculating the Ratio of Total Cholesterol to HDL

1. DEFINE Ratio to hold the rounded result

2. ASSIGN Ratio the value of Cholesterol / HDL

3. One way to achieve one decimal place is to Assign Ratio=Round(CholesterolHDLRatio*10) / 10

4. Another is to convert the number to text as follows Ratio=Format(CholesterolHDLRatio, ##.#)

5. What percent of diabetic patients have a ratio <=4? <=3? How does this relate to risk of cardiovascular events?

Counting Risk Factors

Yes/No variables coded as 1 and 0 can simply be added together to determine the total number of "Yeses" for a patient.

1. DEFINE RiskFactors

2. DEFINE HighCholesterol and assign it a Yes/No value based on reasonable criteria, for example, Cholesterol>

3. RiskFactors=Hypertension+HighCholesterol + Smoke

Finding or Testing Associations Between Variables

1. Is Stroke_TIA associated with hypertension?

2. Is hypertension associated with BMI and/or Waist Circumference?

Mutivariable Analysis—Adjusting for Effects of More than One Variable

1. If you found an association between Stroke_TIA and other variables, what happens if you adjust for Age?

2. Use LOGISTIC regression with Stroke_TIA as the outcome. Include and as other variables and AGE and any others you found to be of interest.

Saving Commands in a Program (PGM)

1. In order to run the same analysis again, perhaps with different data, SAVE the current program.

2. Click the SAVE button in the program editor.

3. Click Save as Text File, and give a location and name to the program (Audit.PGM, for example)

Repeating the Work So Far by Running a Program

1. Run the program and fix errors, then SAVE again

2. Click the RUN button in the Program Editor

3. If there are errors, edit the program to prevent them. Insert ROUTEOUT 'Diabetes.htm' at the top of the program.

4. SAVE the program again.

5. Now OPEN the saved program and RUN it again. You can also use the RUN SAVED PROGRAM command to do the same thing.

Making a Data Entry View from a Data Table

CAUTION: There is a bug in Epi Info that requires setting the EPI INFO DATABASE VERSION in the Epi Info menu SETTINGS to "Access 97" before carrying out this step. After the View is made, you can set the type back to "Access 2000"

1. In the Epi Info menu, find EPI INFO DATABASE VERSION under SETTINGS and set it to ACCESS 97

2. Run MakeView from the menu

3. Under File, choose New and give MyRegistry as the name of the MDB and viewMyRegistry for the View

4. When you have the blank screen, do not create any fields, but instead use MAKE VIEW FROM DATA TABLE under Tools to make the View from the data table PatientRegistry. Be patient; it takes a while, as it also copies all the data.

Adding Variables to the Dataset

1. Rearrange the variables on the screen, using MakeView, and add some groups by click-drag-selecting several variables and then choosing Group from the Insert menu.

2. Add variables for DKA (episodes of diabetic ketoacidosis), and Acute Myocardial Infarction (AMI) as number fields. Add weight in kilograms as Kilos and height as Centimeters. Create a numeric, read-only field called BMI with the pattern ##.##

Calculating Body Mass Index

Metric BMI = kilos/(meters*meters)

Note: meters=centimeters/100

Implement this formula in Check Code in the field for Centimeters in your data entry View.

1. Be sure that all the necessary values are present before doing the calculation so that errors do not occur

Making a Menu to Make the Audit Process Easy and Repeatable

1. Click the shortcut called Run MakeMenu and use the Tools | Create entries to make a new menu called Diabetes. When instructed, look for the Diabetes shortcut on your desktop and double-click it to run the new menu.

2. Use Edit This Menu and find the command block EnterCases. Change the View to PatientRegistry:Registry. In the RunAnalysisPGM block, change the PGM name to Audit.PGM. Save the file and you should be able to enter and analyze data from the Diabetes menu.

Change the Menu Image

1. Use Tools | Change Picture to change the current sky image to Audit.jpg

2. In the MNU file, find the Button "Intro to Epi Info Via Web" and remove it. Move the Exit button by changing its coordinates until it is in a pleasing location. Make any changes in the ScreenText items or the Menuitems that you think appropriate

This completes the exercise, although there are many possibilities for further analysis

Conversion Values

Total Cholesterol:
1 mmol/L = 39 mg/dL

LDL Cholesterol:
1 mmol/L = 39 mg/dL

HDL Cholesterol:
1 mmol/L = 39 mg/dL

Triglerides:
1 mmol/L = 89 mg/dL

Blood glucose:
1 mmol/L = 18 mg/dL

Imperial BMI Formula

The imperial BMI formula accepts weight measurements in pounds & height measurements in either inches or feet.
1 foot = 12 inches
inches² = inches * inches

Table: Imperial BMI Formula

$$\text{BMI} \; (kg/m^2) = \frac{(\text{weight in pounds} * 703)}{\text{height in inches}^2}$$

Metric Imperial BMI Formula

The metric bmi formula accepts weight measurements in kilograms & height measurements in either cm's or meters.
1 meter = 100cms
meters² = meters * meters

Table: Metric BMI Formula

$$\text{BMI} \; (kg/m^2) = \frac{\text{weight in kilograms}}{\text{height in meters}^2}$$

Targets for parameters of interest

Tests done and desired results

Glucose < 7 mmol/L (<126 mg/dL)

Glucose >4 mmol/L (>72 mg.dL)

Hemoglobin A1c <=7% If no cardiovascular disease <=6

Total Cholesterol / HDL Cholesterol

Risk Factors (desired range)

BMI   18.5-24.9 kg/m^2   desired range

Waist circumference   females <88 (34.6 inches) males < 102 cm (40 inches)

Smokes 0

BP   130/80 or below

Adverse outcomes

Emerg Visits

A1C > 7

Other Chronic Diseases

Resources

Sample and exercise files for this chapter are found in **exClinicalAudit** in the **Examples** folder.

CHAPTER 30: TEACHING INFORMATICS WITH EPI INFO AND OPENEPI

Resources for Teaching or Learning Epi Info
Why Use Epi Info?

Why use Epi Info for a course in Public Health Computing? Here are reasons that may or may not be important in your setting:

1. It is available without charge and can be downloaded or distributed on CD ROM so that students are immediately equipped with the tools they study in class and have a reasonable expectation of obtaining updates in the future

2. It uses Microsoft Windows standards such as Microsoft Access Databases, HTML, and ESRI shapefiles, and can import and export common database formats for compatibility with SAS, SPSS, Stata, ArcView, Excel, and other popular database and statistics programs.

3. Many students find Epi Info easier to understand than larger programs

4. Epi Info and related materials are available in Spanish, Italian, and possibly other languages (See the www.cdc.gov/epiinfo) web site for more information.)

5. Epi Info may have been used to construct permanent applications in the setting from which the students come, thus making these courses particularly relevant

6. Because it is possible to design and implement a new database system in half an hour, Epi Info permits rapid instruction in informatics principles

7. Epi Info integrates database design, data entry, data management, tabulation, a broad range of epidemiologic statistics, nutritional anthropometry, graphing, geographic information systems (GIS), encryption and decryption of files, double data entry and verification, help files, tutorials, and a configurable menuing system, into one (more or less) consistent package.

Epi Info for DOS, or Epi Info 6 was popular during the 1980s and 90s, and is still used in many settings today. It has the advantages of simplicity and reliability and the transparency of a text-based file structure, but is increasingly less compatible with the Windows environments that now dominate public health computing at the desktop and laptop level.

Epi Info for Windows initially acquired a reputation for being "buggy," partially because it was, and partially because early users expected Windows programs to respond like and resemble DOS programs. Over the years since its release, however, most of the bugs have been corrected, and the programs are now comparable in solidity to Epi 6. The author's own experience is that, although the programs could be easier to use, and several approaches to solving a problem may be needed before one succeeds, that, once something works, it continues to work. The exercises and examples represent the results of considerable trial and error in the hope of leading students and instructors past the difficult points.

Some users still regret the choice of the Microsoft Access file format as the standard for Epi Info for Windows, because it is neither transparent nor easily understood. The file format should be explained,, as the concept of Microsoft Database (MDB) or project containing multiple instances of Views and Data Tables is quite different from the REC and QES files of Epi 6.

To the maximum extent possible, a course should be a hands-on, laboratory experience, although classes of students, particularly those from outside the United States, seem to expect a certain amount of lecturing, coordinating, and general hand-waving from the instructor. In teaching a class of 10 to 25 students, it is important to have at least one assistant who can circulate, look over shoulders, answer questions, and alert the instructor when students are having problems. In choosing assistants, extensive knowledge of Epi Info itself--although desirable--is less important than general Windows competence, patience with students, and concepts of public health .

Materials for two courses are provided as Course I and Course II at www.epiinformatics.com. Both courses require a general perspective of public health comparable to that of Public Health Master's candidates, medical students, or those working in medical or public health systems. Course I is designed for students with minimal computer skills, and many students have only used Windows for word processing and perhaps email. Course II builds on knowledge of data management taught in Course I. Students beginning course II should be able to make a questionnaire View in Epi Info and do simple data analysis. If they have not taken Course I, this might be obtained by doing the exercises in the Introduction to Epi Info for Windows available from www.EpiInformatics.com and contained on the CD ROM that accompanies this manual. Exceptions can be made for students with advanced knowledge of other database and statistics programs, particularly if they are quick learners.

Strangely enough, those who seem to have the most difficulty in learning Epi Info for Windows are either Epi 6 users or SAS or SPSS text-oriented programmers. Students who have grown up with Microsoft Windows rather than DOS seem to learn and enjoy Epi Info for Windows quite readily.

Demonstrations

Where possible, the sequence of Introduction, Demonstration, Do-With-Instructions, Do-With-Minimal-Instructions is desired. Depending on the previous experience of the class, demonstrations can be inserted as a quick way of bringing everyone to the same entry point. If the entire class has used Epi Info for Windows previously, there is little reason to demonstrate making a questionnaire View at the beginning of Course II. If half the class, however, has only had experience with SAS or SPSS, then a demonstration can help to provide a solid starting point.

Standard demonstrations, using mostly the tables in SAMPLE.MDB, are found in Introduction to Epi Info for Windows (from www.EpiInformatics.com), which is an enhanced version of what were known originally as Guided Tours.

Compact Disks (CDs)

The courses in this series are packaged in two folders (the Windows name for directories) called EpiInfoCourseI and EpiInfoCourseII. It would be possible to give each member of a classe a CD ROM with the following contents:

- EpiInfoCourseI

- EpiInfoCourseII

- Install Epi Info (Contains the latest Epi Info setup file and README)

- Maps (Contains shape files of the world, downloaded from www.cdc.gov/epiinfo)

- CDC Exercises (The contents of a 5-day course for Epi Info instructors, given by the Epi Info Development Team, downloaded from www.cdc.gov/epiinfo)

- Introductions

- This book as a PDF file

- OpenEpi (A series of epidemiologic calculators from www.openepi.com that is a Windows replacement for Statcalc)

- Epi Info 6, for those who might want it

Obtaining, Installing, and Testing Epi Info

The latest version of Epi Info for Windows is available from www.cdc.gov/epiinfo, and can be downloaded and distributed as a single file on CDROM. With a good Internet connection, it can also be installed directly from the web site. A README.TXT file is usually available at the same site. Additional materials, such as tutorials, are available by perusing the same site. These and other teaching materials are described in the next section.

Epi Info is designed to be run from individual computers and not from a network server, although it can be installed from a server in a computer laboratory, and students can all enter data in the same database (MDB) on the server (but with load limitations that should be tested in advance).

Problems in installation have arisen in the following situations:

1. Failing to uninstall previous versions of Epi Info for Windows, unless the web site instructions say otherwise

2. When disk space or RAM or operating systems vary among computers in a laboratory and this is not discovered early

3. Installing with administrative user privileges and conducting the class in a laboratory that imposes special security restrictions on student use. If this is planned, then it is important to test the programs thoroughly in Student mode, and even then, to have someone with Administrative privileges available to enable problems to be corrected if necessary. We manage to teach in a laboratory where the Administrator goes home for the weekend, and no one has administrative access during the course, but there have been some very close calls and some strange workarounds invented on the spot.

4. Where MDBs are either copied from a CDROM by Windows (not XP) in read-only form, or when installed files are made read-only by security modes in a student laboratory. MDBs will not function as read-only files, and this situation must be corrected before doing the exercises. MDBs cannot be accessed directly on CDROMs; they must first be copied to a hard disk, zip drive, flash drive, or other writable medium. We have taught our courses in a laboratory where we are required to place all the exercises on ZIP drives. Although Epi Info and its SAMPLE.MDB are installed in the hard disk in each computer, these files behave as read-only in Student mode, and SAMPLE.MDB must be copied to the ZIP drive for use in the exercises.

5. There is a setting in the Epi Info menu for the Working Directory. Since this setting is stored in the Windows Registry, it must be chosen while the computer is accessed in Administrative mode. It should be set to a writable directory, where the MDBs for the exercises are easily found. If the exercises are on ZIP drive D:, then D:\EpiInfoCourseII\ would be a good choice for the Working Directory. Since this merely controls the default working directory, failing to set it is not critical, but it makes finding files much easier for the students.

6. Testing should be done under conditions, including security settings, that will be experienced by the class. If at all possible, the entire course should be run as a test. This can be a good way to bring your lab assistant(s) up to speed for teaching the course.

Particularly with Windows XP, installing Service Pack 2 (SP 2) automatically configures the Internet Explorer browser so that popup windows are not allowed, and sometimes so that JavaScript is not allowed to run. This prevents OpenEpi, the extra statistical program provided with these exercises (and even some of Microsoft's own web pages) from running. Try OpenEpi and be sure that the programs work correctly. If not, adjust the popup prevention and other security settings until things work properly. Other popup prevention programs (such as the Google toolbar) can be set to permit popups on designated sites or when running programs from the hard disk rather than the Internet.

Computers

Epi Info for Windows runs on all Microsoft Windows versions except Windows 95 and possibly Windows 98 First Edition. System requirements are given on the Epi Info web site. Any reasonably modern desktop or laptop computer will work, although some computer laboratories may lag behind in providing enough RAM, disk space or processor speed to make learning pleasant. The fact that Windows XP has had only incremental improvements over that past few years has greatly aided teaching, and increasingly Windows XP seems to be the system encountered when teaching courses, a blessing for both classes and instructors.

Resources

See the final chapter in this book for a list of resources, including materials for two 15-hour courses..

CHAPTER 31: INTERNAL DETAILS OF EPI INFO

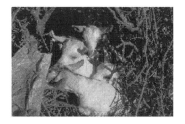 For Visual Basic Programmers

Overview

This chapter provides details on selected parts of the Epi Info internal architecture for Visual Basic programmers who wish to understand how Epi Info 2000 Views are stored or how to write new statistical modules for incorporation into future versions of Epi Info. Views provide metadata about the databases created by Epi Info and also describe the screen appearance of forms sufficiently so that they can be used, for example, to construct an HTML equivalent of an Epi Info View. The Broad Street Library of Statistics is the name given to an anticipated library of statistical routines built around the specification included in this chapter for the IEPI statistical interface. IEPI provides standard means for sending data and settings to a statistical module (a Windows Dynamic Linked Library –DLL, or other ActiveX module) and receiving back the statistical results, both in the form of an HTML string suitable for display and alternatively as a series of named parameters (e.g., "p value") and values (e.g., 0.005).

The Structure of Views

A View is a Microsoft Access file with a structure defined by Epi Info. It contains information on the screen appearance of a database or part of a database. In this sense, it resembles the questionnaire file and especially the header of the REC file in Epi Info for DOS.

Each field in a View is described by a record in the View table. User-generated Check Code and settings for the field are stored in the same record. View records generally contain:

- The Number of the Page where the field is displayed. Page 0 is reserved for special records that pertain to the entire View.

- The Prompt for display on the screen.

- The horizontal and vertical locations of the Prompt and the Field itself, as percentages of screen height and width.

- The Size of the field as displayed (although text fields scroll to accept 128 characters regardless of their size on the screen, and multiline fields will accept almost unlimited amounts of text).

- Check Code for the field.

- Lists of miscellaneous items, such as code files.

- The location where data items are stored or retrieved. The DataTable field contains a reference to a record on Page 0 that contains the actual data table name.

The name of the field is assumed to be the same as the field name stored in the View.

Records with 0 or negative page numbers contain additional information, such as colors and the names of background images that apply to whole pages or to the entire View.

Special field records contain information on Related Views and Grids, which are a type of related View.

Each Data source (Database and DataTable) used by the View has a field in Page 0 of Type SOURCE and a Name consisting of DATA plus a number (1, 2, or 3, for example). The numbers start at 1 and proceed in the order of first use of the data source by the View. The data source fields of the SOURCE records contain the path, filename, and TableName of the data table, using paths relative to the location of the .MDB that contains the View.

Data source fields in each Field record contain the Name used by the SOURCE record, for example, DATA1.

A similar method is be used for Code Tables, storing the location of the Code Table in records of Type SOURCE, with Names CODE1, CODE2, etc. Field records refer to CODE1, CODE2, etc., where the actual names are stored.

Related Views are identified in records on Page 0 with Type SOURCE and names RELVIEW1, RELVIEW2, etc. The same names are used to identify the related views in Field Records of type RELATE.

The effect of these indirect references is to concentrate information on data sources (metadata) in records of type SOURCE. To use a different SOURCE, all that is required is to change the SOURCE record so that it refers to another source. If fields in the source referred to match those in the fields of the View, then the link is successful; otherwise, the fields can be ignored or an error message issued.

Version information for a View should be included on Page 0 of the view (e.g., "Epi Info 2000, Version 1.00").

This process provides a method of substituting new data sources for those in a View. A MetaData table containing the names of SOURCE records in a View will contain references to an alternative set of data sources and the name of the View. MetaData files can be loaded directly into either

Enter or *Analysis* to bring up the relevant View and Data tables. Source records in the View are essentially ignored in favor of the information in the MetaData file (or table). The MetaData information can also be used to generate a description of the database for other purposes, although related Views must be consulted to find information on a complex hierarchy.

Records in the MetaData table are identical to the SOURCE records in a VIEW, with the addition of one more record of Type "VIEW" that identifies the main View to be used with the designated SOURCE files or tables.

The user can OPEN a MetaData table in *Enter* or *MakeView*, and READ a MetaData table in *Analysis*. In *MakeView*, the MetaData table provides only the View. In *Enter* and *Analysis*, the SOURCE records are read from the MetaData table and the information is stored in memory before the designated VIEW is read. SOURCE records in the VIEW are ignored if there is a MetaData table, thus effectively substituting the data sources specified in the MetaData table for those specified in the View table. This allows a single view to be used with as many data sources as desired, merely by making a new MetaData table for each View/Source combination. Views and Sources must "match" to the extent that variables referred to in the View are present in the Source and related tables have appropriate keys.

A Simplified View Table

PageNo	Name	Type	DataBase	DataTable	DataField
0	DATA1	SOURCE	SAMPLE.MDB	recOswego	
0	DATA2	SOURCE	SAMPLE.MDB	recOswego1	
0	CODE1	SOURCE	..\Codes\CODES.MDB	NYCounties	
0	RELVIEW1	SOURCE	SAMPLE.MDB	recContacts	

A Simplified MetaData Table for the View OSWEGO in SAMPLE.MDB

PageNo	Name	Type	DataBase	DataTable	DataField
0	MAINVIEW1	VIEW	SAMPLE.MDB	viewOSWEGO	
0	DATA1	SOURCE	SAMPLE.MDB	recDecatur	
0	DATA2	SOURCE	SAMPLE.MDB	recDecatur1	
0	CODE1	SOURCE	..\Codes\CODES.MDB	GACounties	
0	RELVIEW1	SOURCE	SAMPLE.MDB	recGAContacts	

NOTE: References to a data source outside of the current MDB must be replaced by a reference to an Access Link table within the current MDB.

Fields in a View Table	
PageNo	Number
Prompt	May be very long
Name	Name of field—up to 12 characters
Type	Field type—up to 12 characters *
Index	Type of index if any—Unique, secondary, etc.
DSize	Size of displayed field on screen
FSize	Maximum size of field data
Format String	String of specified types
PlocX	Location of prompt LEFT
PlocY	Location of prompt TOP
FlocX	Location of field LEFT
FlocY	Location of field TOP
TabOrder	Tab order For discussion—page, entire form, or one form
PFont	Prompt Font
PFontsize	Prompt Font Size
PFonttype	Prompt Font Type (italic, etc)
FFont	Field Font
FFontsize	Field Font Size
FFonttype	Field Font Type (italic, etc)
Lists	Legal values, code lists, and special purpose info for some field types, (Very large capacity)
Checkcode	Epi Info Commands for this field
Database	Link to project database (default) or to another database
Datatable	Link to data table
Datafield	Link to datafield

Additional details of View tables can be obtained by making an appropriate View in MakeView and then examining it with the VisData program in the Utilities menu.

Note: The following sections are included for completeness, but may be obsolete, since the source code for Epi Info 3.5.1 has not been released to the public.

The Broad Street Library of Statistics: Specifications for Statistical, Graphing, and Mapping Modules for Epi Info 2000

The statistics, graphing, and mapping in Epi Info 2000 are implemented as ActiveX (formerly OLE) modules. The interface specification used is available for others to use in developing additional modules that could be added to a future version of Epi Info 2000. Communication between a calling module and an ActiveX module such as TABLE.DLL is done through an Interface, which the ActiveX module IMPLEMENTS. The standard Interface Class for Epi Info 2000 is called IEPI (Letter "I" EPI, not numeral "1" EPI)), found in the Visual Basic program file called IEPI.CLS and the Interface Module, IEPI.DLL.

If the ActiveX module is written in Visual Basic, Version 6, the module includes the words, IMPLEMENTS IEPI, in its declarations. Selecting each of the IEPI methods or properties in the programming module of Visual Basic 6 will copy the skeleton of the property or method into the new module, with the addition of "IEPI_" prior to the name of the property or function. Thus GetFunctionNames becomes IEPI_GetFunctionNames, etc. The IEPI.DLL file should be copied to the programmer's computer and registered for use in the system registry, either through Visual Basic or by using a separate program like REGSVR32.EXE.

The IEPI Type Library, Source Code for a DLL Containing Virtual Functions to be IMPLEMENTed by Compatible ActiveX Modules

```
Public Property Get FunctionNames() As Variant
'Returns the names of functions in the module as an array of strings
End Property

Public Property Let NumRows(ByVal vNewValue As Long)
'Set to the number of rows in the dataset by the client that provides the data
End Property

Public Property Let NumColumns(ByVal vNewValue As Long)
'Set to the number of columns in the dataset by the client that provides the data
End Property

Public Property Let NumStrata(ByVal vNewValue As Long)
'Set to the number of strata in the dataset by the client that provides the data
End Property

Public Property Let ColumnTypes(ByVal vNewValue As Variant)
'An array set to the type of data contained in each column
End Property
```

```
Public Property Let ColumnNames(ByVal vNewValue As Variant)
'An array set to the name of each column
End Property

Public Property Let Settings(ByVal vNewValue As Variant)
'Settings relevant to the procedures being requested
'Is an array with two dimensions, (1..2,1..n).  Settings[1,n] is the name of  the setting;
'Settings[2,n] is its value.  Both are variants.
End Property

Public Property Let DataArray(ByVal vNewValue As Variant)
'An array having the dimensions (1..columns,1..rows, 1..strata) containing
'the data.  If the data are not stratified, the third dimension and the value of the index are
'always 1.  If only a single value, such as a Key, is passed, then columns, rows, and
strata 'are all 1, and DataArray[1,1,1) = the Key.
End Property

Public Property Let MoreDataComing(ByVal vNewValue As Boolean)
'A boolean set by the client if more data will follow that is not currently
'in the DataArray.
End Property

Public Property Get Explanation() As String
'Additional explanation, if any, for display
End Property

Public Property Get ResultArray() As Variant
' Results expressed as name of statistic, value of statistic, in a
' two-dimensional array or collection.  May be used as an alternative to the
' string returned by DoFunction
End Property

Public Function DoFunction(FunctionName As String) As String
'Calls on the stated routine.  Note that routines must be
'Public functions so that they remain in memory while
'needed; this routine allows them to be called
'by passing the string name of the routine.  Returns
'Resultstring if successful; otherwise, an error code.
End Function

Public Property Get Settings() as Variant
'Settings relevant to the procedures being requested.  This should be implemented as a
2-'dimensional array (1..2, 1..n) with the first item being a string "setting name" and the
'second the default value of the setting.  This allows the client program to discover or
'display the setting possibilities even without documentation of the server module.
```

End Property

Interaction of the Client (e.g., *Analysis* or *StatCalc*) with the Server (e.g., STAT01.DLL, containing Fisher Exact and Odds Ratio Functions) proceeds as follows:

- Client checks the FunctionNames property of the STATXX module (say, Fisher Exact, for example) to get a list of available methods.

- *Analysis* then constructs an SQL query that includes the SELECTS, IF's, and other conditions prescribed by the user, and places the data in the DataArray property, specifying the number of Rows, Columns, and Strata in the corresponding properties. Setting, or the name of a settings file, can be passed in the SETTINGS property.

- The client program, *Analysis* in this case, then calls the statistical function.

- The Statistical Server (User-supplied function) checks for essential parameters (data, for example) and if some are missing, pops up a user dialog to get those needed.

- The Statistical Server (User-supplied function) does appropriate calculations and returns results as:

A string (up to 32 K), with results suitable for display on the screen or for printing. This can be in plain text format, but the preferred format is HTML, so that the result displays nicely in a browser. Strings suitable for translation into non-English languages should be enclosed between tags with the name "tlt" (for "TransLaTion"), as follows: <tlt>Confidence Limits</tlt>. These tags are not displayed by common browsers, but can be used by Epi Info programs *Analysis* and *StatCalc* to identify items requiring translation. Each item is sent to the language translation module before being sent to the HTML output file in the *Analysis* or *StatCalc* program.

An array containing:

Name of Statistic	Value
etc.	

for the statistics produced.

Analysis or *StatCalc* formats and displays the results that are returned as a string or array. If the module has its own display, as for Chart, Map, and Summary, the user interacts with the server module until he/she wishes to return to the client.

Common Features of IEPI Modules

These are ActiveX modules that are callable from *Analysis* or *StatCalc*, and use the IEPI interface to obtain data from the calling program

Each module has a number of properties by which it is configured, that can be set from dialogs (property pages) within the module and then saved. The name of the saved properties can be passed in the SETTINGS property of IEPI when the module is called. Note that this resembles the mechanism by which .MAP files store the properties of *Epi Map*, allowing one to recreate the map merely by referring to the name of the .MAP file.

The name of the data file or an SQL string to read it may be passed to the module, or a complete set of instructions may be stored in a .MAP or .CHT file for use by the module.

Acknowledgment:

This chapter is taken in its entirety from the manual for Epi Info 2000, published in the public domain by CDC.

CHAPTER 32: TIPS AND TRICKS

Here are some suggestions for performing tasks that are not always easy in Epi Info.

Inserting the Value of a Variable into a Program (PGM)

In Analysis, you can use the DIALOG command to present a choice of fields or values in a field to the user, set a variable to the chosen entry, and then use the variable as part of a SELECT statement, for example. The Epi Info help file for the DIALOG COMMAND gives more details.

Unfortunately it is not possible to use a global variable in a READ command, for example, so that the location of a dataset can be set from a menu. Since the menu program has location variables like MenuDir, and InstallDir indicating where things are, you can insert these values into a PGM using the menu's REPLACE command. If your PGM is called MonthlyReport.pgm, for example, you can place a command like READ %DataLocation% \MyData.MDB:viewData1 into a file called MonthlyReport.SRC and then use REPLACE to change "%DataLocation%" to a value derived from @@menuDir within the menu. The use of the "%" signs is merely to make the phrase unique; you can use any unique identifier as a target for replacement. AAABBBCCC would work just as well.

Consult the REPLACE command in the help file for more information, and check the index of this book for an example.

Inserting a Carriage Return into a Text String Assembled in Check Code

There is no symbol that substitutes for a carriage return or paragraph marker that can be inserted into a series of text phrases to make them appear on separate lines. Suppose that you have a multiline text field called MyText in a View and you wish to assemble several lines as a message., as follows:

MyText="This is line 1" & "This is line 2" & "This is line 3"

This will appear as

"This is line 1This is line2This is line3".

But now, we add another multiline field into the View, naming it CR and checking the REPEAT choice in the field dialog, and, in the first record entered, we press the Enter key once. Then we can change the assignment statement to:

MyText="This is line 1" & CR & "This is line 2" & CR & "This is line 3"

Now MyText will appear as:

This is line 1

> **This is line 2**
> **This is line 3**

After all this is working, you can use the HIDE command to make the CR field disappear.

Stopping an Analysis program that has errors

The most common error in Analysis is that the READ statement fails to find a valid database and View or data table. This causes a series of errors for the commands that follow because they cannot find the variables to which they refer. To prevent this use the RECORDCOUNT variable as follows:

```
IF RECORDCOUNT=0 THEN
  Dialog "The data records were not found; exiting from the program"
  Exit
End
```

To prevent other errors, you can insert DIALOG commands in the PGM that give the user a choice of continuing or exiting from the program.

Translating the Contents of an MDB

If you have developed a View in one language (say, English) and want to translate it to another (say, Spanish), you can change the prompts that appear on the screen in the View merely by double- or right-clicking the prompts in MakeView and making changes. The mask of a date field can be changed in MakeView, from dd/mm/yyyy to mm/dd/yyyy, for example, without causing problems.

Using the Enter program, data in the database can be stored in any language that your computer and keyboard will allow. In the Enter program, the values for "Yes," "No", and "Missing" can be set to those of another language, since they are stored as zeroes and ones in the data.

Changing Field Names

If you want to change the field names and have already entered data, the choices are to delete the data table in MakeView, after which you can change the View any way your like, or to make the changes using Search and Replace in the View table and Data table using Microsoft Access. If you are careful, this will make the necessary changes in Check Code that resides in the View. Note that the field name in a View table must match that in the Data table, and that neither can have spaces or punctuation. The structure of Views is described in detail in the chapter on Internal Details, and can also be seen by opening the database and View table in the Visdata (Visualize Data) program, available on the Utilities menu of .Epi Info. Be sure to make backup copies of your database before attempting this digital surgery.

Copying a View to a New MDB

The COPY VIEW feature in the FILE menu of MakeView is quite flexible and will allow you to copy a view with or without its data table and code tables. If you copy to a non-existent MDB, it will make a new MDB. The Visdata program on the Utilities menu of Epi Info will also copy individual tables from one MDB to another, and may be useful, for example, to copy an individual code table, or to delete unwanted tables.

Deleting a Table

Individual tables in an MDB can be deleted with the DELETE FILE/TABLE command in Analysis. If you prefer to use Visdata, you can open an MDB, display its tables, and right-click on a table to bring up a menu containing a Delete option.

Password Protecting a Database

If you have Microsoft Access, you can password protect an MDB database using the Access feature in DATABASE TOOLS called SET DATBASE PASSWORD. Opening the database in Epi Info will require the password. Since it applies to the entire MDB, you may want to structure your MDBs so that the protected dataset is contained in an MDB by itself.

File Servers and Local Area Network servers have methods for limiting access with passwords, and these can be employed in addition to those from Access or Epi Info.

See "Encryption" in the index for another way of protecting a database.

Preventing Changes in a View and in Check Code

In the Enter program, the FILE menu contains an item called EDIT VIEW that runs the MakeView program with the current View. You can return to Enter with the ENTER DATA feature of the MakeView FILE menu. Although this is a convenience while designing a View and programming Check Code, it allows any user of the View to make changes, whether intentionally or not.

If you are developing a View for distribution to others and do not want them to have access to the MakeView program, you can disable this feature by renaming MakeView.exe in the Epi_Info folder to, for example, "xMakeView.exe".

If you are developing a system with a menu and want to to keep the user out of MakeView. You can run Enter from a batch file or menu with your program, and have the same batch file begin by renaming MakeView.exe to something else, like xMakeView.exe. Then, after exit from the Enter program, your batch file can rename xMakeView.exe back to MakeView.exe. Administrative privileges will be necessary for this to work, but you can have the user right click on your script or menu icon and choose "Run as Administrator" to make things work for some.

If you have Microsoft Access, you can open the MDB file and set properties that prevent editing of the table called viewXX, where XX is the name of your dataset (Oswego, for example) without a password.

These solutions will protect your Views and Check Code. To protect Analysis PGMs, keep a backup copy in text format and have the menu copy it over for use when you run the program.

Displaying a Variable on More Than Page in a View

The MIRROR field type is designed to do this. If you have a variable called NAME on the first page of a multi-page View, you can create additional fields called NAME1, NAME2, etc. on subsequent pages of the View and designate their type as MIRROR. As you do so, the field dialog will ask what field they are to mirror, and you choose NAME. Then Name will appear on each page of the View and will be automatically updated if you change the NAME field.

Sharing Variables with a Related View

From a related view, you can access variables that are defined as GLOBAL in the parent view. This whole process is rather awkward (wouldn't it be nice just to refer to them as parent.Address, for example, a feature that IS NOT available). See the chapter on the Complete Clinical System for a detailed description and example.

CHAPTER 33: THE FUTURE

Epi Info has had more than two decades of evolution. The DOS version, starting in 1985, demonstrated the usefulness of free software in public health and clinical medicine, and its text-based features were popular among those who developed programs for use by others. It was programmed in Turbo Pascal, and the source code was made available to a number of interested parties, but, because it used several commercial programming libraries, it could not be considered truly open source.. The idea to put Epi Info in the public domain originated with federal laws forbidding copyrighting "works of government." Since that time many other programs have been released as "freeware", and the Open Source movement has become a major trend in computer software release (www.opensource.org).

The advantages of a database that could be examined in a simple text editor were used by a program called EpiData, which carried the Epi Info file format into the Microsoft Windows environment (www.epidata.dk).

The Windows version of Epi Info, originally called Epi Info 2000, used the nearly universal Microsoft Windows standards such as the Access database engine and the graphic Windows interface. It was programmed in Visual Basic, a reasonably easy-to-understand language. Although it, too, made use of commercial add-on modules, these were kept separate from the CDC-written source code that depended on them. Although Epi Info for Windows requires Windows, it produces output in HTML, the universal language of Internet pages.

Both the DOS and Windows versions of Epi Info allow more than one user to access a database at the same time, with automatic record locking to prevent conflicts and data corruption. Epi Info for Windows also has the EpiLock utility for encryption of files being sent to another location, but this process requires either manual intervention or additional menu programming to make it automatic.

CDC has recently rewritten Epi Info in the Microsoft C# language and placed what is termed the pre-beta version on a public website as the "Community Edition." (http://www.codeplex.com/EpiInfo). It is said to run under the Linux operating system (in Ubuntu) as well as in Windows, but it is not yet complete.

OpenEpi takes another step toward the Internet in being a completely Internet program. It runs in browsers on Windows, Macintosh, and Linux systems, but only saves output in Windows systems. The next steps will be to enable saving on any system, and to provide a database and the means to enter and summarize data from individuals as well as summary data. OpenEpi is written entirely in HTML and Javascript and all of the code can be obtained from the Download OpenEpi item on the menu.

So much for evolution up to the present time. Some suggestions for the future are found in a blog at www.epiinformatics.com. It seems fairly clear that the Internet, or a future version of the Internet, will be the basis for further progress in epidemiologic and clinical software. Both clinical and community epidemiology, being the study of disease and risk factors in populations, depend on aggregation of data. Up to the present time aggregation of data has depended on collecting it in central locations, usually in files or databases. Collection may be by means of case-by-case interviews ("shoeleather epidemiology") or by telephone or email reports to a central location (traditional surveillance systems).

The Internet offers that possibility of receiving data directly from affected individuals. CDC and Google have recently experimented with a system that uses queries about "influenza" as a possible reflection of the number or timing of real cases. Given the possible disjunction between the urge to google and the presence of a real case of influenza and the influence of press reports on influenza diagnosis, this must be considered an experiment, but Google has gone on to add more specificity by asking users submitting such queries to indicate if they have knowledge of actual cases. Regardless of the success of these experiments, the ability to analyze hundreds of millions of Google queries per day, and extract meaning is a technical achievement that opens new possibilities for future epidemiology.

The tools for high-powered aggregation of data depend on 1) Instantaneous or rapid storage of data in a large, possibly global, database, now known as a "cloud". Although a "cloud" actually consists of thousands or millions of computers linked together, this makes little difference as long as the data can be accessed and analyzed. 2) Analytic capacity that can be provided by the managers of the "cloud", but configured by users.

It follows that future epidemiologic programs will make use of facilities on the "cloud" to make sense of the cloud's contents. So far, the (Google, Microsoft, Yahoo) clouds contain web pages and queries about web pages, and other clouds contain information about commercial transactions (Amazon), weather, gene sequences, NASA's view of the universe, and increasingly precise and recent pictures of the earth's surface. So far the clouds containing medical record information are well protected, administratively separated, and probably not entirely current. But the technology exists to do extensive analysis if the problems of confidentiality (proprietary and patient-oriented), ownership, and access can be solved.

For medical and public health professionals with less global interests, what are the advantages and disadvantages of storing data "on the cloud"? Despite occasional outages and local interruptions in Internet service, the cloud is probably a much safer place to store data than one's personal or even corporate computer. Storing both locally AND on the cloud is no doubt even safer and psychologically satisfying, as long as precautions are taken against a corrupt version updating a healthy version of the data, and against invasion of privacy or violation of data management laws.

One problem to be solved is the authentication of those accessing data in a confidential part of the cloud. There is a secondary problem of identification of subjects whose data is stored but may originate from different sources at different times. Solutions to both problems will undoubtedly excite privacy advocates, for both good and bad reasons. Ultimately the problem will be solved technically when it becomes easier to log into a computer by looking it in the eye and saying "hello" than it is to type an easily counterfeited username and password and have the luxury of wrecking havoc on 10000 users in another part of the world in the name of "free speech." Eventually, the confusion between free speech and anonymous and irresponsible speech will be clarified, either by splitting the Internet into secure and insecure domains, or by recognizing that every user and every computer should be traceable. You can't walk into a bank wearing a mask or drive a car without a license plate; why should you be able to sign on to a worldwide public utility without proper authentication and localization?

For a while, cloud based computing will have to limp along with the best means of identification available, until science catches up and facial recognition, fingerprints, and voice recognition, and/or DNA make anonymity ludicrous. This could be hard on fraud artists and fugitives in the database who would like to have separate personas in New York and Chicago, but they will doubtless find new frontiers.

What kind of features are desirable in future software for clinical and public health epidemiology? Here's a wish list for future developers:

Wish List for Future Software

General Features

- A general purpose, free and open source data entry, database, and statistics program for use by individuals with desktop, laptop, or hand-held computers, and smartphones, on and off the Internet.

- All the programs are entirely Internet based, consist of HTML and Javascript, and therefore function in any operating system with a browser, without proprietary tools or components

- User can construct a questionnaire or form, a spreadsheet view, a menu, and data processing programs easily in the field. Processing can be interactive or programmed.

- Translation and operation in many human languages

- Fun to use for public health and medical professionals, students, and experienced programmers.

- Open Source, with worldwide participation in brainstorming, development, testing, translation, and distribution

- Assured of long-term development, distribution, and support

Data entry

- Comparable to Epi Info for Windows, with optional programming to guide the process, but completely browser based

- Form views and spreadsheet (grid) views selectable with a mouse click

- Input from a wide variety of data formats, by file, cut-and-paste, URL, and other means

- Every record has a permanent and unique global identifier (GUID or UUID)

- Check Code is based on Javascript and stored as an editable Javascript file

- Menus are data-entry forms with menu controls

Data Storage

- Secure storage both locally and on servers, the latter optionally on "cloud" facilities like Amazon Web Services or Google.

- Able to read files on local computer and on remote servers

- Automatic synchronization of local and server-based data.

Analytic Features

- As in Epi Info, processing can occur interactively or through programming.

- Analysis of both remote and local databases

- Programs can be extended with other languages such as Javascript and the "R" statistical package

- Simple commands similar to those of Epi Info, automatically assembled into a program as they are issued

- Revision of commands by clicking on a program line

- Geographic Information System (GIS) based on free public facilities

- Graphing

Security

- Excellent authentication and identification features, able to evolve as technology progresses

- Logging of changes and who made them

- Secure transfer of data during acquisition or sharing

- Security understandable and easy to configure by user

- "Public" and "private" level variables

Support

- Email support in more than one time zone

- Manual both printable and searchable, without flashy features

- On-line users' forum

CHAPTER 34: RESOURCES

Software Examples for This Book

The examples from this book can be downloaded from www.epiinformatics.com as a file called Examples.zip. After downloading the file, unzip it to a convenient folder like C:\EpiBook\Examples\, leaving the directory structure as it is represented in the zip file. The Examples folder should look something like this:

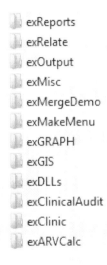

Chapters with examples will refer to one of the example folders with instructions, often to click or double-click on an icon in an example folder. Epi Info must first be downloaded and installed as described in Chapter 4 for most of the examples to work.

The Epi Info Website at CDC

The web pages at http://www.cdc.gov/epiinfo offer not only downloads of the latest released version of Epi Info, but links to the necessary files and instructions to make it operate in non-English languages, including Spanish, French, Italian, and Portuguese.

A collection of map shape files is offered directly and via links to other sites. There are two rather extensive tutorials in addition to the three that are installed with Epi Info.

Take the time to explore this site, as it has many useful resources.

Help, Support. And Communication

CDC offers an email and telephone help line on the Epi Info website with a telephone number of : 1-(404) 498-6190 and an email address of epiinfo@cdc.gov. Since there is often only one person assigned to the help line, the volume of responses is necessarily limited.

There is an unofficial discussion forum and help facility at

http://www.phconnect.org/group/epiinfo/forum

that was started by the Epi Info development team.

Here is the statement of purpose for phConnect:

> **phConnect is an online collaboration tool built to support geographically dispersed professionals working in the field of public health informatics. phConnect provides an environment for collaborative work, professional networking, and moving the field of public health informatics forward. By joining phConnect, you will be connected to passionate people engaged in shaping the future of public health informatics. You can connect, learn, share expertise, solve problems, and take advantage of innovative new approaches of working together.**

Another discussion resource is a Google group called ElFriends at

http://www.google.com/group/ElFriends

As of January 2010, anyone can join the group. Its purpose is stated as:

> **The group is open to anyone interested in Epi Info, and has no official government connection or restrictions. It provides a forum for ideas, expression of needs, suggestions, and news related to Epi Info. It is not intended to carry out the function of a helpline, but please use your own judgment concerning what content to include. All it takes to start a new topic is to send an email with a title not already listed and your idea or comment. We would be delighted to hear about applications you are developing or supporting with Epi Info, for example, as well as ideas for the future.**

It is not clear whether the two forums will somehow merge in the future, as they appear to have similar purposes and roughly the same number of members..

Searching

As with many topics, an Internet search is the quickest way to start looking for resources. Searching with Google.com or other search engines reveals thousands of sites that refer to Epi Info or OpenEpi. To find them all, it is important to use "Epi Info" with and without a space between the words and with and without a hyphen, as it is often misspelled. If possible, add search words that describe specifically what you want, such as "tutorial", "surveillance exercise", "advanced course", or "Greek". Many of the tutorial exercises and investigations will apply to Epi Info for DOS, or Epi Info, Version 6, but could be performed in Epi Info for Windows (Epi Info 2000) as well.

The Epi Info and OpenEpi HELP files

The Epi Info HELP files are found on the HELP menu under CONTENTS. Although they cannot easily be printed as a whole, the help files derive from over 1000 files, and are an extensive reference to the details of Epi Info commands They should be consulted whenever there is a need for more information. Searching in the index and search tabs is the best way to find an item, but many commands have identical titles for the Check Code, menu, and Analysis versions; be careful that you find the right ones.

Unfortunately, the help files are sometimes wrong, and they contain many grammatical errors. Don't be afraid to experiment with syntax when that recommended does not work (for example, putting single quotes around a file name sometimes fixes an Analysis command).

OpenEpi has exercises and documentation available within each module. The exercises are translated automatically into French, Spanish, or Italian (and soon, Portuguese), and can be printed out to form the basis of a course in statistics.

Other Resources

1. Three interactive TUTORIALS in the HELP section of Epi Info's main menu. These include the classic Oswego foodborne outbreak, a postoperative outbreak of surgical wound infections with Rhodococcus bronchialis, and a surveillance exercise.

2. Exercises of a one-week course for Epi Info instructors, taught by the Epi Info development team at Emory University. Download from www.cdc.gov/epiinfo/tutorials.htm

3. A 37-page Introduction to Epi Info for Windows, giving a tour of major functions of each of the Epi Info programs, at http://www.epiinformatics.com/ .

4. A 94-page Introduction to Analysis, with instructions and examples for the advanced statistical functions, from www.sph.emory.edu/~cdckms/

5. Epi Info Course I -- A 15-hour introduction to public health informatics with Epi Info, concentrating on epidemiologic investigation and ad hoc analysis. Case control study of anthrax bioterrorism in New York City, hospital infections, mortality analysis from El Salvador, making maps, graphs, and tables from surveillance data. Download from http://www.epiinformatics.com/

6. Epi Info Course II – A 15-hour, intermediate to advanced course focused on problem solving in a community health department or clinic. Nine data managment problems, stratified analysis, logistic regression, survival analysis, relational file handling and analysis, the SUMMARIZE command, an automatic menu generator program, and Geographic Information Systems(GIS) exercises. Download from www.epiinformatics.com

7. Cholera Outbreak in Rwenshama: Using Epi Info for Windows in an Outbreak Investigation at http://www.cdc.gov/epo/dih/materials.html#EpiInfo . Self-study or classroom-based

introduction to Epi Info, for individuals with strong basic computer skills. It provides 12-16 hours of instruction.

8. Tutorials in Epi Info from the veterinary point of view, from the University of Nebraska, at http://gpvec.unl.edu/StudentRounds/multimediapages/epi-stats.htm

9. The Italian website for Epi Info at http://www.epiinfo.it/casa.asp

10. The Spanish website for Epi Info at http://www.cica.es/epiinfo/ . Note that the latest Spanish translation is included with Epi Info downloaded from CDC.

11. The Portuguese website for Epi Info at http://www.epiinfo.com.br/

12. The Epi Info Norwegian Homepage (Norwegian): http://www.gruk.no/epi-info/download.htm

13. An introductory course in statistics by Bud Gerstman, using Epi Info and EpiData: http://www2.sjsu.edu/faculty/gerstman/EpiInfo/

14. Tutorial introduction to Epi Info by Vic Sahai, http://www.nhip.org/Learning%20Module/Epi2000/epiinfo2000.html

15. Approximately 10,700 other references in a Google™ search on Epi Info Windows Tutorial, give a starting place for further exploration.

Epi Info™ - Community Edition

A new version of Epi Info is being developed, with the following description:

Epi Info™ Community Edition is the open source project to reproduce the popular Epi Info™ suite of tools in C#, with the goal of developing a data collection and analytics system for public health that is highly scalable, platform independent, and database agnostic. While the Community Edition is still in its early stages (pre-1.0 release), public health professionals looking to perform critical activities are highly recommended to continue to use the closed-source but feature-complete version of Epi Info™ available from the CDC's Epi Info™ website.

It will be an open source product, available to all, with information and files available at

www.codeplex.com/EpiInfo

Quick Summary of Epi Info Commands

Check Code	*Analysis* PGMs	Functions/Operators	MNU Programs

ALWAYS / END (run Check Code all the time)
AUTOSEARCH
ASSIGN
CLEAR
DEFINE
DEFINE DLL OBJECT
DIALOG
ENDBEFORE
 	
EXECUTE
GOTO
HIDE
HELP
IF THEN ELSE
RECORDCOUNT
UNHIDE
 	
Field Properties
CODES
COMMENT LEGAL
LEGAL
MUSTENTER
RANGE
REPEAT
REQUIRED
SOUNDEX
 	
RELATE
	Data
	  READ (IMPORT)
	  RELATE
	  WRITE (EXPORT)
	  MERGE
	Variable
	  DEFINE
	  UNDEFINE
	  ASSIGN
	  RECODE
	  DISPLAY
	Select/If
	  SELECT
	  CANCEL SELECT
	  IF
	  SORT/CANCEL SORT
	Statistics
	  LIST
	  FREQUENCIES
	  TABLES
	  MATCH
	  MEANS|
	  SUMMARIZE
	  GRAPH
	  MAP
	Advanced Statistics
	  LINEAR REGRESS.
	  LOGISTICREGRESS
	  KAPLAN--MEIER SURV
	  COX PROP HAZARD
	  COMPLEX SAMPLE
	Output
	  TYPE
	  ROUTEOUT
	  CLOSEOUT
	  PRINTOUT
	  REPORTS
	  STORING OUTPUT
	User-Defined Commands
	  DEFINE COMMAND
	  USER COMMAND
	  RUN SAVED PROGRAM
	  EXECUTE FILE
	User Interaction
	  DIALOG
	  BEEP
	  HELP
	  QUIT PROGRAM
	Options
	  SET
		Operators
		  (+ - * / ^ MOD)
		Comparison
		  (> >= = <> < <= LIKE)
		Booleans
		  (AND OR XOR NOT)
		Numeric
		  EXP
		  SIN, COS, TAN
		  LOG
		  LN
		  ABS
		  RND
		  TRUNC
		  ROUND
		  NUMTODATE
		  NUMTOTIME
		Text Functions
		  TXTTONUM
		  TXTTODATE
		  SUBSTRING
		  UPPERCASE
		  FINDTEXT
		  FORMAT
		Date Functions
		  YEARS
		  MONTHS
		  DAYS
		  YEAR
		  MONTH
		  DAY
		Time Functions
		  HOURS
		  MINUTES
		  SECONDS
		  HOUR
		  MINUTE
		  SECOND
		System Functions
		  SYSTEMDATE
		  SYSTEMTIME
		  ENVIRON
		  EXISTS
			Commands
			ASSIGN
			BROWSER
			BROWSERSIZE
			BUTTON
			CALL
			DEFINE
			DIALOG/MESSAGE
			EXECUTE/RUN/LINKTO/ACTIVATE
			EXIT
			FILEDIALOG
			GETPATH
			HELP
			IF THEN ELSE
			LINK
			LINKREMOVE
			MENU
			MENUITEM
			MOVEBUTTONS
			PICTURE
			PICTURESIZE
			REPEAT UNTIL
			REPLACE
			SCREENTEXT
			SETBUTTONS
			SETDBVERSION
			SETDOSWIN
			SETINIDIR
			SETLANGUAGE
			SETPICTURE
			SETWORKDIR
			SYSINFO
			UNDEFINE
			WAITFOR
			WAITFOREXIT
			WAITFORFILEXISTS
			
			Special Command Blocks
			SHUTDOWN
			STARTUP
			Functions
			EXISTS
			System Variables
			COMPDATE
			INIDIR
			INSTALLDIR
			MENUDIR
			SYSTEMDATE
			WORKDIR
			
			Value of Variable @@

Alphabetical Index

4610849

Made in the USA
Charleston, SC
19 February 2010